Cosmetic Surgery For Dummies®

Important Questions to Ask Your Surgeon

✔ **Are you a board-certified plastic surgeon? (If not, are you board eligible or does your training and certification include the procedure I'm considering?)**

Board certification by the American Board of Plastic Surgery ensures the highest level of training. Call 866-ASK-ABMS (275-2267) or visit www.abms.org to verify.

✔ **Do you have privileges to perform my surgical procedure(s) at an accredited hospital?**

Hospital privileges ensure that other physicians have checked out your doctor for you and determined that he is suitably trained and has demonstrated skill to perform your procedure in their hospital.

✔ **Are you a member of one or both of the two prestigious societies for plastic surgeons: American Society for Aesthetic Plastic Surgery (ASAPS) and American Society of Plastic Surgeons?**

These self-governing societies have high standards and do your homework for you regarding your surgeon's continuing education compliance and facility accreditation.

✔ **Do you devote a significant portion of your practice to cosmetic surgery?**

You're more likely to get the positive surgical result and patient experience you seek when your surgeon focuses on cosmetic surgery.

✔ **How many times have you performed the procedure I want? How often do you perform it? Do you have before-and-after photos?**

Generally, the more experience a surgeon has, the more consistent his results. But, you still have to like the results. Before-and-after photos are a great way to find out if you share the surgeon's aesthetic.

✔ **What is your patient-education philosophy?**

You should be a partner in your care. That means you need to find a doctor who is committed to proactive communication and quality educational materials.

✔ **Will you perform all of my surgery? If anyone else helps you, what will they do?**

You're paying for the surgeon to do your surgery—the entire surgery. You should be told who will assist and how. Some procedures, such as breast reduction, require two surgeons, but you'll be told in advance.

Asking about the Surgery Facility

✔ **Is my surgery going to be performed at the hospital or an ambulatory outpatient surgery center?**

These facilities have to adhere to the highest safety standards. If your surgery will be performed at one of them, you probably don't need to investigate further.

✔ **Is my surgery being performed in an office-based surgery suite?**

If so, you want to know the surgery suite has current accreditation. Ask to see the current license and check out the organization on the Web.

✔ **What type of anesthesia do you recommend for the procedure(s) I am considering?**

You need to understand the risks and benefits of each type and why that type is suggested for your particular procedure.

✔ **What are the qualifications of the person who is providing my anesthesia? Will I be able to meet with my anesthesia provider?**

I recommend using board-certified MD anesthesiologists or certified registered nurse anesthetists (CRNAs).

Cosmetic Surgery For Dummies®

Cheat Sheet

Looking for Red Flags

If you run into the following situations, you might want to continue searching for a surgeon.

During an appointment or pre-consult

- The phone isn't answered promptly or is answered by a machine.
- No one takes time for your call; the doctor's staff is abrupt or downright rude.
- You don't receive promised information materials before your consultation.
- You can't get your questions answered because the staff isn't knowledgeable or says "the doctor will tell you everything at consult."
- You can't find out a ballpark fee. How can cost be a secret?
- You find out you won't be meeting with the surgeon at your consult. Don't waste your time.

At the consultation

- You wait too long, which can be a sign that the physician doesn't respect your time. If this happens, you must decide whether you can add an hour of waiting to every visit. If a physician is running late but apologizes because it's unusual, then you don't necessarily need to be concerned.
- You feel like just a number. Neither the doctor nor his staff is friendly or taking time to get to know you. You feel like you're known only as the breast aug in Room 3.
- Your doctor isn't listening to what bothers you or adds procedures that you're not sure you want. He's giving you one-size-fits-all answers when you want a tailor-made surgical plan.
- The practice can't show you before-and-after pictures, or if the doctor is in a group, the staff can't tell which doctor did the surgery pictured.
- You don't receive a written fee estimate at consult, or the practice doesn't have written policies for costs related to secondary surgery.
- You feel negative energy in the facility. You see examples of disinterest in you by the doctor or staff or notice unrest in their interactions with each other. Staff members contradict the surgeon's recommendations for you.
- You feel pressured into scheduling surgery that day. This is a big decision, so you need time for reflection.

When making your decision

- If something about the technique or recovery is sounding too good to be true, it probably is, especially if other surgeons disagree.
- The practice does nothing to follow up after your consultation—no phone calls, no letters. Do they care?
- Your gut is telling you no. If something doesn't feel right, trust your instincts. Second consults may help you feel more comfortable. Or continuing until you find the right surgeon and staff may be the best solution.

For Dummies: Bestselling Book Series for Beginners

Cosmetic Surgery

FOR

DUMMIES®

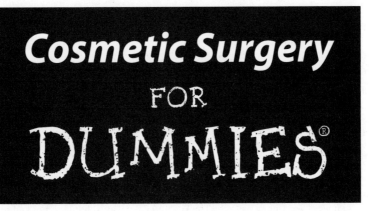

Cosmetic Surgery FOR DUMMIES®

by R. Merrel Olesen, MD
Marie B.V. Olesen

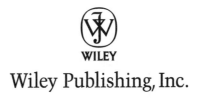

Wiley Publishing, Inc.

Cosmetic Surgery For Dummies®

Published by
Wiley Publishing, Inc.
111 River St.
Hoboken, NJ 07030-5774
www.wiley.com

For general information on our other products and services, please contact our Customer Care Department within the U.S. at 800-762-2974, outside the U.S. at 317-572-3993, or fax 317-572-4002.

For technical support, please visit www.wiley.com/techsupport.

Wiley also publishes its books in a variety of electronic formats. Some content that appears in print may not be available in electronic books.

Library of Congress Control Number is available from the publisher.

ISBN: 0-7645-7835-9

Manufactured in the United States of America

10 9 8 7 6 5 4 3 2 1

1B/SR/QT/QV/IN

WILEY

About the Authors

R. Merrel Olesen, MD, is medical director of the La Jolla (Calif.) Cosmetic Surgery Centre, which he founded in 1988. Dr. Olesen, the former head, Division of Plastic Surgery at Scripps Clinic and Research Foundation, holds dual board certifications from the American Board of Medical Specialties in plastic surgery and otolaryngology (head and neck surgery). Dr. Olesen completed surgical residencies at Columbia Presbyterian Medical Center, NYC, and the University of Michigan Medical Center. He has over 35 years of surgical experience. Dr. Olesen is a member of the American Society for Aesthetic Plastic Surgery (ASAPS) and the American Society of Plastic Surgeons (ASPS).

While Dr. Olesen's busy cosmetic surgery practice attests to his surgical skill, he is known among his plastic surgery colleagues for his industry-transforming work in patient education. He authored patient-friendly informed consent and patient education materials that are used by over 950 plastic surgeons and have been translated into five languages.

As a double-boarded plastic surgeon, Dr. Olesen hopes that he has represented facial plastic surgeons fairly in this book, as he loved practicing ten years as a head and neck surgeon before training to become a plastic surgeon.

Marie B.V. Olesen is the vice president of Inform Solutions, a cosmetic surgery consulting company that is a subsidiary of Mentor Corporation. She is a national speaker and plastic surgery practice consultant. Marie teaches innovative customer service principles that enable plastic surgery practices to better serve cosmetic surgery patients. She has worked in healthcare management for over 25 years and holds a degree in public administration from San Diego State University.

In the late 1980s, Marie began surveying cosmetic surgery patients and found that they wanted better information and higher levels of participation in their surgical experience. She created a patient communication system that greatly enhanced patient satisfaction and developed metrics to measure practice success.

To enable other practices to use the patient education materials and systems they developed, the Olesens founded Inform Solutions, where Marie was the architect of Inform&Consent and Inform&Enhance, two software programs used by plastic surgery practices to communicate with their cosmetic surgery patients.

Both Olesens are extremely concerned about the inherent dangers to the consumer in the current cosmetic surgery marketplace. These feelings have been a powerful stimulus toward the writing of this book. They are donating 50 percent of the proceeds of this book to charitable causes.

Dedication

We want to dedicate this book to our beloved mothers. Sally Bonvillain, who died recently after a wonderful life, was an incredibly positive person who always encouraged us in our work and our life. Lucile Olesen, who at 93, retains all of her mental, visual, and writing skills, is a world-class human being, adored by everyone who knows her.

Authors' Acknowledgments

Traci Cumbay, project editor, and Tina Sims, copy editor, at Wiley Publishing have prodded and pushed us into writing a book that we hope will be useful to anyone considering cosmetic surgery. As nonprofessional writers, we have found the process harder than it looks. Their efforts have made a real difference.

A number of colleagues have contributed significantly to the medical information in this book. All busy with their own practices, they took time to heed our calls and to help make this a better book. Some of them already work in our practices, and we wish that they all could. Kudos to Lori Saltz, MD; Michael Roark, MD; Robert Kearney, MD; Johan Brahme, MD; Louis Bonaldi, MD; and Joe Bauer, MD — all plastic surgeons. Special thanks to Richard Fitzpatrick, MD, dermatologist, and to Gary Williams, MD, PhD, rheumatologist. We especially wish to give recognition to the members of Anesthesia Medical Group, who contribute so much to the care of patients in our practice and added their expertise: Andrew Heinle, MD; Gerald Haas, MD; Stuart Young, MD; Dayle O'Conner, MD; and Peter McElfresh, MD.

Others who have contributed in very intelligent and hard-working ways are Michele Ellingsen, Melissa Callahan, Monique Ramsey, Fredda Morgan, Annette Segal, and Donna Cook, RN. They have contributed ideas, grammar, photo organization, and logistical support. This book would not exist without them. We also wish to acknowledge and thank all the staff at La Jolla Cosmetic Surgery Centre, who on a daily basis embody the patient care values we commend in this book.

We would like to thank the patients who so generously shared their personal stories. Marie wishes to thank her corporate bosses at Mentor for giving her permission to work on this book. Lastly, we would like to thank (we think!) Judi Strada, coauthor of *Sushi For Dummies,* who first suggested this book.

Publisher's Acknowledgments

We're proud of this book; please send us your comments through our Dummies online registration form located at www.dummies.com/register/.

Some of the people who helped bring this book to market include the following:

Acquisitions, Editorial, and Media Development

Project Editor: Traci Cumbay

Acquisitions Editor: Stacy Kennedy

Copy Editor: Tina Sims

Technical Editor: Donald R. Nunn, MD

Senior Permissions Editor: Carmen Krikorian

Editorial Manager: Jennifer Ehrlich

Editorial Assistants: Hanna Scott, Nadine Bell

Cover Photo: © Ron Chapple/Alamy Images/ ThinkStock

Cartoons: Rich Tennant (www.the5thwave.com)

Composition Services

Project Coordinator: Maridee Ennis, Emily Wichlinski

Layout and Graphics: Carl Byers, Andrea Dahl, Stephanie D. Jumper, Clint Lahnen, Heather Ryan, Brent Savage

Special Art: Illustrations by Kathryn Born, M.A.

Proofreaders: Leeann Harney, Jessica Kramer, Carl William Pierce, TECHBOOKS Production Services

Indexer: TECHBOOKS Production Services

Special Help: Elizabeth Rea

Publishing and Editorial for Consumer Dummies

Diane Graves Steele, Vice President and Publisher, Consumer Dummies

Joyce Pepple, Acquisitions Director, Consumer Dummies

Kristin A. Cocks, Product Development Director, Consumer Dummies

Michael Spring, Vice President and Publisher, Travel

Kelly Regan, Editorial Director, Travel

Publishing for Technology Dummies

Andy Cummings, Vice President and Publisher, Dummies Technology/General User

Composition Services

Gerry Fahey, Vice President of Production Services

Debbie Stailey, Director of Composition Services

Contents at a Glance

Table of Contents

Introduction

· ·

Cosmetic surgery is a hot topic! These days, every daytime talk show, popular magazine, late night show, salon conversation, daily newspaper, lunch with the girls, locker room discussion, fashion magazine, and yes, even reality TV show covers the subject, sooner or later.

Most likely you're also aware of someone — even if it's a television commentator — who's had cosmetic surgery. Procedures that once were limited to people in the entertainment or television industry are now being performed on plenty of people who aren't celebrities. You may have friends, colleagues, or acquaintances who have had cosmetic surgery. People from all walks of life — teachers, golfers, grandmas, and computer programmers — are doing it. As the statistics prove, more and more women and men — yes *men* — are having cosmetic surgery. If you're thinking about becoming one of those people, *Cosmetic Surgery For Dummies* is for you.

About This Book

Science is making cosmetic surgery safer, easier, and more effective. New drugs, new techniques, and new training are all evolving to make these procedures more affordable and available across the country and around the world. As you consider cosmetic surgery for yourself, I give you advice in this book that can help you make informed decisions about your key choices — your surgeon, the operating facility and anesthesia provider, and the surgeon's patient-care team. If you want to take advantage of all the advances in cosmetic surgery while avoiding the pitfalls that could compromise your safety or the quality of your result, reading this book can help you do just that.

As you read the information in this book about cosmetic surgery procedures and treatments, you can assume we made every attempt to give you the most current information available when we wrote the book. However, medicine and medical techniques evolve constantly. Surgeons are always looking for better ways of doing things. Rules and regulations by the federal government, states, credentialing organizations, and medical specialties change as well. Our bias as authors is that surgical training and certification are important safeguards that put the odds in your favor.

If you're looking for answers to your questions about cosmetic surgery, this book is for you. If you're considering cosmetic surgery, wondering how to pay for it, or asking yourself whether it's safe, this book is for you. If you're fascinated with the science of the new procedures or the corrections available for problems caused by genetics or gravity, we can help you understand them.

You probably realize that beyond skin deep, cosmetic surgery has both immediate and long-lasting effects on the social, psychological, sexual, and even spiritual well-being of the people having it done. We include many stories of real patients who talk about the wonderful changes that occurred in their lives as a result of making changes to their bodies. We believe that your physical appearance, self-confidence, and mental outlook are interconnected. Changing one aspect of yourself can bring about positive changes that are much more far-reaching than the physical ones you anticipate.

The book is organized so that you can start reading anywhere you want. You don't have to read it from cover to cover. Just pick a topic from the table of contents or index that interests you and jump in.

Conventions Used in This Book

Although this book was co-written by two authors, I (Dr. Olesen) supplied the medical information. The patient references are to my practice and my patients, so that's why you see "I" used in most cases instead of "we." But keep in mind that my wife, Marie, is the driving force behind this book. Her desire to help you make an informed decision about cosmetic surgery is what kept the project (and me) going full steam ahead. She's as familiar as I am with every word on these pages because she's written a significant portion of this book.

To help you navigate through this book, we've established the following conventions:

- ✔ *Italic* is used for emphasis and to highlight new words or terms that are defined.
- ✔ `Monofont` is used for Web addresses.
- ✔ Sidebars, which are shaded gray boxes full of text, consist of information that's interesting but not necessarily critical to your understanding of the topic.

What You're Not to Read

Depending on how much you really want to know, you may want to skip anything marked with a Technical Stuff icon. In those paragraphs, we get specific about procedures or anatomy. If you find this detailed information interesting, by all means, dig in! But if you'd prefer *not* to know the nitty-gritty details, feel free to skip them. You won't miss out on anything you need to know to make informed decisions.

Foolish Assumptions

In order to write this book, we had to make some assumptions about you and your needs. We assume that one or more of the following statements apply to you:

- ✔ You're considering cosmetic surgery and want to know what all the excitement is about.
- ✔ You've decided you're ready for cosmetic surgery and want to be an informed consumer.
- ✔ You have a friend or family member who's considering cosmetic surgery and you want to help them make the right decision.
- ✔ You're looking for cosmetic facial rejuvenation treatments that are alternatives or complement cosmetic surgery.
- ✔ You've had successful cosmetic surgery in the past and you're ready for more.
- ✔ You had a negative outcome from cosmetic surgery and want to explore your options for future surgery.

How This Book Is Organized

We've organized the book into five parts — from considering the idea of cosmetic surgery to recovery issues and everything in between. You can follow the process sequentially or go directly to the issues that most concern you first.

Part 1: Considering Cosmetic Surgery

Start with this part if you want an overview of cosmetic surgery. We deal with the kinds of issues that motivate people to have cosmetic surgery and give you the lowdown on medical specialization and surgical safety issues.

Part II: Preparing for Cosmetic Surgery

If you're a smart shopper and use good consumer principles, you can increase the likelihood of having a wonderful experience and a positive change in your life. In this part, we explain a formal shopping process and suggest shopping criteria that can help you make a wise choice of your surgeon, operating facility, and patient care team. We also give you tips for getting ready for surgery — financially and physically.

Part III: Exploring Your Options

This part gives you the nitty-gritty on most of the cosmetic surgery procedures available to you. We give you details about everything from freshening the skin on your face to giving your butt or thighs a lift. You find all the details you need to determine whether you're a good candidate for a particular procedure, what you can expect if you decide to have it, and how to find the right surgeon for the job.

Part IV: Going for It: Preparation and Recovery

If you opt for surgery, you'll want to understand the risks and plan carefully for your entire surgical and recovery experience. Your activities and attitudes influence the healing process and speed or retard recovery. In this part, we offer strategies for dealing with the outside world before and after surgery, handling any complications that may arise, and moving forward when the result of your surgery isn't what you expected. We also cover what you can do after a positive outcome to go forward and take pleasure in the new you and enhance your enjoyment of your life.

Part V: The Part of Tens

In this part, we give you ten tips for getting the most from your cosmetic surgery, debunk ten lingering myths about cosmetic surgery, and offer questions to ask yourself to find out whether cosmetic surgery really is right for you.

Icons Used in This Book

Like other *For Dummies* books, this one has icons in the margins to help you zero in on what you want to know. The following paragraphs describe the kinds of information each icon highlights.

When something is likely to save you time or money or keep your cosmetic surgery experience running smoothly, we point you to it with this icon.

Cosmetic surgery is complex, so we use this icon to highlight the really essential issues — stuff you'll want to keep in mind as you navigate the maze of options.

Whenever we talk about potential hazards along the road to cosmetic surgery, we use this icon.

If you aren't planning on going to medical school, you can skip these details. We use this icon to point out stuff that goes deeper into the topic than you may care to go.

We use this icon to share personal stories of real cosmetic surgery patients.

Where to Go from Here

Start anywhere you like. Read the sections that most intrigue you; skip those you know you aren't interested in. If you're just delving into your options and haven't decided whether cosmetic surgery is for you, we suggest you start with Part I. If you're ready to shop, you'll likely find Part II has the information you want. Check out Part III for information about specific procedures.

However you choose to approach this book, just remember that behind all the glitz and glamour, this is real surgery, and details make a difference. Don't stop looking for information until you feel comfortable with every aspect of your decision.

Part I
Considering Cosmetic Surgery

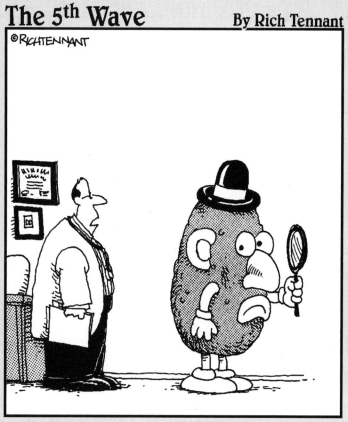

"We can try another set of ears, fix the eyes, stick on a new nose, but eventually you're going to have to accept the fact that you're always going to have a potato for a head."

In this part . . .

Cosmetic surgery is growing by leaps and bounds as medical science progresses and more and more people decide to do something about outsides they don't feel match their insides. In this part, I tell you about the current cosmetic surgery boom and fill you in on making the very big decision to take the leap. Because cosmetic surgery is real surgery and comes with the risks that are part and parcel of going under the knife, I also tell you how to keep yourself as safe as possible.

Chapter 1

Entering the Golden Age of Cosmetic Surgery

*L*ike any golden age, cosmetic surgery's golden age is flourishing and creating happiness among its devotees. The combination of science, society, and psychology has created this renaissance. New techniques, improved materials, and better training have catapulted cosmetic surgery (once reserved for the famous, the brave, and the rich) into the mainstream.

Cosmetic surgery is now safer, easier, and more affordable than ever before. Out of the closet, it has taken center stage in the self-improvement world and is being embraced by millions every year. Some patients are choosing facial surgery — eyelifts, facelifts, nose reshaping, and chin implants. Other patients are changing the contours of their bodies with liposuction, breast surgery, tummy tucks, and other even arm and thigh lifts.

Cosmetic surgery is real surgery, so you need to be an informed consumer. We cover the subject from A to Z. You can benefit greatly from approaching your decision as a serious one and taking the time to fully use the tools presented in this book.

Putting the "Plastic" in Surgery

You've heard the terms *plastic surgery*, *cosmetic surgery,* and *reconstructive surgery* bandied about, and you're confused. No wonder. You'll see both medical and marketing uses of these terms and when you see them, you need to know what they mean.

When you hear the word *plastic*, you probably think of the modern material that's molded into myriad products — patio chairs, kids' toys, kitchen glasses, and airline knives and forks. The list goes on and on. This plastic isn't what we're talking about. Actually, the word comes from the Greek word "plastikos" or the later Latin word "plasticus," both of which mean "to shape or mold." Plastic surgeons shape or mold your body into new and more pleasing forms.

Another form of this word, the suffix *-plasty,* is used in the names of many plastic surgery procedures. In the mid-1800s, the medical term for nose reshaping came to be *rhinoplasty* — *rhino* (for nose) plus *plasty* (to describe the shaping technique). Other examples include *abdominoplasty* (reshaping of your abdomen), *mammoplasty* (changing the shape of your breasts), and *blepharoplasty* (reshaping of your eyelids).

As defined by the American Medical Association, the medical specialty of plastic surgery includes two subcategories of procedures:

- ✔ **Cosmetic:** Cosmetic surgery is performed to reshape *normal* structures of the body to improve the patient's appearance and self-esteem.

- ✔ **Reconstructive:** Reconstructive surgery is performed on *abnormal* features of the body (usually caused by congenital defects, developmental abnormalities, infection, tumors, or disease). It is generally done to improve function, but may also be done to approximate a normal appearance.

Cosmetic surgery improves form, whereas reconstructive surgery improves function.

Defining cosmetic surgery

The primary purpose of cosmetic surgery is to improve your form, or appearance. In cosmetic surgery (sometimes called *aesthetic surgery*), you take a normal or near-normal part of the body and alter it to make it look better. For example, a young man with a weak chin line seeks cosmetic surgery to alter his profile. Or a 60-year-old woman with a face that is normal for a 60-year-old decides to get a facelift to improve her appearance.

The most common cosmetic surgery procedures are the following:

- ✔ Liposuction
- ✔ Breast surgery
- ✔ Nose reshaping
- ✔ Eyelid lift
- ✔ Tummy tuck
- ✔ Facelift

The rate at which these procedures are performed has been growing exponentially for many years. From 1997 to 2003, the number of surgical and non-surgical cosmetic procedures grew from 2.1 million to 8.3 million, according to the American Society for Aesthetic Plastic Surgery. If this keeps up, you won't have a neighbor or coworker who hasn't has something lifted, tightened, augmented, or filled.

Cosmetic surgery and cosmetic surgeons are not synonymous. If you or a loved one is considering a cosmetic surgery procedure, you really need to know whether the surgeon you're consulting is trained in plastic surgery. Some doctors, even good ones in other fields, hoping to blur the boundaries of training and experience, run ads calling themselves cosmetic surgeons. This is perfectly legal in many places. They may be wonderful physicians, dermatologists or OB-GYNs, for example, but they never had specialized training in plastic surgery, never did a residency, and so are not as qualified to give you the best result. (Chapter 3 tells you more about this topic.)

Ask, ask, and then ask again to verify that the person who will do the surgery you want is trained in the specialty of plastic surgery or a surgical specialty that includes training in the procedure you want.

Understanding reconstructive surgery

During reconstructive surgery, the surgeon works with a body part that is not within a range of normal appearance to make it look more normal. Generally disease, deformity, or trauma prompts patients to seek reconstructive surgery. The repair of a cleft lip or reconstruction of breasts after cancer is considered reconstructive surgery, not cosmetic surgery, because the body part that is being improved didn't start out in a range of normal appearance; rather, it's being brought back to a normal appearance or function.

Other common reconstructive procedures include facial reconstruction after serious accidents and hand surgery for work-related injuries or degenerative diseases such as arthritis.

Blending cosmetic and reconstructive techniques

Sometimes the cosmetic and reconstructive techniques are combined in one procedure that improves both appearance and function. An example is a rhino/septoplasty, in which the rhino portion of the surgery shapes the outer nose and the septo portion improves the breathing function of the inner nose.

Looking Into Cultural Ideals about Looks

Cosmetic surgery deals primarily with the "ideal" appearance, which is shaped by the culture and the time in which you live. Right or wrong, our modern culture places enormous emphasis on youth and appearance. People who don't embody the ideals often feel inferior or left out. Children who don't fit within the norms are often teased and sometimes shunned.

Many people think this view is shallow, that it ought to be different — that the prevailing cultural emphasis on youth and appearance is wrong. They may be right. But it's almost impossible to be part of a society and not be affected by the expectations and views of the people around you. Your views of beauty are defined, reinforced, or challenged by the world around you.

For centuries, people have been working to change the way they look to meet cultural ideals of beauty. They've used cosmetics, costumes, and accessories and even changed the shape of their bodies. Chinese mothers bound their daughters' feet from birth to keep them tiny. People across the ages and across cultures created all kinds of techniques and used many types of materials to improve their appearance.

Plastic surgeons didn't invent the concept of enhancing personal beauty; they just took it to another level. The modern version is that advances in medicine, including the discovery of antibiotics, now make cosmetic surgery solutions a safe option for the general public.

Tapping Into Cosmetic Surgery's Popularity

You may wonder how surgery, once thought of as risky, at best, and dangerous, at worst, attracts millions of people. Cosmetic surgery is pervasive in the media and becoming more so in daily conversation and daily life. You can't escape the news surrounding this topic, especially in the Information Age. You may occasionally retreat from the world, but unless you've chosen to live as a recluse, hidden in a cave, you'll be exposed to cosmetic surgery — and often.

It's not only Las Vegas showgirls, actors, and entertainers who seek help when they want to change their appearance. Programmers, professors, secretaries, and pop stars do it, too. You may notice your grocer or hairdresser looking different. At a college reunion, you may find classmates who seem to have changed a lot less than you expected. Seeing results everywhere may make you yearn for a personal change. Finding out about advances in medicine can help you decide to go for it.

As people find out who is having surgery and how these people look afterward, cosmetic surgery's popularity increases. Results are becoming more natural and easier to obtain. If you're considering surgery yourself, finding out that science has made leaps and bounds in anesthesia, antibiotics, and surgical techniques is reassuring. Learning about the training and specializations that plastic surgeons undertake helps you understand that it works and why it works.

Living dangerously for beauty?

If you read about fashion and surf the 'Net, you may have read that the first cosmetic surgery was performed on Victorian women who underwent surgical removal of their ribs in order to conform to the Victorian emphasis on small waists. This is a myth. Fatality rates for amputations performed in the mid-1800s were high. With odds like these, it's hard to imagine anyone voluntarily having surgery:

- **Forearm:** 13 percent
- **Arm:** 52 percent
- **Leg:** 50 percent
- **Thigh:** 85 percent

Finding Out Who's Going under the Knife

Although cosmetic surgery used to be for the rich and famous, now everyone is doing it. From school teachers to trial lawyers to real estate agents, all kinds of people are opting for cosmetic surgery. If your job puts you before the public, you may be particularly interested in cosmetic surgery.

With such a surge in popularity of cosmetic surgery, it may be easier to put your finger on who's *not* going under the knife than who is. Certain religions or sects frown on personal adornment, let alone cosmetic surgery. And if you have certain health problems — you're a smoker or diabetic, for example — having cosmetic surgery may not be possible. (Chapter 7 tells you more about which conditions make surgery risky.) But if you've got the desire and have the money and the time, options abound for fixing pretty much whatever bothers you about the skin you're in.

Men get into the act

If you think only women are interested in improving their appearance, you're a little off base. Statistics show that 82 percent of all cosmetic surgery consumers are women. That's still pretty high when compared to men, but 18 percent is nothing to sneeze at. Business, a longer life span, public acceptance, and more openness about the subject all combine to make many men comfortable with an exploration of cosmetic surgery.

Many men want the same procedures as women. Rhinoplasty, eyelid lifts, and liposuction are popular. Generally, cosmetic surgery for men is modified from the female version of the same procedure. Often that means less extreme. In facial surgery, the placement of incisions is different because men need their scars hidden behind a male hairstyle or receding hairline.

Young people take the leap

If you think cosmetic surgery is only for the 45-and-above crowd, think again. In 2003, almost 336,000 teens 18 or younger had some kind of cosmetic surgery or procedure, a 50 percent increase over 2002. The most popular procedures for this age group were facial peels and nose reshaping. Breast augmentation and liposuction were way down on the list. Naturally, parental consent is needed for patients under 18.

Cosmetic surgery among those between 19 and 25 years old also is exploding. Young women seeking breast augmentation and liposuction, as well as nose reshaping (rhinoplasty) are heading to their plastic surgeons in droves and getting the inside scoop on what's possible. Although many still turn to older adults for support and money, this group is completely comfortable with the idea of aesthetic improvement. Young adults read the magazines and view the shows that deal with this topic. They are also seeking romance, so how they look and feel about themselves is an important concern. They're not going to suffer in silence; they're going to get it fixed.

Surgery for the older set

Clearly, both men and women want to look good at any age. Today, even many older people — people who are capable and fit and often still employed — don't want to look their age. They know that modern culture and the business world are often prejudiced against them. A youthful appearance can often be the key to keeping a job, and cosmetic surgery is the way to achieve that look.

The good news is that cosmetic surgery done by a qualified and trained plastic surgeon in a good facility is generally safe at any age. Age is no barrier to someone healthy, but surgeons may adapt or modify surgeries for people past age 65. For example, most anesthesiologists begin to set limits on the amount of surgery that can be performed, and surgeons would perform less-extensive body contouring procedures for this age group. Happily, older people are more concerned with how they look in clothes rather than out of them, so this approach a good match.

More and more of the over-65 group — including people in and out of the workplace — are also seeking solutions to issues with their appearance, regardless of whether they feel discriminated against or not. When these people start feeling a disconnect between what shows up in the mirror and they way they feel, many consider doing something about it rather than coping, as their parents did. This age group is more active and vital than ever. Aided by medications and living a longer life span, most want to enjoy their golden years. For some people, looking more in tune with how they feel helps makes the rewards of a long career and success even sweeter.

Investigating Issues for Kids and Teens

You probably remember or may have even experienced yourself how unforgiving children and teens can be to the kids that don't fit it. Although cosmetic surgery can't change your kid's IQ or height, it can solve some issues that can significantly change appearance — protruding ears, large noses, or weak chins. In cases of severe acne, teens and their parents often decide on laser peels that make high school social life easier.

Popular procedures for teens

According to the American Society of Plastic Surgeons, patients 18 or younger had the following procedures in 2003:

- Chemical peel: 126,327
- Microdermabrasion: 74,722
- Nose reshaping: 42,515
- Ear surgery: 15,973
- Botox injections: 5,606
- Collagen injections: 4,094
- Sclerotherapy: 4,002
- Breast augmentation: 3,841
- Male breast reduction*: 3,033
- Liposuction: 3,017

* Breast reduction in women is considered reconstructive surgery.

If you're a parent who wants your child to avoid the stigma of these issues, you may be open to having whatever concerns your child has surgically corrected. You need to be particularly sensitive to your child's own desires and dig deep to find the real problem. Foisting a surgical procedure on an immature young person (even for his benefit) is a recipe for disaster. It's best if your child or teen expresses the desire first. Then you want to be sure he or she is engaged every step of the way and fully understands what is involved before, during, and after the surgery. The child also needs to fully understand and be realistic about outcomes. If you're considering helping your teen through this process, ask your child for his or her opinion and then listen carefully to his or her responses.

You need to be careful when deciding upon surgery for a teenager. Teens are still growing, so their bodies continue to develop and, in some cases, develop a lot. Hormonal activity continues to shift. Maturity and clearheadedness about expectations are other issues to consider. You need to be cautious when choosing a surgeon. You'll want someone who is sensitive to these issues and develops rapport with your child or teenager.

More than for any other age group, if you are considering cosmetic surgery for your child or teen, you want to consult with several qualified surgeons and be sure that everyone agrees about the best course for your child.

Evaluating Your Motivations

So you may be you are asking yourself, "Do I *need* cosmetic surgery?" My answer is that no one *needs* cosmetic surgery. You may *want* to have it, but don't kid yourself: If you decide to have surgery, it's because you've identified it as something you *want* to do.

Ultimately, only you can decide what's best for you. You do have some things to consider when making the decision. Evaluate what you consider to be your flaws. Sure, other people may identify as flaws the very things that irk you, your quirky and unique features, but *only* if you're bothered by them, really bothered, should you consider doing something. Keep track for a while of how often these flaws surface in your mind.

If you think of them every day, you have more reason to go forward than if you remember a flaw once a year when you pull a particular outfit from the closet. Journaling or even keeping a notepad where you tick off the times during a day or week when your mind lingers upon what you don't like about your appearance will help you evaluate how important this concern is to you.

Maybe some mornings you're brushing your teeth or hair and notice that you just don't look as good as you feel. Or a snapshot shows up those things about your appearance you'd rather not see. You may be shopping for clothes and suddenly realize you've got to do something after you see yourself in a full-length, three-way mirror. You may shrug and say, "Oh well, I'm getting older" and go on about your life. Or you may think, "Maybe I can improve upon Mother Nature, but more along the lines of a tune-up and oil change." Or you may want a complete overhaul — your own *Extreme Makeover.*

You may not want to be a fashion model, but you may want to wear the current fashions. You may not want to look like an actor but still want to look as successful as you feel on the job. Go through the process of evaluating carefully. Get real with yourself. After all, surgery is never something to be taken lightly. You may realize that you're okay with your looks — or you may really want an improvement.

If you discover through tracking and asking the hard questions that you really do want to make a change, grant yourself permission. Check out Chapter 2 for more details about making your decision.

Depending on your philosophy, comfort level, desire for change, budget, and willingness to take risks, you will decide if, how much, and how extensively you want to change your appearance. You may be one of those people who, after making sure you can afford it, decide to "go for the gold." If you're like these folks, you decide that if you're going to have surgery, then you want to correct all the things about your appearance that bother you. Or you may instead choose to take things more slowly, focusing on one procedure to see what kind of difference it makes in how you look and feel. If you have a great experience, then you may want to go back for more.

Shopping for Cosmetic Surgery

If you're thinking about having cosmetic surgery and starting your shopping process, you're going to be confronted with a lot of acronyms and you may feel like you've been dropped into a bowl of alphabet soup. Trying to make sense of who is who and what is what in the wide world of cosmetic surgery isn't easy. Between your friends, advertising, and the popular press, you can gather lots of good information, but unfortunately, you'll hear some things that are either misleading or downright wrong. Misinformation abounds in the field of cosmetic surgery. You need to play detective to get to the truth. Chapters 3, 4, and 5 give you all the information you need to shop for — and find — the right surgeon.

Shopping may or may not be your thing, but when you're shopping for cosmetic surgery, you better know what you're doing or you could really endanger yourself. You need to shop intelligently after first finding out how to proceed. You need recommendations or leads, and you must get estimates of the cost so you can budget. (Chapter 6 discusses the financial issues.) You have to find a good surgeon and explore your surgical options (which you can read about in Part III). This may sound like a lot of work, but spending your time finding out how to shop for a surgeon is a lot better than spending time regretting your decision.

If you want to find a good surgeon, you have to educate yourself. You have to make sense of certification (see Chapter 3) so that you can evaluate the doctors you'll visit. Be on the lookout for someone well educated, properly trained, board-certified, and experienced in the procedure you've decided on. You want to be sure that your surgery is being performed in a safe setting with an appropriate anesthesia provider. You also want to choose a capable patient-care team to see you through the preparation and recovery process.

More importantly, you'll have to determine the risk-to-benefit ratio. It sounds scientific and tough to do, but really it isn't. Every surgery has risk factors, but every surgery also benefits the patient in some way. As an intelligent person, you'll want to know about the risks (which I discuss in Chapter 17) and weigh the benefits — in other words, become an informed consumer — before finally making your decision.

PERSONAL STORY

Finding Dr. Right

Beverly, a 60-year-old retired elementary principal with seven grandchildren, inherited her mother's and grandmother's tendency to wrinkle and decided to pursue facial surgery. She felt that as a professional woman she needed to look younger and healthier.

She approached the process of choosing a surgeon seriously. Beverly wanted to know their skills, so she did her Internet research. She developed a group of questions to compare surgeons and facilities. She decided to have consults with three surgeons, all of whom were board-certified plastic surgeons with accredited facilities. She determined that the three surgeons produced similar quality results.

Beverly based her ultimate decision on a variety of factors she could discern only in on-site consultation visits. Here's what she had to say about making her decision, "Actually, I liked another surgeon's personality better, but the surgeon I chose recorded his thoughts and assessments and sent a follow-up letter. He was professional and knowledgeable. The nurses and front office staff were professional, reassuring, and knowledgeable. They really were the deciding factor with my list of pros and cons for surgeons and facilities."

Her advice if you're considering cosmetic surgery: "Do research, ask questions, and go into surgery with total confidence in the surgeon, facility, and the staff — especially the nurses. Go for it! This is one area I would never look for a 'bargain.' While cost is a factor, it is better to save for a few more months than accept anything but the best surgeon."

And did her system work? Here's what she has to say about her ultimate result and the impact on her life: "My eyes look livelier, and the forehead wrinkles have decreased. I have more self-confidence that people will see the *real* me when they look at my face. I recently interviewed for a job, knowing that I looked my best, and I was hired. My life hasn't changed — I have an active, fun, interesting life. What has changed is that my face matches my energetic youthful feeling."

Being Realistic about Recovery and Results

Sometimes being realistic is a challenge, but if you're considering cosmetic surgery, you'll need to know what's possible and more likely to happen. Aligning your expectations with what is really possible makes for a successful surgery. An obese person who wants liposuction to substitute for dieting and good health habits isn't being realistic. If he imagines that he'll suddenly have the smooth body of a weightlifter, he'll be terribly disappointed. But someone who's already lost massive amounts of weight and wants a body lift to remove the extra skin is more realistic and may be very happy so long as he understands the scarring involved. Be fully informed and accept what your surgeon can and cannot do. Yes, lots of patients call their procedures "miracles," but remember these are scientific miracles, limited and on a human scale.

You also need to be realistic about your recovery (see Chapter 18). You can take steps yourself to positively affect your recovery, including being in great physical shape and creating the necessary time and conditions to rest and heal. Don't imagine that recovery is instantaneous. Your recovery will take time, so plan for it.

Life is unpredictable, and sometimes, even with the best of surgeons, things can go wrong or complications arise. You'll want to know how the practice you've chosen handles these situations. Find out what to expect from the doctor, the nurse, or other team members. Also find out in advance what complications are normal for this procedure and whether there's anything you can do to help prevent them. For example, you'll want to be completely honest with your surgeon about your health history, the medications you take, drug allergies, other sensitivities, and specific health conditions. Although you may think these things may be unrelated to plastic surgery, let the doctors — the surgeon and anesthesiologist — work with the most information to get you the best result. Many offices handle complications well, wholeheartedly support their patients, and fully resolve any problems. Look for a practice with that motivation and reputation.

If you go by the numbers, your surgical experience will be a happy one. You'll come through surgery with a normal healing phase and reenter your life feeling better about your appearance and with a better self-image — like you've had an emotional facelift.

Chapter 2

Making a Decision about Cosmetic Surgery

Cosmetic surgery used to be for the rich and famous and sometimes for the self-centered and vain. Today, however, most cosmetic surgery patients are average, everyday people who wish to improve their lives in a positive, happy way. We're presuming that if you're reading this book, you're looking for good information to help you evaluate the many implications of this important choice and make a more informed decision. Ultimately, it doesn't matter what other folks are doing or why. You must make an intensely personal decision and decide whether cosmetic surgery is right for you.

Finding Out whether Cosmetic Surgery Is Right for You

Cosmetic surgery can be one of the most life-changing and positive experiences over which you have control. Although cosmetic surgery brings happiness to millions of people, your chances for success are much greater if you begin from the right emotional and psychological place. If you're healthy (physically and psychologically) and can afford it, then you may well choose to consider cosmetic surgery.

When you're facing a decision of this importance, introspection is a good thing. Spend more time exploring your concerns and understanding your motivations. If your concerns are real and your motivations are emotionally sound, then you may well give yourself the green light to change some aspect of your physical appearance. But, if you're looking to cosmetic surgery to change your life and resolve significant social or psychological issues, then your first visit should be to a psychologist rather than a plastic surgeon.

Assessing what bothers you

Not everyone who looks in the mirror sees flaws. A lot more people live comfortably within their skin than choose to change their appearance surgically. Unlike the wicked queen in *Snow White,* most cosmetic surgery patients are not seeking to be "the fairest one of all." They're more likely to say, "I just want to look like myself, only better."

As you think about your motivations and concerns, you want to be sure that you know exactly what's bothering you and can describe it clearly to someone else. See Chapter 21 for a list of questions to ask yourself before having cosmetic surgery.

One way of measuring how important the physical changes are to you is to assess how often you think about them. Do your concerns bother you daily or weekly? If you experience top-of-the-mind awareness, then it's probably time to start your research.

The following factors motivate many patients to pursue cosmetic surgery:

- ✔ **Genetics:** You can choose your friends but not your relatives and certainly not your genetics. You look in the mirror and see your Italian grandpa's big nose staring back at you. Your Irish freckles may appeal to your mother, but not to you. Your family origins — be they Asian, African-American, or Italian — dictate physical characteristics, including body fat distribution, that you may not want to live with.

- ✔ **Aging:** Even if you like your basic looks, Father Time still chases you. Your wrinkles appear without permission, and it isn't just because you've been laughing a lot. Gravity has its uses, like keeping your feet on the ground, but it takes a toll on your body. The loose skin around your eyes or chin and neck may connote wisdom and longevity to some minds, but not to yours.

✔ **Sun damage:** You may be one of the many people who didn't even know UV rays caused skin damage — you just thought you were basking in the sun, getting a great tan. Maybe you know about UV rays now but don't care, and you're still frolicking outdoors or playing golf or tennis without SPF skin protection. But the day of reckoning comes when you look in the mirror and see leathery skin staring back at you, or that first basal cell grabs your attention.

✔ **Post-traumatic injuries and scarring:** You may have hit your cheek on the corner of a table when you were a child and have a depressed scar that bothers you. Or you may have very noticeable scars from previous surgery or a burn. Once you have a scar you'll always have a scar, but you'll be happy to know that cosmetic surgeons have at least partial solutions for almost all these problems.

✔ **Physical conditions:** A variety of physical conditions have unpleasant symptoms that prompt people to consider cosmetic surgery. Eyelid surgery can correct limits in peripheral vision; nasal surgery can reduce or eliminate breathing problems. Body reconstruction can take care of many of the physical symptoms that follow massive weight loss (see Chapter 13.) Breast reduction surgery can relieve back and neck pain and chafing under the breasts (see Chapter 16).

✔ **Smoking-induced premature aging:** Smoking compounds and accelerates the effects of aging on your skin. Both first- and secondhand smoke can be detrimental to your skin. If you smoke, you may not be a candidate for certain cosmetic surgery procedures. See Chapter 7 and the individual procedure chapters for more information.

Determining why you want a change

Whatever you hear, see, and encounter in your life becomes part of who you are. You can't get away from the world you live in, and it's only natural to want to fit in with your friends, families, and co-workers and to achieve whatever you can be in your personal life or career. Cosmetic surgery can really help you make changes in your physical appearance that enhance your self-image and enjoyment of life, and plastic surgeons feel that motivations like I describe in the following sections are valid reasons for having surgery.

Being career-minded

Sometimes having cosmetic surgery is a business decision. If you have a job that involves meeting the public, your appearance may be of special concern to you. Looking good and projecting confidence are assets to any career. When you walk out your door in the morning, you want to look and feel your best.

More and more people from all walks of life are coming to plastic surgeons citing workplace issues as a primary motivator. Our culture places enormous emphasis on youth, and older workers can feel threatened or disadvantaged in the workplace. Repeatedly, patients tell me versions of the following: "All the salespeople in our company are young, and I'm beginning to look old. I'm worried about keeping my job."

Looking old and feeling young

One of the most common concerns boomers and preboomers describe is the dissonance between how they feel internally and how they look in the mirror. If all else in your life is in order, then cosmetic surgery may be a means to reconcile the differences you perceive. A new and younger-appearing you can make you feel better not only about yourself but also about life in general. As people begin to live healthier, longer, and more active lives, this concern and a cosmetic surgery solution are more and more common.

Fitting in

You live in today's world, and the fact that voluptuous ladies were Reuben's ideal doesn't help you when you see today's cultural ideal walking down a fashion show runway. As much as you may not like these icons and don't seek to look exactly like them, you're still likely to be somewhat influenced by glamorous celebrities and fashion models, whose well-proportioned bodies and perfect facial features attract media attention every day. Whether you like it or not, society's views of these people aren't going to change any time soon. Surgery isn't a simple solution, but it is certainly an option if you want to more closely approach the cultural definition of the ideal body.

Helping your child avoid stigma

Cosmetic surgery isn't only for adults. Maybe your child has some slight cosmetic abnormality that could influence his successful socialization. Examples include young children with protruding ears, early teen-agers with abnormal appearing noses, or girls with significant breast asymmetry, overly large breasts or no breast development at all. In these cases, parents can intervene on the child's behalf to avoid permanent social consequences.

Plastic surgeons are happy to address these kinds of issues. Where they draw the line, even with parental consent, is when a young person wants surgery that is not based on genetic or post-traumatic issues but is socially motivated. For example, a 16-year-old girl, who is not completely developed physically or psychologically, wants to enlarge her otherwise normal breasts from a B cup to a full C. In these cases, I encourage the patient and her parents to wait until her physical development is complete.

Maintaining attitude

Christine, a 63-year-old civil servant, first started considering cosmetic surgery about two years ago because she "wasn't getting any younger" and didn't like what age was doing to her. After doing her homework and finding a qualified plastic surgeon, she decided to give herself a lift of her face, neck, and eyes. Christine describes herself as having an outgoing personality and positive outlook on life, and she was "determined to do something that would help me maintain that attitude."

According to Christine, "The results have far exceeded my expectations. I had no idea how well it would turn out. My husband likes it and is always telling me how good I look. I'm nine years older than he is, and now I look years younger than I did before."

Coping with life changes

Lots of things in life come our way that we don't expect — some are positive, and some are negative. You may be dealing with a major lifestyle change, such as divorce or the death of your spouse. You or your child may be about to get married. These and many other types of lifestyle changes prompt people to consider cosmetic surgery as a positive and restorative choice. There are as many stories as people, and you may have a story of your own that motivates you at some point in your life to think about cosmetic surgery.

Getting your body back after childbearing

You may identify with the young mothers who come to plastic surgeons complaining about the changes in their breasts and tummies. Childbearing takes its toll, and exercise and dieting can only do so much. Today's fashions emphasize breasts and tummies, and if your breasts are saggy and your tummy skin is wrinkled, then you may want to do something about it.

Wanting to be rid of excess fat and skin

You may exercise and eat right, but no matter what you do, you can't get rid of pockets of excess fat or excess skin. This is where cosmetic surgery really shines. Both male and female patients come to plastic surgeons with these issues. If your issue is localized fat deposits, liposuction can be very helpful. If you're concerned about excess skin, common procedures for women are breast and tummy surgery. Women and an increasing number of men are seeking eyelid and facial/neck surgery to remove excess skin and to give them a fresher, younger look.

Dealing with excess skin after massive weight loss

More and more people are having gastric bypass surgery or losing massive amounts of weight. If you lose 75 to 100 pounds or more, you may well be able to hide the excess skin under some clothes, but you'll probably never be happy until the unwanted skin is removed. Sometimes losing as little as 10 or 20 pounds can cause severe skin excess in your breasts or abdomen. Exercise almost never helps shrink the skin following large weight loss. And the more weight you lose, the greater the excess skin problem. Turn to Chapter 13 to find out more.

Wanting to restore your self-esteem and sexiness

You may be dealing with changes in your body that affect your feelings about yourself and find that these feelings carry into your sex life. You're less willing to be seen or touched. Your enjoyment of intimacy is reduced, and you don't like feeling that way. Any number of issues can stimulate these feelings, but certain cosmetic procedures, including breast surgery, body contouring procedures, and facial procedures, may help restore your self image and your enjoyment of sex. Patients who have cosmetic surgery for this reason often say, "I'm so happy with how I feel about myself, and now the romance is back in our relationship."

Looking at how much the problem bothers you

Physical issues can also impact the quality of your life or lifestyle choices. If you're limiting your life because of physical issues that can be changed, then you may well want to live your life to the fullest by either considering cosmetic surgery or accepting who you are now and getting on with your life.

Cosmetic surgery isn't a substitute for healthy living, wise food choices, or sound emotional decisions. But if something about your body gets in the way of your enjoyment of your daily life — maybe you hide from the camera, avoid wearing shorts or sleeveless tops, or steer clear of social situations — acknowledging and thinking about the problem should be another step of your decision-making process.

Listening to others

Whether those close to you support or reject the idea of cosmetic surgery in general or for you specifically, you need to consider their feelings and opinions. You can certainly expect encouragement and support from your circle of friends and family who have had positive cosmetic surgery experiences.

They'll enjoy the mentoring role — giving helpful advice and useful observations. But despite their positive experiences, you should be prepared for the fact that they may not agree with you about what you envision.

You can also expect some friends and family to express justifiable personal concerns about the idea of your having cosmetic surgery. When dealing with the concerns of people close to you, you need to think seriously about their objections. Are their concerns justified or are they objecting because they don't have the problem and don't know how it feels? You need to integrate their opinions with all the other factors you consider as you make your decision. Don't be afraid of naysayers, because they'll help you sort through important facts that need to be considered.

As you think about whom to tell, you need to start with your spouse or significant other, especially if you expect objections. Even if you believe you need a facelift, your spouse may think you look great and have other thoughts about how to spend the money. This topic can be emotional or unpleasant to talk about, but you should work through these issues *before* surgery. If you value your relationship, this isn't a time for unilateral action.

Communication and shared commitment are important. If your spouse or significant other has concerns or serious objections to your having cosmetic surgery, one way you can come to a joint decision is to ask him to come to the consultations with you so he can hear what surgeons think about your issues, ask questions himself, and understand the risks, recovery, and costs associated with your potential decision.

Think carefully about the other people you plan to tell. Potential supporters could become detractors if they find out after the fact. You also need to think about whether you're going to share your thoughts with friends and family who you know won't support you in this decision. If your aunt is a Christian Scientist or an Orthodox Jew, her religious beliefs preclude her from ever supporting such a decision. Maybe it's a conversation not worth having at this point along the way. Alternatively, you could tell her in advance and acknowledge her beliefs but let her know that you're seriously considering taking this course. Give her the opportunity to explain her objections. Maybe you'll learn something important that you hadn't considered.

Watching for red flags

Sometimes people want to have cosmetic surgery for reasons that should send up red flags. If any of the following sections apply to you, then you need to be very cautious about having cosmetic surgery at this time. If you identify with one of the following situations, a better approach is to solve this primary issue and think about cosmetic surgery later when you're at a better place in your life.

Thinking you have a problem but no one else sees it

You may occasionally become fixated on some portion of your anatomy that you think is abnormal. Yet when you seek verification from friends, family, or cosmetic surgeons, they don't see anything wrong. A good plastic surgeon doesn't want to operate on an area that he perceives as completely normal.

When no one else in your life can see the problem that you see, you may be dealing with body image issues. At its most extreme this is a mental health diagnosis called body dysmorphic disorder (BDD), and requires psychological or psychiatric help rather than cosmetic surgery.

Feeling depressed

You may definitely feel better about yourself after cosmetic surgery, but it's not a substitute for good mental health care. If you're depressed, you should seek professional help for your depression first. Then, after you're well on your way to overcoming that problem, you can consider cosmetic surgery.

As long as your reasons for seeking cosmetic surgery are sound ones, your mental health professional can help you to analyze your motivations and determine when the time is right within the context of the treatment you're receiving for depression.

Solving a relationship crisis

If you're in the midst of a marital or relationship trauma, don't expect cosmetic surgery to solve interpersonal relationships. You don't want to make such an important decision because you feel you may lose a spouse or partner. Changing your appearance may be an important and positive step forward for you, but you never want to look back and think that you wouldn't have had surgery if you hadn't been in a fear-of-loss situation.

Both you and your spouse or significant other may agree that you want/need a cosmetic procedure, but do it when your emotional life is stable. Your chances for a positive outcome are much better when your environment for surgery and recovery is as stress-free as possible.

Recovering from the death of a spouse

Don't make a decision to have cosmetic surgery while you're in the midst of major stress, such as grieving. Undergoing surgery involves physical, emotional, and psychological factors, so you want to be sure that you're fully prepared on all fronts. Give yourself time to grieve so that you can reach the place where you can optimally prepare for and recover from surgery as well.

You also need time to heal so that you can make a totally rational decision. Wait a while and allow time to mourn. If you take this approach, doing something for yourself also seems much more palatable to those around you.

Feeling bored or restless

Cosmetic surgery does wonderful things, but every procedure is real surgery with real risks. If your motivation is boredom and restlessness, try a new hobby or exercise program, not cosmetic surgery, which is something that requires serious thought and planning. You want to consider cosmetic surgery because of real physical, emotional, or social issues that inhibit your enjoyment of your life. If you're thinking about surgery because you're bored or restless, seeking professional guidance may be your best first step.

Acknowledging eating disorders

If you suffer from an eating disorder, such as bulimia or anorexia nervosa, you don't want to have surgery, and besides, your surgeon won't want to operate on you if it puts your life at risk. All these problems relate to body image issues, and resolution of these concerns should take precedence over cosmetic surgery.

If you're otherwise healthy and under treatment for an eating disorder, cosmetic surgery may be appropriate. You must reveal your problem to your surgeon, and if you're under care, bring a note from your psychologist or psychiatrist that explains why you can proceed with surgery. You want to be sure that whatever concern brings you to the plastic surgeon is appropriate from a physical and mental health perspective. If its not, then this is not the time to be having cosmetic surgery and your surgeon will not go forward without a psychiatric clearance.

Having surgery because of outside pressure

The first and most basic rule of cosmetic surgery is that you do it for yourself and not for someone else — especially not to please a boyfriend or girlfriend whom you may replace in several months. Although appearance is something that can cause pain or give pleasure, be very careful when you hear messages from a boyfriend or girlfriend that suggest that you'll be acceptable, attractive, or loveable only after cosmetic surgery changes.

Ultimately, you and you alone subject yourself to the real risks involved, and you're the one who has to live with the outcome. Don't make a decision of this importance unless you're personally driven by a real need to fix something that bothers *you.*

Determining whether You Are Right for Cosmetic Surgery

Only when you are realistic about the real risks of having cosmetic surgery, the costs, and the recovery can you make the best possible decision for yourself. Remember, you're in the driver's seat here, and the choice is yours. You can say "aye" or "nay" to cosmetic surgery. One thing is certain: You'll be the one who has to live with the consequences, whatever you do.

Different people have different triggers that turn dissatisfaction into action. At some point, something happens that tilts you over the edge — one way or another. Your decision-making process may lead to one of three conclusions: go forward, stop, or postpone your decision. Understanding your motivations is an important step toward making your final decision.

Getting to the heart of your motivations

When considering having cosmetic surgery, you want to be sure that your motivations are personal and positive. When you're in control of your life and are a positive and happy person, cosmetic surgery can be a wonderful way to improve some imperfection that is bothering you. You're not looking at cosmetic surgery as a panacea for your problems but as an enhancement of your nice life.

PERSONAL STORY

Saying good riddance to a complex

Nancy, a 22-year-old cosmetologist, is surrounded by the world of beauty. She first considered cosmetic surgery when she was only 14 years old. "I started having a complex about my nose, and knew I eventually wanted to do something about it."

She says that what finally prompted her to call was that a friend was having her nose done. Although she visited three surgeons during her research, Nancy said that she wouldn't have changed a thing about the surgeon or the facility and staff that she eventually chose. "The staff was very important and always made me feel like I was getting the best care possible."

Nancy is very pleased with her results and says that her surgical experience was "ten times easier than I had expected, and my results came out perfect to my expectations. My confidence has gone way up."

If you're thinking about having cosmetic surgery to solve some life crises or heal a sick emotional relationship, think again. The very fact that you are dealing with significant emotional or psychological issues should be a warning flag to you to wait. If you don't have any emotional or relationships issues but are facing significant financial or health issues, then you also want to wait until those issues are resolved. This is a significant personal decision, and you want all your ducks in a row. This decision isn't one in which you simply hope for the best or plunge ahead.

Assessing your health

Surprisingly, most people who function normally are able to have surgery, but it requires complete honesty, many precautions, and careful planning. A careful medical workup reveals whether cosmetic surgery is safe for you.

Some conditions definitely make it too risky to have certain procedures. See Chapter 7 for more information on this important topic. Understand that you must be candid with your surgeon — you may have health conditions (obesity, for example) or personal habits (such as smoking or drug use) that make surgery impossible.

If you want to ignore sound advice and withhold pertinent medical information, you may be able to keep shopping until you find a surgeon who will operate on you, but at what risk? What will be the impact for you and your family should you follow this course and something really unfortunate happens? If your medical and surgical specialists tell you that you're not a safe candidate for surgery, then you need to listen.

Checking your finances

One very practical reason for deciding to go ahead with the cosmetic surgery that you've been wanting is that you can finally afford it. Cosmetic surgery is rarely covered by insurance, so you have to be prepared to pay for it yourself.

If you're like some patients, you prepare in advance and have the total amount of money you need for the procedure in your checking account. Fewer than 50 percent of patients fall into that category. An increasing number of patients are using creative ways to realize their cosmetic surgery dreams. You don't want to be financially irresponsible, but if you find that you can afford it, then you may decide to "go for it." Chapter 6 covers this topic in more detail.

Your desire to have cosmetic surgery can't supersede rational financial planning. Out-of-control finances can do permanent damage to your financial future. Get your financial life in order before you go forward with the surgery. Never forget that healing is optimized when you're calm and stress free. Being in severe financial trouble can cause emotional distress, which can impair healing and recovery.

Accepting cosmetic surgery's limits

The mirror may reflect something you want to change, but you must be realistic about what's achievable. Ultimately, you need a consultation with a surgeon to determine whether your desires are fully compatible with your body type. The best surgeon can't change your genetic makeup. You'll find more details about this subject when you read the procedure information in Part III. The happiest patients are those who accept the changes that are achievable and don't expect those that aren't possible. They aren't trying to look like someone else or become someone else — they just want to be the best they can be.

Cosmetic surgery doesn't absolve you of the responsibility to eat and exercise responsibly. Liposuction is a good method of changing contours, but it's not a substitute for weight loss. Liposuction is a wonderful procedure for the person who is within normal weight ranges but who can't diet or exercise away certain genetic contours that can be truly troublesome. The single exception is surgery after massive weight loss (see Chapter 13).

Finding Out What to Expect

In 1990, I wrote patient education and surgical information that is now used by more than 950 plastic surgeons. One reason for providing this material was that I believed that patients entered the surgical experience without really understanding what was going to happen — they didn't know what to expect as far as risks and complications and what was normal during recovery.

The information I gave then is just as valuable today. If you decide to have cosmetic surgery, you'll be a lot happier because you fully investigated the potential consequences and made an informed decision. You may also decide that the risk-reward ratio is one that you can't tolerate. In either case, read the following sections with an open mind.

Acknowledging the risks

As you think about having cosmetic surgery, you must acknowledge that all surgery involves some degree of risk, and you must accept those surgical risks — however small the percentage. If a surgical procedure has a 2 percent or even 20 percent risk factor, then the percentages of positive outcomes are in your favor. However, if you end up having a problem, then the 2 percent or 20 percent becomes a 100 percent risk factor to you. So don't skip over the discussions of general surgical risks in Chapter 17 or the specific risks discussed in the various procedure chapters in Part III. You have to decide — going in — that emotionally, financially, and physically, you can deal with a potential worst-case scenario.

Being realistic about the pain

The amount of pain you experience relates to a number of factors:

- ✔ **Type of surgery:** Generally, the more minor the surgery, the less the likelihood of significant pain. In general facial surgery also has less pain than body contouring surgery.

- ✔ **Your own pain tolerance:** As you can see in patient comments throughout this book, some people report almost no pain, while others for the same procedure report serious pain. Pain tolerance varies greatly from person to person.

- ✔ **Gender:** Any nurse will tell you that men have a lower pain tolerance and less patience for the recovery process than women.

Fitting recovery into your lifestyle

For some reason, many cosmetic surgery patients seem to think that they aren't really going to have to consider a real recovery phase. Not true (see Chapter 18 for more details on recovery).

If plastic surgeons could figure out who would have faster and easier recoveries, they would do so. Like the issue of pain, people's individual responses to surgery vary greatly — from quick and easy to slow and hard. Following your surgeon's instructions is the best option. Take it easy and let your body heal. If you're too active too early, you can cause a complication that will throw your recovery schedule to the wind and possibly involve additional surgery and additional costs.

Plan for the worst-case scenario and be happy if things go better than expected. Beware of the surgeon who promises fast and pain-free recovery while other doctors are describing recovery processes that are longer and more limiting. There is a definite relationship between the extent of surgery you have, the corresponding recovery, and your ultimate results.

Being prepared for additional costs

Another factor to consider is that you may need more money than the cost of the surgical procedure you're considering. You need to be prepared for a worst-case scenario that would increase costs or decrease income: if you have to be away from work longer than expected because of healing delays or if you need secondary surgery. Wait until you're ready financially and then proceed. Chapter 7 gives you the lowdown on financial preparation.

Getting acquainted with the new you

One possibility that you must consider is that you'll have a negative postsurgical reaction to the new you. Although most patients are very happy with their results, a small minority is thrown into an emotional tailspin by the changes they see. They no longer see themselves in the mirror and can't identify with the changes. If this occurs to you, keep in mind that most patients are able to work though this reaction, but it's an important reason why you must always have surgery because *you* want it and not because others wanted you to have it.

Letting the Decision Be Yours Alone

Ultimately, this decision rests with you. It reflects your needs and desires. You'll reap the benefits and cope with any potential consequences. You need to give yourself permission to do this if it's really important to you. You don't need to suffer in silence when a solution is readily available.

If you're like many cosmetic surgery patients, you've been considering having cosmetic surgery for years. Then one day, you finally decide to go for it. You've finally overcome your embarrassment and nervousness about picking up the phone and telling a stranger something intensely private — what you want to have fixed about your body. Lest you change your mind, you call a plastic surgeon immediately and want surgery instantaneously — *yesterday* or *tomorrow* at the latest. My office lovingly refers to these calls as requests for emergency cosmetic surgery.

Returning to the real me

Unhappy with her neck and feeling like she always looked tired, Priscilla, a 58-year-old teacher, decided to do something about it. "I saw photos of myself from a family wedding and thought, 'This does not look like me.' I tore them up. My husband suggested I go ahead and do something, but he also said it was totally up to me."

She made two consultations but ended up canceling the second after feeling completely comfortable with the first surgeon and his staff. "My physician did not push additional surgeries . . . he gave me options." Priscilla said that her results are "all and more" than she expected and would urge people considering surgery to "explore your options. Don't be too critical about yourself afterwards and be sure you are doing it for *yourself,* not someone else."

Whatever your choice, be sure to allow yourself adequate time to do your research and implement the shopping process I urge you to go through. You'll hear a lot of advice and opinions, and you'll need to be at the top of your game to sort through the complexity of this subject. Use your intuitive and intellectual powers and make the best decision possible.

If you think you're ready to go forward with cosmetic surgery, ask yourself the following questions. Chapter 21 also contains some important questions to help you assess your readiness and check your decision-making process.

- ✔ **Am I doing it for me or someone else?** Your primary motivation must be for yourself. Don't do it because someone else is pressuring you.

- ✔ **Am I the only one who sees the problem?** If everyone in your life — friends, family, and consulting surgeons — doesn't agree with your assessment, then perhaps you need counseling rather than surgery.

- ✔ **Is my timing right?** Remember, it isn't just about wanting surgery *now,* but about a myriad of factors, including finances, general health, recovery time, family support, and work issues.

- ✔ **Am I ready for all the potential consequences?** Although most cosmetic surgery turns out well, you need to be prepared for all eventualities. Make sure you're really ready.

- ✔ **Do I have a plan about how to proceed with clear criteria that will optimize a good decision?** You want to thoroughly research your options as explained in Chapter 3 and use the shopping process described in Chapter 4. You also need to exercise due diligence in a way that increases the likelihood that you'll make the best decision possible.

You can freely choose to have cosmetic surgery. Cultural acceptance increases daily. As I often tell patients, "If this is something you want to do for yourself and you aren't taking food from the mouths of your children, then go for it. It's not immoral, illegal, or fattening."

Chapter 3

Looking Out for Your Safety

In This Chapter

▶ Making choices that ensure your safety

▶ Becoming an expert in board certification

▶ Understanding specialization

▶ Making sure the operating suite is accredited

▶ Finding out your anesthesia provider options

▶ Taking the right steps to finding a surgeon and surgery site

*W*ithout a doubt, this is one of the most important chapters in this book. It gives you the information that you need to make wise choices involving your surgeon, the surgery suite, and the anesthesia provider.

In the past, virtually all surgery was done in the hospital, so you didn't have to concern yourself with whether your doctor was qualified or the operating room had the right equipment and personnel. The hospital medical staff and facility certification processes took care of all that for you. Over the past 30 years, much has changed. Today about 75 percent of all surgery is performed on an outpatient basis. You can still count on medical staff surveillance and specialization protocols to protect you if your surgery suite is going to be at a hospital or independent outpatient or ambulatory surgery center (ASC).

Most cosmetic surgery is performed in an office-based setting (a surgical suite in a doctor's office), and depending on your doctor's surgical specialty or the state where your surgery occurs, you may have to make sure that your surgeon is qualified to perform your surgery and that your surgery takes place in a safe environment with all the needed patient protections in place.

Protecting Yourself

With all the different types of consumer protection in this country, you may be shocked to know that the government offers very little protection if you're having surgery in an office-based setting. Federal laws allow anyone with an MD (medical doctor) degree to perform cosmetic surgery in an office-based setting. At its most absurd, that means that so long as a doctor is operating in his or her office, any doctor could do heart surgery or brain surgery on a patient foolish enough to allow it.

This state of affairs means that you must be very careful to protect yourself if you're thinking of having surgery in an office-based setting. Legislation to protect medical consumers varies by state, which makes it even more important that you understand how to find out which doctors are qualified to perform cosmetic surgery.

For some reason, the U.S. government wants to make sure that free competition exists in the field of medicine. Having free and open competition may protect you from price gouging, but it fails to protect cosmetic surgery consumers in the office-based surgical setting. Unfortunately, the free market enables any MD — including general practitioners, internists, gynecologists, oral surgeons, general surgeons, radiologists, otolaryngologists (head and neck or facial plastic surgeons), dermatologists, ophthalmologists, and so on — to perform cosmetic surgery.

The money that consumers around the world spend on looking better is staggering. Cosmetic surgery by itself is a multi-billion-dollar industry. At the same time that the growth of cosmetic surgery has exploded, Medicare and other third-party payers (insurance companies) have decreased what they pay doctors and dentists for providing needed medical and dental care. In many areas of the country, insurance reimburses only 25 to 40 percent of what a doctor charges.

As a result, plenty of practicing physicians would be glad to exchange incomes with a plumber in their community. Instead, they look at the areas of medicine where the consumer pays directly, and cosmetic surgery is one of the most lucrative of these areas. Because of limited consumer protections, these doctors, regardless of whether they have had specialty training or not, can perform cosmetic surgery in an office-based surgery suite.

If you choose to ignore these issues, you put yourself at risk unnecessarily. Things can go wrong even in the most ideal situation. Why put yourself in a position where you're more likely to end up in the hands of a doctor who doesn't actually have the training and experience she claims?

Sorting Through Board Certification

You've probably heard that you need to find a doctor who is *board certified* (vetted by their specialty board) to perform your cosmetic surgery. And you'd think that having gone through at least 13 years of schooling beyond high school, surgeons would automatically become board certified upon completion. But that's not the way it works. They still have some very big hurdles, including spending a specified time in practice, demonstrating surgical quality, and passing comprehensive written and oral exams.

Doctors are certified by the American Board of Medical Specialties (ABMS). According to the ABMS, about 89 percent of physicians are certified by one of its member boards. For more details, see the section "Relying on the American Board of Medical Specialties," later in this chapter.

Understanding medical specialization

Medicine is so complicated that all doctors can't possibly know everything about every topic. So doctors *specialize,* or focus on narrower areas of medicine and surgery. For instance, internal medicine is a medical specialty, and plastic surgery is a surgical specialty. To become a surgical specialist, a candidate must first graduate from college and then spend four years in medical school. After that comes the specialty training (residency), which involves a several-year commitment during which the young physician works at a hospital with senior staff and progresses from minimal responsibility to eventually having essentially complete responsibility for the care of patients.

Becoming a plastic surgeon requires six to eight years of training beyond medical school. Becoming a facial plastic surgeon requires five to seven years, and dermatology training can range from three to five years.

When doctors complete their training, they must apply to the state in which they practice for a license to practice medicine. That's a different process from board certification, which, once achieved, is a specialty status that is recognized in all states.

Checking out the process for certification

After doctors complete their residencies, they can enter practice but still aren't considered board-certified. For a specified time (one to several years, depending on the specialty), doctors are designated as "board eligible." Board-eligible surgeons have completed all their training, but they're not yet able to "sit" (qualify) for their boards.

Boards are usually a combination of written and oral exams focused entirely on the combination of medicine and surgery knowledge associated with a particular specialty. Passing the boards is a very big deal. For essentially all surgeons who have completed their surgical training, passing the boards is a matter of medical life and death. Not everyone passes. Some good plastic surgeons are not board certified, but I recommend going with the odds and choosing a board-certified surgeon.

To become board-eligible, surgeons must begin to practice on their own, operate on patients, and keep records of the results in order to be able to prove their competency in a wide variety of surgical cases. A board-eligible surgeon has completed all her training but hasn't met the time-in-practice or experience criteria required before she may take her boards. She may be the best or the worst surgeon in your community. If you wish to use her services, you need to check on her skills in other ways (see Chapter 5).

If you think about it another way, all board-eligible plastic surgeons have had more training than any of the surgical specialties that require only one residency. So a board-eligible plastic surgeon may be as good or better for your surgery than a board-certified head and neck surgeon who has met the time-in-practice criteria but has one less surgical residency.

How some doctors fudge a little on board certification

Several surgical specialties have board-certified members who perform cosmetic surgery procedures. What you, as a consumer, want to know is whether their training programs prepared your potential surgeon to perform the specific procedures you want.

Sorting through all this isn't easy. For instance, the ABMS specialty of oto-laryngology is variously called ENT (ear, nose, and throat) and head and neck surgery. Surgeons trained in this area have also created a board that they call the American Board of Facial Plastic and Reconstructive Surgery but which is not recognized by the ABMS. For more on that, read on.

What commonly happens is that you go for several consultations to inquire about a facelift, for example. You may find out that one surgeon you meet with was trained in ENT (head and neck surgery) and became board certified in ENT, so she can discuss your options about facial surgery and also state that she is board certified. If she's totally ethical, however, she'll explain that her board certification is in otolaryngology and she hasn't been trained to perform any procedure below your neck. She may even say she is a facial plastic surgeon, which is not a board certification that is recognized by the American Board of Medical Specialties. If you aren't careful, this doctor may allow you to leave her office believing that she is a plastic surgeon.

To be fair to the facial plastic surgeon in this example, she may have had training in facelifts. She may even be the best facial surgeon in your area. But, if she allows you to believe that she's a plastic surgeon and has completed two surgical residencies when she has not, then her behavior is devious at best and, at worst, borders on fraud.

A dermatologist may be the best person to see about a peel or some types of laser treatment. Both plastic surgeons and head and neck surgeons may be equally prepared to perform nasal surgery. Problems occur when the facial plastic surgeons start doing breast augmentations or tummy tucks. Their specialty training didn't include those procedures. Likewise, a general surgeon who wants to do cosmetic surgery has had no training in cosmetic surgery of the face and probably had no training in cosmetic procedures of the body either. She is trained to remove your gall bladder, though.

Clearly, gynecologists, emergency room doctors, and general practitioners have had no plastic or cosmetic surgery training at all. These specialists, if performing cosmetic procedures, have usually learned one type of cosmetic surgery, such as liposuction or perhaps breast augmentation. Although you may find a rare instance of one of these "specialists" performing quality cosmetic surgery, I don't recommend that you choose such a doctor for your cosmetic surgery. They're not trained or certified for those operations, and they likely have failed to complete the educational requirements to get such training or certification.

Relying on the American Board of Medical Specialties

Wading through the ins and outs of medical specialization is too tall (and too boring) an order for most prospective patients. Fortunately, an organization known as the American Board of Medical Specialties (ABMS) takes care of this step for you by determining who has the appropriate education and training to practice which forms of medicine.

Only 24 specialties are recognized by the ABMS. In addition, there are over 180 self-designated medical boards in the United States, some of which have applied for ABMS membership and have not met the criteria and many others that have never applied for approval.

Understanding the ABMS

The job of the ABMS is to act on the public's behalf and to ensure that physicians have met educational and professional standards that merit board certification. The subject is so complex and the turf battles so intense that consumers should be very glad that the ABMS exists.

The ABMS is actually an organization of 24 approved medical specialty boards, each of which has its own name and supervises the activities of its specialty, including training, assessment of professional patient care quality, and the right to set requirements and grant board certification.

Each of the member boards is called the "American Board of (insert name of specialty)." For plastic surgery, the ABMS certifying agency is called the American Board of Plastic Surgery. For anesthesiology, the ABMS certifying agency is called the American Board of Anesthesiology.

Benefiting from insider knowledge

Even though more than 100 boards have applied for formal approval, the ABMS has certified only 24 specialties — meaning that their training and testing processes merit recognition by the ABMS. You can see that the ABMS has done a great job of saying no, but, unfortunately most of the public doesn't know what they've said yes to!

Your first assignment, if you choose to accept it, is to look at the following list and become familiar with the 24 medical specialties approved by the ABMS. Here they are:

- ✔ Allergy and immunology
- ✔ Anesthesiology
- ✔ Colon and rectal surgery
- ✔ Dermatology
- ✔ Emergency medicine
- ✔ Family practice
- ✔ Internal medicine
- ✔ Medical genetics
- ✔ Neurological surgery
- ✔ Nuclear medicine
- ✔ Obstetrics and gynecology
- ✔ Ophthalmology
- ✔ Orthopedic surgery
- ✔ Otolaryngology
- ✔ Pathology
- ✔ Pediatrics
- ✔ Physical medicine and rehabilitation
- ✔ Plastic surgery
- ✔ Preventive medicine
- ✔ Psychiatry and neurology
- ✔ Radiology
- ✔ Surgery, general
- ✔ Thoracic surgery
- ✔ Urology

Perfectly clear, right? But you're thinking about having cosmetic surgery. Well, where's the cosmetic surgery specialty? It's not there. Cosmetic surgical procedures are hidden within this list and mostly under the specialty of plastic surgery, which includes both cosmetic surgery to deal with changes in form and reconstructive surgery to deal with changes in function, as I explain in Chapter 1.

Not one of the 24 boards approved by the ABMS has the word "cosmetic" in its title. So if you hear that a doctor is board certified in cosmetic surgery, then you know that surgeon is not board certified by the ABMS. That means her training and board certification may be in question. Your first rule must be that you will choose a surgeon who is board-certified in a specialty recognized by the ABMS to perform the procedure you're considering. So you need to keep looking for a surgeon who has been trained and certified to perform your cosmetic surgery.

Recognizing sound-alike boards

Muddying the waters further, some doctors have created their own boards that sound a lot like they're part of the ABMS but aren't. These doctors may be great, but they have been trained and certified by an entirely different process, which isn't as thorough as that set forth by the ABMS. If they could earn ABMS approval for their specialty, you can be certain that they would have done so.

Checking with the ABMS first

Kelly described her shopping process when she decided to entertain the idea of cosmetic surgery. She spoke to several friends and got the names of three doctors, "The first thing I did was to call the medical board (ABMS) to inquire about their qualifications and to be sure they were plastic surgeons. Then I made my appointments."

Because they were quite different, her consultations with the surgeons helped her decision process. "Two of them suggested only specific procedures with NO other options. It seemed they wanted to redo my entire face instead of focusing on my problem areas. One of them did not have any before-and-after pictures to view. He said he did not need to prove his work to anyone else because he knew he did good

work." Another doctor had several photos but was extremely expensive. The doctor she chose "had several books to show his work. I was very impressed; before-and-after photos played a huge part in my final decision." One week later, she decided to have both her eyes and nose done. "I thought if I was going to go through a surgery, I should do it all at the same time . . . money and healing being an issue."

Kelly describes her recovery and result: "After the bruising and swelling had gone, I felt like Cinderella. I didn't mind looking in the mirror again. I used to dread seeing those bags and large nose. The bags are completely gone, and my nose is cute. People I knew said I looked 10-plus years younger."

If, for example, your doctor says she's board certified by the American Board of Facial Plastic and Reconstructive Surgery (ABFPRS), you may think she's been approved by the ABMS. Sounds a lot like it, right? Go back to that list of specialties. You can see that the ABMS doesn't recognize facial plastic and reconstructive surgery as a specialty. Although the American Board of Plastic Surgery (ABPS) is one of the 24 specialties approved by the ABMS, the similarly named American Board of Facial Plastic and Reconstructive Surgery is not. It's just a bunch of doctors — some of whom may be very good — who made up their own board in 1986.

So you can see that what's an "American board" to one set of doctors is an "American non-board" to another. Trust me. Leave this matter to the folks in the know — the ABMS. You want to find board-certified surgeons who tell you truthfully which ABMS board certifies them to perform your surgery. If any doctors say that they're board certified by any board other than one of the 24 specialties listed above, then you need to ask yourself why they want to misrepresent their education and training.

Many of the 100 "boards" that applied for ABMS status (and were rejected) went outside the ABMS system and started unofficial or uncertified boards. Thus, a very pretty and official-looking document can be issued by a group of physicians who make up the governing body and have formed such a medical board. They do this because, according to the rigorous standards of the ABMS, they don't have the specialty training required to perform the procedure and earn board certification by the ABMS. And, worst of all, in my opinion, they're unwilling to go back and go through the training process that would enable them to ethically perform the procedures they want to.

The question you have to ask yourself is why would you want to have your surgery performed by someone who took a beginner training course at a weekend seminar. No matter how charming the surgeon is, you deserve better. There are real risks to having surgery — even with a qualified plastic surgeon in a certified facility. Don't submit to surgery from a virtually untrained person or someone who is operating outside of her specialty training.

Facial plastic surgeons are not trained or board certified in surgical procedures of the body, such as breast augmentation, tummy tucks, breast reductions, body lifts, and so on. Don't let a head and neck or facial plastic surgeon do any of these procedures on you. And remember that their ABMS specialty is otolaryngology (ear, nose, and throat), which means they aren't trained to do surgery below your neck.

Asking about board certification

Almost all physicians who market or advertise cosmetic surgery services state that they're board certified. The $64,000 question is, "In what specialty?" You want to be sure the answer is a board recognized by the ABMS.

Look for the surgeon's board certification certificate on her office walls. If it isn't clearly displayed, ask to see it. If it doesn't say that the surgeon is certified by the American Board of Plastic Surgery, the surgeon isn't a legitimate plastic surgeon. Those of us who are plastic surgeons are very proud of the name and the level of training and commitment that it represents; we don't enjoy others borrowing it for purely monetary reasons.

If you're in doubt about whether your surgeon is certified by an ABMS board, it's easy to check. Go to your computer or the telephone and contact the ABMS at `www.abms.org` or `www.certifieddoctor.org`, which has a link to the ABMS site. You can call the ABMS, too: 866-ASK-ABMS (275-2267).

Wonderful and skilled physicians in all specialties have an interest in cosmetic surgery. In your particular area, the best noses or faces may be done by a board-certified ENT surgeon. The most knowledge about laser treatments or peels may be found at a cosmetic dermatologist's office in your community. I didn't write this book to persuade all patients to go to plastic surgeons for all problems. Statistically however, I feel that you probably have the best chance of getting the best skill set and experience level if you choose a plastic surgeon who is active in the cosmetic surgery field.

Understanding How Hospitals Handle Medical Specialization

Medical specialization defines what a doctor can and cannot do — this is referred to as "scope of practice." Hospitals across the country have systems in place that protect the public from doctors doing procedures that they haven't been trained to do. When a new physician moves to your community, she needs to join a hospital staff where she can admit patients who need hospitalization. If hospitals allowed any doctor, regardless of qualifications, to take care of sick patients in their hospital, care would deteriorate, and eventually something would go wrong and a patient would be injured or die. Hospitals therefore take great pains to ensure that the doctors they work with are qualified to practice the kind of medicine they're trained to perform and remain within their scope of practice.

Legislating cosmetic surgery

Interested medical and dental organizations have now taken the scope-of-practice fight to the state legislators to try to solve their problems on a global scale. Scope-of-practice bills are designed to give various non-plastic surgery specialties the legal right to perform cosmetic surgery in any hospital in that state. If these bills pass, those surgeons can have their own certified operating rooms or work in outpatient surgery centers or hospitals.

In 2004, a scope-of-practice bill that would allow oral surgeons to practice cosmetic surgery in California was passed but wasn't signed by Gov. Arnold Schwarzenegger. Similar bills are being considered across the country. The arguments for such bills are that oral surgeons treat facial injuries and broken jaws in the hospital and that barring them from doing other facial procedures is unnecessarily restrictive.

Similar arguments can be made for dermatologists who have some training in dermatologic surgery and ophthalmologists who have extra training in eyelid plastic surgery procedures.

These issues will be fought in the coming years. The oral surgery bill in California will be considered again in 2005. Gradually, more and more non-plastic surgeons will be allowed to provide cosmetic surgery. That's why you, the consumer, must be sure that you make the right choice amidst the politics of self-interest.

Suppose that an ENT physician (head and neck surgeon), Dr. X, finds the workload increasing but her income diminishing because of third-party payer issues. Cosmetic surgery procedures pay 150 to 200 percent more than what she's trained to do. Because a portion of her residency training included rhinoplasty, a cosmetic procedure, she decides that she'll start doing other cosmetic procedures, including facelifts and perhaps even breast augmentations.

The problem for Dr. X is that in order for her to perform cosmetic procedures in a *licensed* facility — a hospital or outpatient surgery center — she needs to have permission to do those same procedures in the hospital.

Hospital committees that govern medical care in hospitals are composed of physicians. If the appropriate committee decrees that Dr. X didn't have enough training during residency to qualify her to do facelifts at the hospital, committee members won't give her privileges to do so. She has had no training that justifies her doing breast augmentations. Dr. X is at an impasse unless she operates in her own office-based surgery suite.

The hospital recognizes that facelifts don't fall into Dr. X's scope of practice. Dr. X can try to influence the doctors on the committee, go to the hospital administration, or threaten to sue. These issues have created serious tensions among hospital staffs for years. Thirty years ago, Dr. X had no chance of doing facelifts. Times have changed however. At this time, in many hospitals, head and neck surgeons who can demonstrate that they were trained to perform facial cosmetic surgery procedures have gained the right to perform those operations, so Dr. X may now be happy. Fortunately for consumers, her ability to get privileges to perform breast augmentation is still highly unlikely.

Determining whether a surgeon has hospital privileges to do your procedure has been a consumer protection in the past. Because of legal issues, rather than medical protections, it may become less so in the future. Scope of practice battles are being fought all over the country. Take my advice and choose a plastic surgeon for your plastic surgery.

Certifying Surgery Centers

After you're sure that your surgeon is certified, the next step is to be sure that the operating facility is also certified. This topic is also complicated, but one of extreme importance to you.

If you choose a board-certified plastic surgeon who is a member of the two most prestigious professional societies for practicing plastic surgeons, the American Society of Plastic Surgeons (ASPS, which represents 97 percent of board-certified plastic surgeons) or the American Society for Aesthetic Plastic Surgery (ASAPS), the matter has been decided for you. You can be sure that you have chosen a board certified plastic surgeon who has hospital privileges to perform your procedure and that your surgery will occur in a certified operating room. ASPS and ASAPS require their members to operate in certified facilities, either at the hospital, in accredited ambulatory surgery centers, or in their own accredited office-based surgery suite. The only exceptions are minor cases using local anesthesia.

Understanding surgery center choices

Your surgery can be performed in a hospital, independent surgery center, or office-based surgery suite. According to ASPS statistics for 2003, 25 percent of cosmetic surgeries were performed in hospitals, 23 percent in independent surgery centers, and 52 percent in office-based surgery suites (up 7 percent from 2002).

At both the hospital and at the surgery center, three levels of protection occur. Mandatory federal oversight in the form of Medicare/Medicaid certification is combined with state licensure. Both involve strict regulations and routine inspections and may include unannounced inspections. Both hospitals and surgery centers also voluntarily submit themselves to the inspections of independent accrediting organizations that set and measure against performance standards. Both of these types of organizations have medical staff committees to be sure that doctors stay within their scopes of practice.

In most states, federal or state licensure at the office-based surgery suite is purely voluntary and relates to insurance and reimbursement issues rather than to patient safety. Some states, California and Florida for example, require office-based surgery suites to be accredited (check out the upcoming section, "Using an office-based surgery suite"), but they leave the accreditation and inspection process up to the independent accrediting agencies, which I discuss later in this chapter. The problem comes in the office-based surgery setting, where the doctor is the medical staff and may not be following the same set of rules that apply in a hospital or surgery center setting.

Use a local hospital or accredited outpatient surgery center. As long as you have surgery in an independent surgery center that many surgeons in your city or community use, or in a hospital, you can be sure that the safety issues relating to operating facilities and anesthesia providers have been addressed. These facilities can't operate and collect money from third-party payers without being certified by Medicare, which has the most stringent facility regulations.

Just as important, if your surgeon is on the staff at one of these facilities, she has had her background and training checked and is doing a procedure within her scope of practice. That means the surgeon has been trained properly and her skills have been vetted by the medical staff of the surgery center or hospital. This doesn't necessarily mean your potential surgeon is perfect, but it does mean she is at least very good.

Having surgery at the hospital

Most cosmetic surgery is outpatient surgery, meaning that you don't spend the night in the hospital. That doesn't mean that you can't have surgery at the hospital. Many hospitals have outpatient departments for cosmetic surgery.

If you have cosmetic surgery in an accredited hospital, you don't have to concern yourself with whether the surgeon is qualified. The medical staff makes sure that surgeons function only within their scopes of practice and are trained and qualified to perform your surgery. Similarly, if you choose to have surgery in the hospital, you can be sure that the personnel and systems in place protect you. You don't have to concern yourself with whether the operating room conditions are ideal or wonder whether the equipment and protocols are in place to ensure your safety. Hospitals are accredited, and the accrediting agency sets standards to protect you.

Going to the surgi-center

Another safe option is to go to an independent ambulatory surgery center (ASC), which deals only with outpatient surgery, including cosmetic surgery. These facilities have medical staff requirements and generally follow scope-of-practice protocols. They are like the hospitals in terms of equipment, safety, drugs, crash carts, personnel, and so on. Each year, millions of patients undergo outpatient surgery in these facilities. These independent organizations have all of the advantages of the hospital in terms of medical staff and safety, but generally you can't stay overnight should you need or want to do so.

Many plastic surgeons prefer to use an ASC rather than a hospital because the ASC staffs are more familiar with outpatient surgery and the special needs of the cosmetic patient. The advantages to the patient in terms of surgeon vetting and safety are obvious. Many surgeons who use an ASC do so because they practice alone or feel that they want to focus on being a surgeon rather than running a surgery center in their offices.

Using an office-based surgery suite

With the large increase in cosmetic surgery and the strong need for patient privacy, many plastic surgeons and other surgeons doing cosmetic surgery have constructed surgery suites in their own offices. You'll find such suites more common with groups of surgeons who are busy enough to need multiple operating rooms on a daily basis.

When one of the accrediting agencies certifies these office-based suites, you can be sure that the facilities are sophisticated and up-to-date and contain the same equipment and trained staff you'll find in good hospital or ASC operating rooms.

Nurses certified for advanced cardiac life support (ACLS) provide postsurgical recovery staffing. The suites have the same safety levels as hospital operating rooms, with similar equipment, staffing, and emergency drugs and procedures. Like the ASC, the biggest physical and functional difference is that you can't be admitted onto the hospital floor after your surgery is complete.

Office-based outpatient operating facilities have many advantages. Use of these centers virtually always saves you money. The surgeon who owns the facility staffs the operating room with technicians and nurses who are or who become cosmetic surgery specialists. Your comfort level is usually higher, and you usually feel more comfortable with office staff that you probably already know.

 If your surgeon suggests using her office operating suite, ask to see the suite before making your final decision. Is it certified? Does it look clean and professional? If you have any doubts but you like the surgeon, ask her to operate on you at the surgi-center or hospital instead.

Finding out about certifying agencies

If you're considering surgery in an office-based surgery suite, then you must be sure that the facility is accredited. An office-based surgery suite offers the advantages of privacy and specialization, which are the reasons so many patients are opting for this choice.

Accreditation is the facility equivalent of board certification. A third party, in this case an accrediting body, aims to optimize patient safety by enforcing standards of patient care and surgical and safety protocols.

If you choose a surgeon who is not a plastic surgeon or not a member of ASPS or ASAPS, then you must take responsibility for ensuring that your surgery takes place in an accredited operating suite. The following organizations certify hospitals, ASCs, and office-based operating suites:

- ✔ **Joint Commission on the Accreditation of Healthcare Organizations (JCAHO):** Evaluates and accredits over 15,000 health care organizations and programs in the United States, including an estimated 1,200 hospital-based ambulatory surgery centers (ASCs), several hundred ASCs, and a small number of office-based surgery centers.

- ✔ **Accreditation Association for Ambulatory Health Care (AAAHC):** About 80 percent of its approximately 1500 organizations are ASCs, and the remaining 20 percent are office-based surgical facilities. AAAHC does not certify hospitals.

- ✔ **American Association of Accreditation of Ambulatory Surgery Facilities (AAAASF):** Over 90 percent of the 800 AAAASF-accredited facilities are office-based surgery suites, and the remainder are ASCs. AAAASF does not accredit hospitals.

The area of greatest risk to patients is in the unaccredited office-based surgery suite. Don't have surgery in any operating room that isn't accredited unless your surgeon is doing a minor procedure under local anesthetic.

Understanding Your Anesthesia Options

If you're like a large number of cosmetic surgery patients, your potential fears about cosmetic surgery center more on anesthesia risks than on the surgery itself. Anesthesia has become very safe over the years. Today, you have a 1 in 250,000 chance of dying in surgery from an anesthesia death. Thirty years ago that number was 1 in 5,000.

Despite these incredible advances, you want a good person supplying that care and taking responsibility for your safety when you have general anesthesia or are heavily sedated. You need to know the qualifications of that person because he'll be the one administering your medications and monitoring your vital signs. Anesthesia training ranges widely — from medical specialization after earning a medical degree to nursing training only.

The following professionals may administer anesthesia and/or sedation:

- **Anesthesiologist:** This doctor has been to medical school and received additional specialty training enabling him to earn board certification from the American Board of Anesthesiology.

- **Certified registered nurse anesthetist (CRNA):** A CRNA is a registered nurse (RN) who has completed at least two additional years of training in anesthesiology. A CRNA is licensed to administer general anesthesia; her certification is overseen by her state's board of nursing.

- **Registered nurse:** Each state has its own board of nursing with similar standards. An RN is licensed to administer intravenous sedation at the direction of a physician and to monitor your vital signs.

- **Certified plastic surgical nurse (CPSN):** These nurses specialize in the field of plastic surgery and have a minimum of two years of experience to qualify for the national certifying exam. Their role in administering sedation is the same as that of a registered nurse.

- **Surgeon:** In some cases, your surgeon may be the person administering the medications to sedate you and make you drowsy during your surgery. Usually in this case, your vital signs are monitored by a nurse while your surgeon operates.

In the hospital or ASC setting, a higher authority determines who provides your anesthesia. Your anesthesia provider will be either an anesthesiologist or a CRNA, who provides anesthesia under the supervision of an anesthesiologist.

Using the Internet to get the skinny on surgeons

Essentially everything you want to know about any surgeon is available on the Internet. I once consulted with a woman who had seen several other surgeons about facial surgery. When she told me their names, I mentioned that two of them were probably not plastic surgeons. She became a little testy and assured me they certainly were. If she had looked them up on the Internet, she would have found they were ENT physicians (otolaryngologists).

All you have to do is type the name of any potential surgeon into Google or another search engine, and you'll get more information than you probably want.

If you're not computer literate, one of your near friends probably is. Take advantage of this astounding technology to help you make smart decisions about your cosmetic surgery wishes.

Only in the office-based setting do you need to check on who is going to provide your anesthesia.

Many plastic surgeons employ nurse anesthetists, and the reported safety records for both the physician and nurse anesthesia providers are similar. However, there is at least one recent study that finds that in the event of a life-threatening emergency, there is greater success with anesthesiologists than with CRNAs.

The type of anesthesia available to you varies according to the type of procedure you're having. Table 3-1 shows you your options. I tell you more about anesthesia for each procedure in Part III.

Table 3-1	**Anesthesia Options**			
Procedure	*Local*	*Local with Sedation*	*General*	*None*
Abdominoplasty (Tummy tuck)		X	X	
Breast augmentation		X	X	
Breast lift		X	X	
Chemical peel		X		X
Collagen injection	X			X
Fat injection	X			
Dermabrasion	X		X	
Blepharoplasty (Eyelid surgery)		X	X	
Facelift		X	X	
Facial implants		X	X	
Brow lift		X	X	
Laser facial resurfacing		X	X	
Liposuction	X		X	
Gynecomastia (Male breast reduction)	X		X	
Rhinoplasty (Nose surgery)		X	X	

Source: American Society of Plastic Surgeons, www.plasticsurgery.org

Getting the Best Results with Minimal Hassle

If you really don't want to become a Certified Cosmetic Surgery Shopper (CCSS), use the following approach. This method applies to any surgeon you choose for cosmetic surgery procedures, but it's especially important when surgeons perform all their surgery in their own office-based surgery suites.

Find an ASAPS member

Choose a surgeon who is a member of the American Society for Aesthetic Plastic Surgery (ASAPS).

ASAPS's 2,100 members are all board-certified (by the American Board of Plastic Surgery in the United States and, in Canada, the Royal College of Physicians and Surgeons of Canada) plastic surgeons who have been in practice at least five years and have significant cosmetic surgery experience. Their surgical results, medical ethics, and continuing education are all monitored. ASAPS has stringent criteria for membership. It doesn't accept new members casually, and society standards are very high. Good surgeons are refused for issues of ethics or medical judgment.

PERSONAL STORY

Making the decision

Bridgette gives this explanation for her decision to have cosmetic surgery: "I think my personality and outlook on life played a big role in my decision to have surgery since I believe in looking my best and am not concerned with what others may think. I did keep my decision private and felt it was a gift I was giving myself, and it was nobody else's business. I believe in pursuing solutions instead of issues, so when I realized there were a few things about my appearance that I really wanted to improve, I pursued a reasonable and hopefully long-lasting solution, which was cosmetic surgery."

Bridgette gives the following advice to people considering surgery, "I think it's important to do your homework and know what questions to ask before and after your surgery. As a patient, you must take responsibility for the process, especially since each individual has different needs, a different healing timetable, and different concerns." Here's what other advice she offers:

✔ Do it only for yourself; don't do it for someone else. At the end of it all, you're the one looking in the mirror, and your satisfaction with your appearance is what matters most.

✔ Do your homework, talk to people who have had work done, and go on the Internet and research doctors you're considering.

✔ Have a lot of patience with the healing process and appreciate the daily improvement to your appearance.

Investigate hospital privileges

Ask all surgeons you're considering whether they have privileges in an accredited hospital to perform the surgery you're considering. If the answer is yes, you can be sure that the surgeon has been through a significant review process by the hospital medical staff to review the surgeon's training and ability to perform the procedure you're considering. If a doctor doesn't have hospital privileges, don't even consider hiring her! Such a doctor may tell you that she's trained to perform the procedure you want, but the medical staff is saying that she's not. If you're in doubt, call the hospital and ask.

Check for facility accreditation

Ask whether the surgeon you're considering operates in a surgical suite that meets at least one of the following criteria:

- ✔ Is a state-recognized accrediting organization
- ✔ Is state licensed
- ✔ Is Medicare certified

Because currently most states don't require cosmetic surgery to be performed in accredited facilities, this question is especially important. Most surgeons who accredit their office-based operating suites do so voluntarily at great effort and expense. To optimally protect their patients, they make application to accrediting bodies such as the American Association for Accreditation of Ambulatory Surgery Facilities (AAAASF). If the surgeon's facility meets these strict standards, it denotes a high standard of safety, equipment, and surgical processes. As of July 2002, all ASAPS and ASPS members were required to operate in accredited surgical suites.

Ask about board certification

If your potential surgeon is not a member of ASAPS or ASPS, then you want to make sure she's a board-certified plastic surgeon (see the section "Relying on the American Board of Medical Specialties," earlier in this chapter). You want to be sure that you choose a board-certified surgeon whose training and boards included the procedure you're considering. When a doctor tells you she is board certified, ask which board. The ABMS recognizes only one board to certify doctors in the specialty of plastic surgery: the American Board of Plastic Surgery.

Part II
Preparing for Cosmetic Surgery

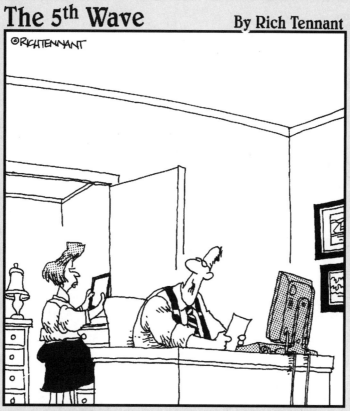

The 5th Wave   By Rich Tennant

©RICHTENNANT

"I see you had some cosmetic surgery done. I always wondered how much a wallet peel cost."

In this part . . .

Deciding to have cosmetic surgery means deciding to take on a host of responsibilities to ensure that your experience is the best it can be. First and foremost, you need to find the right surgeon to do the job. I tell you how to sort through the often confusing information and find someone who is qualified, competent, and caring. I also give you the details you need to make sure you're prepared financially and physically for cosmetic surgery.

Chapter 4

Prequalifying: Beginning Your Search for a Surgeon

. . . .

. . . .

You need to be prepared to spend a lot of time shopping for a cosmetic surgeon. When looking for something that involves your looks, health, well-being, and a sizeable chunk of your bank account, you need to know exactly what criteria to base your decision on. You want to focus on the key issues that you know will produce the positive outcomes you seek — a great surgical result and a wonderful emotional experience.

Searching for a surgeon becomes more manageable when you use a clearly defined system to make the choice. You want to consider all your options and weigh them cautiously. In this chapter, I show you what to look for in a cosmetic surgeon and how to whittle down the list of possibilities.

Creating a Solid Game Plan

When you're looking for something as important as a surgeon, you need to create a game plan so you're sure to consider the myriad factors involved. You're trusting someone with your body and your health, and you want to make sure that trust is warranted. I recommend a two-step process:

✔ **Prequalifying:** During this stage of the game, you start looking around at your options to determine which surgeons meet your needs. This stage includes the following steps:

- Getting recommendations from those in the know or using the Internet and advertising sources to find out what your options are

- Calling the offices of surgeons who seem promising and gathering information about certification, education, and experience

- Whittling your original list to no more than five surgeons whose qualifications meet your expectations

✔ **Qualifying:** During this part of the process, which I cover in Chapter 5, you want to take a close look at the surgeons on your short list. You do that by scheduling consultations, typically one-to-two-hour visits to the office during which you talk with the surgeon and his staff to assess his experience, results, and fees and evaluate the caring and competency of the entire practice team.

Schedule at least three consultations but no more than five. You don't want to spend more time than necessary, but you also want to make sure you're getting enough information to make the right decision. If you use the right criteria (see the section "Defining your search criteria") to make these selections, you can optimize your time and still make the right choice.

Certainly the most important decision you'll make is your choice of surgeon. But you have other important factors to consider. Your best outcome occurs when you thoroughly review your options for three key factors:

✔ **Expertise:** Choose an expert surgeon with proven experience and consistent results.

✔ **Safety:** Look for a certified facility that offers broad anesthesia options.

✔ **Support:** Be sure that your choice offers a supportive environment with a pro-active patient care team.

All sorts of doctors, even dentists in some states, perform cosmetic surgery. Some have no training in plastic surgery, but current law allows them to advertise a certification (in another field) without specifying the field. You can easily be confused or even misled by advertising unless you're careful in the early stages of shopping. Be on the lookout for those doctors who are certified, specially trained, and experienced in the procedure you want.

You can find a way through the maze of certification in Chapter 3, but for now, be prepared to ask the right questions during your first contact with a surgeon's office. Asking questions on the phone *before* you make an appointment will certainly save you time, and maybe a lot of trouble and even your life, later on.

Defining your search criteria

One of the most difficult aspects of shopping for plastic surgery is that more than likely you're not a medical professional. That makes it hard to know what's important and what's not. Figure 4-1 shows you a sample shopping chart that assigns points to each factor you need to consider. This shopping chart provides you with a system that helps you focus on the important shopping criteria and provides an easy way to keep track of what you learn about each surgeon you're considering.

Category	Area of Concern	Maximum Points	Dr. A	Dr. B	Dr. C
1. Verifying Your Surgeon's Credentials & Experience					
Board Certification	Board-Certified **Plastic** Surgeon	4			
	Board-Certified **Cosmetic** Surgeon	-4			
	Other ABMS Board Certification	2			
Medical Specialization	Hosptial privileges for procedure	4			
Training	Medical school, 1 point per year	4			
	Dental school	2			
	Surgical residency including plastic surgery, 1 point per year	8			
Professional Societies	FACS, Fellow American College of Surgeons	1			
	Member ABMS Speciality Society: ASPS, ASAPS, 2 points each	4			
Expertise	Demonstrated skill	2			
	Proven experience	2			
	Sub-Total Surgeon	33 points			
2. Finding Your Team					
Staff	Quality initial phone call	2			
	Appointment at convenient time	1			
	Staff: friendly, knowledgeable	3			
	Follow up after consultation	1			
	Presurgery patient education visit	2			
	Office staff includes RN or PA	2			
Doctor	Reasonable waiting time	1			
	Consult with surgeon	3			
	Good rapport developed	3			
	Shown quality before and after photos	2			
	Meet staff who had surgery from doctor	2			
Practice	Recommended by friend or family	2			
	Informative and helpful materials	3			
	Facility: attractive, neat & clean	3			
	Offered sizing or imaging, if appropriate	1			
	Written fee estimate	2			
	Fees discussed in private setting	1			
	Sub-Total Practice	34 points			

Figure 4-1a: Use this chart to prioritize as you shop for a surgeon.

Source: La Jolla Cosmetic Surgery Centre

3a. Making Sure You're Safe — Hospital or Ambulatory Surgery Center (ASC)					
Hospital or ASC	Hospital or Independent Ambulatory Surgery Center (ASC) If not, go to 3b. Office-based Surgery Suite	30			
Anesthesia	MD Anesthesiologist	3			
	Certified Nurse Anesthetist	2			
Sub-Total Facility Safety		**33 points**			
3b. Making Sure You're Safe — Office-Based Surgery Suite					
Office-Based Surgery Suite	Surgery facility certified for general anesthesia	6			
	Anesthesia	2			
	Uncertified	Just say No			
Anesthesia or Sedation	MD Anesthesiologist	3			
	Certified Nurse Anesthetist	2			
	Sedation by Registered Nurse	1			
	Sedation - Surgeon only (unless minor)	0			
Clearances	Lab work required	3			
	EKG, over age 40	3			
	Medical clearance, if needed	3			
Monitoring	Monitoring in operating room: EKG, pulse oximetry, blood pressure, Capnograph (CO2)	3			
	Monitoring in recovery room: EKG, pulse oximetry, blood pressure, temperature probe	3			
Recovery	Nurse in recovery with no other duties: ACLS (Advanced Cardiac Life Support), CPR	3			
	Crash cart	3			
Emergency	Transfer privileges to hospital in emergency	3			
Sub-Total Facility Safety		**33 points**			
Total		**100**			
Making Your Choice					
List recommended procedures					
Enter fee estimate					

Figure 4-1b:
Use this chart to prioritize as you shop for a surgeon.

Source: La Jolla Cosmetic Surgery Centre

Each section — surgeon, practice, and facility — is subdivided into components that have different point values. For instance, each doctor receives points for board certification (see Chapter 3), surgical training, and hospital privileges. The patient care team criteria include point values for quality patient information, good rapport with the surgeon and staff, and good before-and-after pictures. You can rate facility safety by such things as level of certification, emergency equipment, and transfer privileges to the hospital. This chart allows you to evaluate three surgeons as well as their operating suites and offices. You should be able to get most of the information about the surgeon and facility from your telephone calls, practice materials, and other research. Some information can be gathered through your consultation appointments.

After you've found the information you need, add up the point value for each section and compare it to the fee quote each surgeon has given you. If your highest quote comes from the practice with the lowest point value, then you may want to find a better value for your money. On the other hand, if a quality plastic surgery practice with good communication and high safety levels has a moderate price, you have an opportunity to save money without compromising quality.

Shopping must be a dynamic process. Be ready to make adjustments as your knowledge base increases. Don't hesitate to raise the bar rather than lower it.

Your search process begins and ends with your search criteria. You'll have more choices, obviously, if you consider anyone with an MD degree rather than only board-certified plastic surgeons. But you also face greater risks that the doctor isn't as well trained or experienced. Agreeing to have surgery in an uncertified operating room may save money, but doing so means you may have concerns about safety. If you choose to ignore warning signs of uncaring or disorganized offices, then you can't be surprised if they don't support you before surgery or abandon you after surgery.

As you shop, you may encounter things that prompt you to remove a surgeon or office from your list of top choices. When you do so, turn to your list of runner-up choices and move a doctor from that list to your A list.

As you use the shopping chart, you gain experience and effectively evaluate surgical quality and patient care attitudes in your community. If you like what you find, then you can choose your surgeon. Otherwise, depending on where you live and the number of options available to you, you may want to broaden your search beyond the group of doctors you originally considered or expand the geographic area you're considering.

Beware of surgeons who promise that the operation will be scar free or pain free or have minimal recovery. If it sounds too good to be true, it probably is. The extent of your ultimate results from cosmetic surgery is usually in direct proportion to the extent of surgery that is done.

Focus your allocated shopping time on those surgeons who qualify for your consideration. Certainly there may be an occasional doctor who can provide a good result and great experience without meeting your criteria, but they are the exception. For the best results, stick to your criteria.

You may want to shop with a friend or relative who is also considering having cosmetic surgery. Ideally, this person wants the same procedure you do, and you can shop together. If you shop for a surgeon this way, one of you may see or hear some information that the other person missed. Recovering together can actually be fun, and you may be able to share or even avoid some caretaker expenses.

Taking the show on the road

You may decide to schedule your surgery where you live, or you may want to have the surgery in another location. Before you shop, determine how far you're willing to travel and how you'll find a surgeon in another neck of the woods. If you're shopping from afar, the Internet makes doing so much easier than it used to be.

Several factors can prompt you to opt for surgery out of town:

- ✔ **A good support system:** You need time to recover after cosmetic surgery, and the more involved the surgery, the more important your recovery plan. In many cases, the best support system is your family, so you may opt to schedule your surgery in the city where your mom or cousin lives, for example. Think about your supporting cast and shop accordingly.

- ✔ **More options:** If you live in a town with just two plastic surgeons, you may need to go to a larger city to find a surgeon with extensive cosmetic experience. Depending on the difficulty of the procedure, you may need to put quite a few miles on your car to get a competent, experienced surgeon.

- ✔ **Privacy:** If privacy is important to you, go out of town for surgery. You're less likely to meet acquaintances and business associates in a plastic surgeon's office in another city. You can go out in public wearing bandages without a worry or put on sunglasses to hide bruising and go out to lunch.

- ✔ **Denial:** If your plan is to deny having cosmetic surgery, get out of town! You can go off to the "spa" and come back after liposuction with a valid reason for looking better. Combining surgery with a California or Florida vacation explains why you're looking so rested after a facelift. A New York shopping trip combined with a new hairstyle can explain away an eyelid lift.

- ✔ **Superstar surgeon:** You may also need to hit the road if you want someone famous to do your surgery so you can enjoy the bragging rights that go with higher fees. But don't go with stars in your eyes. Use your shopping criteria and be sure that the doctor's superstar status doesn't blind you to any possible warning signs of a disinterested surgeon or uncaring staff.

If you choose to leave town for surgery, you need to modify your shopping process. You can either take a shopping trip to the city where you plan to have surgery and proceed conventionally, or you can surf the Web or let your fingers do the walking.

After you've settled on the surgeons you want to consider in another town, my best advice is to plan a trip and conduct on-site interviews. When distance is involved, your communication and education needs are much greater, and you want to be sure you won't be forgotten when you return home after surgery.

Generally, the more out-of-town patients that a surgeon serves, the better the practice is at addressing your unique needs. As an out-of-town patient, you'll need the staff's help with all kinds of arrangements, including hotels, car services, and after care. Be sure the surgical practice you choose is ready to provide the help you need.

Setting aside time to shop

Don't expect to find a surgeon in the same amount of time you found your last frying pan. Shopping for cosmetic surgery is time consuming and rightly so. You're looking for someone to make you look and feel better, and that's a job worth doing right. Skimp on the shopping process, and you may make a bad decision that actually costs more time (and money) than getting the job done right in the first place.

Factor the following time guzzlers into your total shopping time:

- **Surgeon's availability:** Depending upon your community or choice of surgeon, you may have to wait weeks for a consultation.

- **Research:** You'll spend roughly one to two hours in the doctor's office for every consultation. During this time, you talk with the surgeon, fill out paperwork (of course), and talk with a patient coordinator about fees, scheduling, and any other general information you need. On top of that, you need to factor in your time to get there and back, which can vary widely depending on where you live.

- **Your schedule:** Depending upon the doctor you choose, you may have to wait weeks or months for your surgery date. If you want surgery within 30 days, there's no point in interviewing a doctor who doesn't have operating time available for three months. When you call for an appointment, ask about the surgery schedule. If it's not a fit, ask if they can adjust their schedule to the date you want. Be clear that if they can't accommodate your schedule, you're going to have surgery with someone else. If they can't accommodate you, move along to the next name on your list or, if this is the surgeon you really want, adjust your time frame for surgery. You can also ask to be put on a waiting list for cancellations.

- **Recovery:** Remember the old adage, "If you don't have time to do it right, when will you have time to do it over?" If you don't allow enough time to recover, you may unintentionally cause a complication that delays healing or necessitates secondary surgery and extends your recovery even further. The time frame for an optimal result after surgery varies depending on procedure. You need to know this time frame before you finalize your decision, and then count backwards and plan accordingly. If you absolutely cannot cope with a longer recovery time, then postpone your decision until your time frame is not so tight.

Assembling Your List of Prospective Surgeons

Finding your surgeon involves gathering information from a number of sources. You need to begin creating a list of prospects from the pool of surgeons available. Some of these physicians will not be appropriate for the procedure you have in mind, and even fewer will provide top-notch work and give you excellent care before, during, and after your procedure, so you want to make your initial list as strong as possible.

Asking around is a great way to kick off your search. The best starting point for finding a good surgeon is referrals from physicians. Friends or acquaintances who have had cosmetic surgery can be also be excellent sources. Other medical professionals, such as nurses, hospital administrators, or staff from physicians' offices, can give good advice.

Because you're seeking cosmetic surgery advice, you can also think outside the medical box and ask people who work in the beauty or fashion industry, including hair stylists, aestheticians, and people who work at a department store makeup counter or in the lingerie department. They all have professions that put them on the front line with people who've had cosmetic surgery, so they can certainly be a source of prospective surgeons' names.

Using multiple sources is a good idea. If you hear about one surgeon from your doctor, a friend, and the administrator at the hospital, then you can be pretty sure that you may want to consider this surgeon. The more open you are about your intentions, the easier it is to solicit advice from multiple sources. If you're new in your community, your resources may be more limited, making your shopping criteria even more important.

Checking with friends and acquaintances

Many women enjoy talking about topics related to cosmetic surgery, so you may find great resources anywhere you go, from your hair salon to your health club and all points in between. Not only can you hear the straight skinny on complications, results, and scandals, but you can also get recommendations from those who've boldly gone where you plan to go.

Talk to friends and acquaintances about their surgery experiences, look at their results, and pick their brains about their shopping process. They may tell you that their surgeon is the best, or they may say, "If I had to do it again, I'd choose Dr. X." One of the best referrals in my practice was a woman who had gone to another surgeon and regretted her choice. She sent all her friends to me.

For traditional medical procedures, you probably want to ask a doctor for a recommendation and weigh that advice highly in your analysis. But for cosmetic surgery, patient referrals are very valuable and extremely important. Patients know the inside scoop, especially about service and attitudes.

As you gather names, you may hear that someone had a great experience with a surgeon who doesn't meet your criteria. Don't get sidetracked. Don't let a friend's enthusiasm cloud your thinking.

Asking Dr. Welby

Who better to give sound medical referrals than those in the medical community? If you have a primary care physician or specialist that you like and respect or if one of your friends or neighbors is a doctor, call and ask him, his head nurse, or his office manager whom they would recommend. Dig deeper with the following questions:

- ✔ If your wife, mother, or child were having the procedure I'm considering, whom would you choose?
- ✔ Is this a professional recommendation or have you had personal experience with this surgeon? (You can probably put more stock in a recommendation based on personal experience.)
- ✔ Why do you think this surgeon is a good choice?
- ✔ Is there anyone you would add or delete from the list of surgeons I'm considering? Why?

You never know where a good MD recommendation may come from. An internist who sees many mature women patients may be a great resource for a facelift recommendation; an OB-GYN may be helpful if you're considering a tummy tuck or breast augmentation recommendation. Just beware if the doctor you call for a recommendation offers to do the surgery for you. Stick to your shopping criteria and choose a surgeon whose training and board certification includes your procedure.

If you're lucky enough to know an anesthesiologist who works in a surgery center or hospital where a lot of cosmetic surgery is performed, ask his advice. Anesthesiologists see a lot of surgery being done and know who the good (and nice) surgeons are. You may also want to ask your cosmetic dentist or orthodontist for referrals, because they're also in the medical beauty biz.

Be careful when asking a doctor in a large multi-specialty group for a cosmetic surgery referral. Often multi-specialty groups have "closed" referral systems, meaning that doctors refer only to the group's physicians and surgeons. They can't refer outside the group to another surgeon. As a result, they may not be able to tell you who they really think is the best plastic surgeon in your community because that doctor isn't a part of their group.

Some communities have annual surveys in which physicians are surveyed by a third party (often a local magazine) who solicits their opinion about the best specialists. The doctors are asked which other doctors they would send their family members to. If your community has such a survey, be sure to take advantage of this resource. Surgeons who have been recognized in these surveys frequently mention them in their brochures or other marketing materials.

Asking nurses and other health-care personnel

When you're trying to find a surgeon, nurses or operating room staff from the hospital or surgery center can be extremely helpful. Nurses are special people who know a lot about who the good doctors are. People who already work in the cosmetic surgery arena, such as cosmetic surgery operating room nurses or operating room technicians, are exceptionally knowledgeable about who's great and who's not.

Many types of medical personnel can give input. If you don't know someone personally, ask around. You may find someone who can give you a name. Here are some places to start looking:

- ✔ **Surgery center:** A good source is staff from a surgery center where a lot of cosmetic surgery is done. The larger the cosmetic component, the better the chances of a good recommendation. Ask operating room technicians; nurses (admitting, circulators, or recovery room); or anesthesia providers, who can be either doctors (anesthesiologists) or nurses (certified registered nurse anesthetists, or CRNAs). Even nonmedical administrative staff should have an opinion or be able to find someone who knows.

- ✔ **Hospital:** The operating room staff is generally your best bet here, but some hospitals have special outpatient recovery units for cosmetic surgery, and the nurses on that floor should be full of helpful information, including insight into how well the surgeon and his staff take care of their patients after surgery.

✔ **Recovery facility:** Some communities have special recovery facilities for cosmetic surgery patients. The owners and staff of these facilities see many immediate post-op patients, and they can certainly tell you which surgeons have patients who have great results and talk about their doctors positively.

✔ **Plastic or cosmetic surgery office:** People who work in the field of cosmetic surgery frequently know the good doctors. They may tell you only about their doctor, and that may or may not be good advice. (Size up the recommendation according to your shopping criteria.) Probe further by asking, "If I don't choose your doctor, who else would you recommend?"

✔ **Other medical offices:** Nurses or office staff in other physician's offices may well know who to suggest. They may know who their doctor recommends or someone to ask at the surgery center or hospital. Just as in every profession, the word gets around — about the good guys and the bad.

When you find someone to ask for a recommendation, be frank. Tell the person you're thinking about having cosmetic surgery and ask the following questions:

✔ If you were considering having my procedure, which surgeons would you consider?

✔ Which surgeons would you avoid?

✔ What is it about this surgeon that you particularly like or dislike?

If you're new in town or never go to the doctor, call the best local hospital and ask for the operating room supervisor. Explain your situation and ask whom he or she would choose if having the type of surgery you're considering.

Taking your search online

If you're comfortable surfing the Web, you can access most of the information you need without leaving your computer. If you aren't used to using the Web, get a friend, student, or neighbor to help you, but don't shirk on this part of your homework. Even if you don't use a Web site for referrals, you can find out the specifics of the various procedures, what makes a good candidate, the training for various specialties, the most common complications or risks involved, and a lot more. For a list of Web sites to help you in your search, turn to the Appendix.

Narrowing your choices

You can find plenty of suggestions for shopping for a surgeon in this book, but here's wise advice from Linda, a patient who had a lower eyelid lift and rhinoplasty. Her shopping method worked well for her and may help you out, too:

✔ Do it for yourself.

✔ Do your homework: Talk to friends. Listen to their experiences with cosmetic surgery. Talk to those who have had the same procedure you want. Don't talk to someone about liposuction if you want your nose done.

✔ Call the medical board to check out the surgeon's background and past records.

✔ Don't go to just one doctor. Get at least three opinions before making your decision.

✔ Take note of how the staff treats you. Do they follow up after your appointment with notes or phone calls? Are they prompt? Do you have a connection with them?

✔ Ask patients in the waiting room how their experiences were.

✔ Look at before-and-after photos. Where are the incisions going to be?

Here's how Linda sums up her experience: "Would I do it again? In a heartbeat. Emotionally, I feel like a new person. I feel and look younger. It was a gift I'll always treasure."

Be sure that no medical board action has been taken against any surgeon you're considering. You also may find in your research that many doctors are known for the articles they've written for medical journals. Although publishing articles or being involved in research is nice, surgical talent is a far more valuable way to gauge a physician's skill.

For more information about checking out a doctor's credentials, see Chapter 3. Be sure to visit www.abms.org, the site of the American Board of Medical Specialties to find out whether a doctor is board certified and in what specialty. You can also contact the local or state medical society, the American Society of Plastic Surgeons at www.plasticsurgery.org, or the American Society of Aesthetic Plastic Surgeons at www.surgery.org.

Virtually every cosmetic surgeon has a Web site of his own or a listing on a society or public information site. These sources vary greatly, so they may or may not meet your needs when you're looking for a surgeon. You can also visit chat rooms to get recommendations from other patients and hear about their experiences.

Taking ad-vantage of the Yellow Pages and media

Maybe you don't have connections to the medical community, don't know anyone to ask, or aren't computer literate. Perhaps you're not ready to openly discuss your thoughts about having cosmetic surgery just yet. If you're in one of these categories, you can always turn to the Yellow Pages. Just remember, the phone book is a place to start, not a place to finish.

Keep your shopping criteria in mind as you leaf through the many pages of ads before deciding which practices to call. Look for the symbols of quality described later in this section and in Chapter 3. In order to find a surgeon qualified to perform the surgery you want, you need to know how surgeons are trained, what credentials to look for, and how to verify their credentials.

Keep in mind that that doctors can list themselves under any specialty heading they like, and they can advertise any services they want to sell, regardless of their training and credentials. You must make sure that the surgeon has the proper credentials that matter for your procedure and that he has hospital privileges to perform your procedure.

When evaluating ads in the Yellow Pages, keep in mind that ad size or design quality doesn't guarantee surgical quality. Also be aware that doctors can advertise their practices in different sections of the Yellow Pages. For example, if you need nasal surgery, check out the plastic surgery section and the cosmetic surgery section. If you're considering dermatological treatments such as skin peels or laser, look in the plastic surgery or cosmetic surgery sections or for dermatologists in the physicians and surgeons section.

You'll probably turn to the Yellow Pages looking for someone who specializes in the procedure you're considering. Unfortunately, most ads aren't designed to help you find an expert. Most physicians' ads display long lists of the various procedures they perform. This doesn't mean these physicians don't specialize in your procedure; it just means that you have to call to find out how frequently they perform the procedure you're considering.

Qualified plastic surgeons are intensely trained and can competently perform many types of cosmetic surgery, and they or their marketing advisors mistakenly assume you want to know *everything* they can do rather than the actual focus of their practice and the essentials about board certification, facility certification, and experience. Don't get turned off by the lists; call and check on the procedure you're interested in.

Increasing numbers of people are using ads in newspapers and magazines and on the radio, television, and the Internet to choose surgeons, especially if they're new to a community. Doctors no longer consider it gauche or unethical to market one's practice. I've advertised my practice for many years, and prospective patients frequently tell us that they found my practice through my advertising or the Internet. Not everyone has the connections to find a doctor in the more-traditional ways.

Don't choose a doctor based solely on media or Internet ads. Many good doctors don't spend a lot of money on advertising, because they have a strong referral-based practice and don't need to advertise. On the flip side, less-capable doctors may spend a lot of money on flashy ads. Somewhere in the middle are good doctors who want to let newcomers to the community know about their plastic surgery choices. There's no proven correlation between ad quality and surgeon capability, however. You still need to see a surgeon's results, both in photographs and, ideally, in person. People have many definitions of beauty, so be sure you agree with the surgeon's aesthetic.

Screening Surgeons

Armed with the information you've collected in your research, put together a list of practices you'd like to screen. Your list should be lengthy enough so that you can create a shorter list from the initial calls you make. You'll also want to keep some names on a backup list to replace the names you delete after the first round of calls. Star the names that particularly impress you so that you know to call them first.

You may be surprised by how much information you can gather just by calling your prospects — and not all of it comes in answer to your questions but from the way you're treated. Some offices answer questions readily during your first call, and others may act like you're an interruption in their day. Others have rules and policies about giving any information away over the phone; instead, you're supposed to come to their office to learn everything, including the price! Every practice has only one chance to make a first impression — make a note of yours.

Some practices gladly follow up after your inquiry with a packet of information that anticipates most of your questions. Many promise to mail something to you and don't follow through. Whether the practice has an information packet to mail to you or not, you should be able to get lots of information upfront. If not, move on to your next prospect.

Don't hesitate to ask as many questions as you want and call back if you think of something that you didn't ask in the first call. Your goal is to find a practice that prides itself on openness and follows your lead. They shouldn't be hedging or hurrying you through a set process. Some of the information you gather will be a direct response to the questions I suggest, and some of the information will give you a "feeling" rather than a concrete answer.

Use your screening calls to get answers to your important questions about credentials, certification, the facility the doctor uses, who does the anesthesia, what options are available, and the fees involved in your procedure. Also get an idea of the doctor's schedule to see whether it matches yours.

Finding clues in phone calls

Good phone skills on the part of the surgical practice you're calling reflect a degree of organization that bodes well for your surgical experience. You'll notice whether the person with whom you're speaking is knowledgeable, patient, and encouraging. You'll also quickly get a sense of how well an office is run. You deserve a thorough response to every question and issue you raise. Don't settle for anything less.

The following indicators usually point to a well-organized practice with a competent and caring staff:

✔ **Your call is answered promptly:** If the staff members don't have time to pick up the phone, how will they have time to answer your questions? Unless you're in a very small town or the doctor has a very good reputation, go to the next name on your list.

✔ **You're not put on hold multiple times:** Are your needs less important than the person they're leaving you to help? But if you're put on hold because the staff wants to transfer your call to someone who has the time and knowledge to really help you, that's a good thing.

✔ **The staff makes the time to talk:** You want the staff to have time to fully answer your

questions and give you information you didn't even know you needed. You shouldn't feel rushed. A good practice takes your call seriously and won't blow you off.

✔ **The staff offers to send additional information:** You certainly need the information you get from the phone call, but written information that you can review on your own time is also good to have. See who offers and who waits for you to ask. Compare what different practices have available and see who's anticipating your needs and who isn't.

✔ **The staff understands your time frame:** Whether you want surgery now or six months from now, the practice should respond appropriately. Don't be made to feel like you're accommodating the practice's schedule; the staff should be accommodating yours. If someone is pushing you faster than you're comfortable with, scratch that name off your list. If they can't meet your time frame, then that's another reason to keep moving.

A referral to the practice's Web site for more information is also a positive sign. The materials they mail you aren't likely to be as extensive as what you find on the Web site.

Keep your list of questions in front of you when you call. Take as much time as you need to work through your list. Don't let anyone rush you! Remember that an ethical surgeon wants you to be well informed and well prepared. The more calls you make, the faster the process will go. Some practices will volunteer some of this information even before you ask, so all you need to do is check it off on your shopping chart (refer to Figure 4-1).

You want to find out about the following points during screening calls:

✔ **Board certification in a surgical specialty recognized by the American Board of Medical Specialties (ABMS):**

What board certification does the doctor have from the ABMS? (You want a surgeon who is certified in a surgical specialty by the ABMS. (Chapter 3 gives you the complete list of specialties.) For more information, visit www.abms.org or call 1-800-CALL-ABMS.

Does the doctor's certification and training include the procedure I'm considering? (For instance, a facial plastic surgeon who would be wonderful for face and nose surgery may not be certified for breast surgery or a tummy tuck.)

✔ **Accredited surgical suite:**

Do you operate in an accredited surgery center or hospital?

If not, does your office have an accredited surgical suite? If not, can my surgery be performed at an outpatient surgery center or the local hospital?

✔ **Types of anesthesia and providers:**

What types of anesthesia do you offer?

Do you use a board-certified anesthesiologist or a certified nurse anesthetist (CRNA)? If not, does a nurse or the doctor sedate me?

✔ **Surgeon's education and experience:**

Where did the surgeon go to school and how many years of surgical training did he complete?

Has the physician completed residency in an ABMS recognized-specialty that includes cosmetic surgery?

How long has the surgeon been in practice?

Of the procedure(s) I am interested in, how many does the surgeon perform each month? How many has he done total?

What percent of the surgeon's practice is cosmetic surgery?

✔ **Miscellaneous:**

What kind of follow-up care does your practice offer?

How does this office handle a complication or postsurgical problem, if one arises? What are the associated costs?

Does the surgeon have admitting privileges? If so, at which hospitals?

What national, state, and local associations is the physician a member of?

While you're making your initial calls and before you take the time for a consultation, you want to be sure that the surgeons you plan to visit have sufficient cosmetic experience and cosmetic surgery activity to warrant an on-site visit.

Asking the hard questions may be uncomfortable, but the stakes are so high that I strongly recommend that you ask the questions that will really help you make sure you're choosing the best surgeon. Even if the questions were answered at your initial call, it doesn't hurt to verify your understanding during your consultation visit.

Shopping advice from a happy patient

Stacy, who had rhinoplasty, describes her decision-making process: "The first surgeon I contacted was too expensive. Then I went to a second surgeon. The staff was pleasant, friendly, and professional. I did not have to wait long to see my doctor. He took one look at me and said he could fix my nose. He thoroughly explained the process and answered my questions. I felt very comfortable and at ease throughout the visit. They took pictures and electronically altered my nose so I would have an idea of how it would look after surgery. After thinking about it for a few days and discussing it with my family, I decided to have surgery and chose the second surgeon because he fit my criteria."

Stacy offers the following advice to others shopping for cosmetic surgery:

✔ Do your homework. Research, research, research. The Internet is full of a wealth of information. Understand the risks as well as the benefits.

✔ Have specific criteria in mind and don't be afraid to ask questions. Most cosmetic surgeons offer free consultations. My criteria in searching for a doctor were experience, expertise, certification, reputation, hospital privileges, location, cost, and service.

✔ Have realistic expectations. Understand that cosmetic surgery will not solve all your problems or make you look like a supermodel. However, it will change your life for the better. It's a step in beginning to rebuild self-esteem and confidence.

The following list of questions can help you evaluate the extent of the surgeon's experience:

- ✔ **What percentage of your practice is devoted to cosmetic surgery?** If the surgeon is doing more than 50 percent cosmetic surgery, you can probably look at that practice favorably — after you confirm his credentials and assure yourself that you agree with his ideas of a great result.

- ✔ **How many cosmetic surgery procedures do you do each month?** Consider at least 15 procedures per month to be an acceptable frequency.

- ✔ **What procedure do you perform most frequently, and how many do you do each month or year?** If the surgeon's top procedure is your procedure, then that's definitely a good sign — if you like the quality of his results. See the various procedure chapters in Part III for tips about the definition of good results for each type of surgery.

- ✔ **What are the common complications for my procedure?** Ask how big an issue these complications are to resolve and how frequently they occur in his practice. You should hear essentially the same answers from all surgeons. If you have any doubt about whether you're getting an honest answer because one surgeon minimizes risks or his rate of complications, then choose another doctor.

- ✔ **Who pays the costs of a second or third surgery (revision) if it becomes necessary or beneficial?** Every surgery has risks and potential complications, and you need to understand them before you accept those possibilities. What you really want is the assurance that, if something goes awry, the office you've chosen will take care of your problems with good cheer and understanding (and at minimal extra cost, if possible). Chapter 6 has more information on how to prepare yourself financially for surgery.

Chapter 5

Choosing Your Surgeon

. . . .

In This Chapter

▶ Taking a realistic approach

▶ Gauging a surgeon's professional experience

▶ Making the most of consultations

▶ Finding a doctor with the right personal qualities

▶ Reaching a decision

. . . .

*O*f all the choices you make about cosmetic surgery, the choice of your surgeon is the most important. You must take enormous care in this selection because the greatest potential for a positive and safe outcome hinges on this single decision. This chapter guides you through the process of selecting your surgeon by helping you evaluate the information you get in consultations and assess the service quality of the patient care teams at each doctor's office.

If you have trouble sifting through all the various criteria for choosing a surgeon, an abbreviated shopping method is to find a plastic surgeon who is a member of the American Society for Aesthetic Plastic Surgery (ASAPS). The society has already vetted the surgeons for you, requiring them to be board-certified plastic surgeons that have significant cosmetic experience and operate in certified or accredited operating suites. Simply go to www.surgery.org and choose a plastic surgeon in your region.

Setting Realistic Expectations

Many cosmetic surgery patients are searching for the fountain of youth. Yes, it would be nice if such a magical solution existed to take care of aging faces and less-than-perfect bodies, but unfortunately, there are no easy solutions in the very real world of cosmetic surgery. Be wary when a surgeon promises an easy solution to a difficult problem, especially if she's the only one you've heard who would treat your condition in that way.

Your cosmetic result and your recovery occur in direct proportion to the amount of treatment or surgery you choose to undergo. If a doctor promises you a quick recovery, then the procedure or treatment is probably being adjusted in a way that also reduces the immediate or long-term impact of your result. For example, recovering from a skin-only facelift is easier than recovering from a standard facelift (in which the surgeon repairs the underlying muscle), but the skin-only lift won't last as long.

Be skeptical of a surgeon who promotes herself as the "best" or the inventor of a heretofore unknown operation. Self aggrandizement is probably a tip that you don't want to be involved with that doctor. And if a surgeon promises something that sounds too good to be true, it probably is. If it sounds like a magic solution, consign it to the storybook where it belongs. You can't have surgery without scars. You can't have surgery without some form of sedation or anesthesia. And all surgery involves some form of recovery.

Prospective patients frequently diagnose themselves and are disappointed when the surgeon doesn't agree. It's not that she wouldn't like to agree, but even plastic surgeons have to follow certain rules of nature. For instance, many patients want to eliminate excess skin in their neck or faces, but they don't want a facelift or any scars. Mother Nature doesn't enable plastic surgeons to meet these unrealistic expectations.

The greatest danger when you don't follow a qualified plastic surgeon's advice and instead go to a lesser-trained specialist is that the outcome will not be good and you have endangered yourself by being unrealistic. All plastic surgeons tell stories of prospective patients who didn't take their advice, went to another doctor in another medical specialty, and then came back when they needed help to deal with the problematic surgical outcome of making the wrong choice.

Here are some of the common misconceptions patients hold:

- **Treating the surface of the skin solves excess skin problems.** Treatments for the surface of the skin do just that — treat the texture. Wonderful improvements are possible these days with chemical peels and laser peels (see Chapter 8). But if your problem is excess skin, then you probably need some form of a facelift (see Chapter 9).

- **Liposuction of the abdomen can solve excess skin problems after pregnancy or weight loss.** Because liposuction removes fat under the skin but doesn't remove the skin itself, the skin surface may dimple or wrinkle. If you have excess skin, you'll probably be told that you need a tummy tuck (abdominoplasty) to remove it and maybe some liposuction as well to flatten or debulk your hips or abdomen.

✔ **Excess neck skin can be treated without being combined with some form of facelift.** Plastic surgeons are like seamstresses, and whether it's skin or fabric, some of the same principles apply. If you're unhappy with your "turkey neck," then a little microliposuction may offer some help, but it can't resolve problems caused by excess skin. The skin has to be removed surgically, and your surgeon has a limited number of places to hide the incisions (such as in front of and behind your ear.) The only way to go is up. She has to cut away the excess skin, and incisions (meaning future scars) are the way she does that.

✔ **Sagging breasts only need to be made bigger, and all your excess skin problems will be solved.** You may think the surgeon can just put in implants and the additional volume will fill out the extra skin. Unfortunately, what you get are large, sagging breasts, which most women don't want. Again, your surgeon must remove skin to get the best cosmetic result. In addition, whenever skin is removed anywhere on your body, scars are involved, and many women aren't prepared for that result. See Chapter 15 for more information about breast lifts.

Using ASAPS criteria to find your surgeon

From the American Society for Aesthetic Plastic Surgery (ASAPS) Web site (www.surgery.org), you can find all sorts of information about plastic surgeons in your area who focus on cosmetic surgery. The site also fills you in on what it takes to become a member of ASAPS. It encourages application by trained and experienced plastic surgeons who concentrate their practices in performing cosmetic plastic surgery of the face and body. ASAPS membership is an exclusive privilege for those surgeons who possess the necessary qualifications. Only about one-quarter of all American Board of Plastic Surgery certified surgeons have been accepted into ASAPS membership. Physicians who have been trained in specialties other than plastic surgery are not eligible.

To be a member of ASAPS, the surgeon must be board certified in plastic surgery by the American Board of Plastic Surgery or the Royal College of Physicians and Surgeons of Canada and trained and possibly board certified in at least one other surgical specialty. The plastic surgeon also must have been in practice at least five years and have proven experience in cosmetic surgery covering a wide range of procedures. To qualify for membership, surgeons must be sponsored by two ASAPS members and adhere to ethical professional standards. ASAPS members are required to operate in certified facilities.

Evaluating MD Experience

Experience usually makes for a better surgeon. On the other hand, the best surgeon in your area may be the one who has just finished her training and has almost no unsupervised experience. I hope you use all the information in this book to find a surgeon with the best blend of experience and knowledge for your situation. I believe, however, that your best chance of achieving what you want is to find a great surgeon with lots of experience.

Some surgeons subspecialize, or limit what operations they do. For example, Dr. A does only breast surgery and is busy, so she's probably very good because she has been able to attract many patients in a limited surgical area. Most plastic surgeons, however, do the full range of cosmetic surgery very well. Look at their results and keep your criteria in mind (see Chapter 4). I discuss how to evaluate your doctor's work later in this chapter and in Part III's chapters on specific procedures.

Don't be afraid to ask the surgeon (and her nurse when the surgeon's out of the room) about her surgical experience. If she hedges or hesitates, move along to the next doctor on your list. Plenty of surgeons have significant cosmetic surgery experience.

If you have the name of a cosmetic surgeon you plan to see, talk to the office manager or patient coordinator and ask her, "If you wanted procedure X performed and your physician wasn't available, who would you want to perform the surgery?"

Like most things in life, there's a correlation between experience and quality. Ultimately it's about the surgeon's results. They call it the practice of medicine. And while you've heard that "practice makes perfect," only perfect practice makes perfect results.

Getting the Information You Need from Consultations

If you've done your homework well (see Chapter 4), you've generated a list of doctors who have made your short list. Now it's time for the qualifying test run. You visit each doctor's office for a new patient visit, called a *consultation,* during which you qualify a surgeon by meeting the doctor, hearing her recommendations, evaluating before-and-after pictures, getting a sense of the staff dynamics, receiving a written fee quote, and checking out the office itself (for such things as cleanliness and organization). You especially want to verify for yourself that the doctor and her staff seem interested in you, listen to your concerns and needs, and respond appropriately.

Make a commitment to complete all the consultations even if you think you've found the surgeon you want at your first visit. You may discover an even better option if you continue to shop. At the very least, you'll confirm your choice and learn more in the process. I think patients are ultimately happier with their total experience when they're better informed, so I always encourage patients to see several surgeons.

Scheduling your on-site visits

As you talk to the practices and begin making appointments for consultations at the office, you'll want to ask some questions about what you can expect. You want to schedule consultations at offices that have provided good information and followed up with quality materials. As you make your appointments, confirm what you can expect when you visit the office:

✔ Will I meet with the surgeon at my consultation?

✔ Will I be able to see before-and-after pictures?

✔ Will I be able to talk to patients who had the same procedure?

✔ Will I be able to talk to staff members who had the procedure? Can I see their scars?

✔ Do you have a system that enables me to preview the possible results of my procedure? (This may include sizing for breast augmentation or computer imaging for nasal or chin surgery.)

✔ Will I leave with a detailed fee quote explaining the costs?

✔ Will you explain what costs are involved should I need surgery for complications or revisions?

✔ If I decide to have surgery, can you accommodate my time frame?

✔ How long should I plan for the consultation?

✔ Is there a consultation fee? If so, is the fee applied to my surgery should I decide to go forward?

Most practices will willingly answer these questions. If you find a practice that seems resistant or hesitant about providing this kind of information, then don't make an appointment. Spend your on-site time with practices that are trying to help you gather the information you need.

Depending on where you live, practices may or may not charge for cosmetic surgery consultations. Whether surgeons charge or not isn't based on surgical skill but rather on other market factors. Ideally, you shouldn't have to pay to shop, but this isn't always true in medicine.

Finding someone who listened

A 54-year-old teacher and school administrator, Cathleen didn't like what she saw when she looked in the mirror. "I didn't *feel* tired, but when I looked in the mirror, I *looked* tired. My skin was starting to sag, and my desire to maintain a youthful appearance won out over my thought that growing old is just a part of life."

"I spoke to four surgeons before I made my final decision. I wanted a surgeon that I thought would really listen to my expectations. I did not want a full facelift." Although she said her husband thought she was "nuts" for wanting cosmetic surgery, Cathleen said she feels very fortunate to have a wonderfully supportive family. "I have two grown sons who were not in favor of my having surgery, but because of their love for me, they said, 'If that's what you really want, Mom, go ahead.'"

Although she couldn't be more pleased with her result, Cathleen said she was embarrassed for a few days because she thought she resembled a cotton swab because of the postsurgical head dressing. "Maybe my desire to work until I drop led me to make the decision about keeping the outside looking as young as I feel in my heart."

Factor shopping costs into your budget. Don't stop shopping just because surgeons charge for consultations. In the big scheme of things, the cost of consultation fees is minor when making a major investment in your appearance. If you decide to schedule surgery with one of the doctors you visit, most practices credit your consultation fees toward the surgery. Your worst-case scenario is that you pay some consultation fees to be sure that you visit enough surgeons and gather enough information to make the best possible choice.

Don't exclude a quality surgeon just because he or she charges for consultations. Sure, you may save a small amount of money, but you may also make an expensive wrong choice. In some cases, by explaining that you have already paid a fee elsewhere, you can ask the patient coordinator if the office will waive the fee.

Setting up your consultation goals

Aside from your research, your consultation visits are one of the most important steps in your decision-making process. Therefore, you want to be sure that you have a game plan and know what you want to accomplish during the consultation. Here's what you'll do:

✔ **Spend time with the doctor.** Be sure you have an opportunity to spend enough time with your doctor and don't meet only with the nurse, patient coordinator, or patient counselor.

✔ **Evaluate whether the surgeon listens to your goals.** You want the surgeon to find out what concerns you have and make recommendations that solve the problem you've defined. She needs to understand your issues and suggest solutions that produce the result that you're looking for. Surgeons have a tendency to try to solve the problems they see, so they'll suggest all kinds of things if you don't make your intentions clear.

✔ **Determine whether she understands your motivations.** You really need to tell your potential physician what's motivating you. If you aren't sure what your motivations may be, check out Chapter 2. Your concerns give your patient-care team good insights into how best to help you. For example, if you want surgery in preparation for your wedding or high school reunion, the doctors and staff will be excited about helping you prepare for the big event. It creates a bond that can actually help your recovery process.

✔ **Ask questions until you're satisfied with the answers.** Make sure your doctor answers all your questions thoroughly and in a way that makes sense to you. She needs to explain things in layman's terms so you know what she's talking about. Ideally, you want the practice to help you navigate your surgical course by providing detailed patient information at every step of the process. You should have received materials after making your consultation appointment and have a good idea from your initial call about how helpful the practice is going to be and whether your questions are welcomed or not before you even set foot in the office.

✔ **Discuss alternatives.** If you choose not to have the procedure you're considering or even not to have surgery at all, find out whether other treatments can solve the same problem. Ask about the benefits and issues related to these alternatives. Ask for fee quotes for these other alternatives if you're considering them seriously. Remember, you always have one alternative — not to have surgery.

✔ **Ask about the surgeon's training and experience.** You need to ask some hard questions, especially about qualifications, board certification, experience, costs, payments, and complications. A good surgeon isn't bothered by any of this; one who isn't open about these factors may be hiding something.

✔ **Look at before-and-after pictures.** No matter how well trained and experienced the surgeon is, you have to like her results or she simply isn't the surgeon for you. Do the patients for your procedure look like you'd want to look? You can find more detail about what to look for in the upcoming section "Evaluating before-and-after photos" and in the chapters that deal with each procedure.

✔ **Talk about your likely result.** Some procedures, such as noses or chin implants, can be shown with imaging technology. This aids communication and helps clarify your goals and the surgeon's understanding of them. See the procedure chapters for more on this topic.

✔ **Be open with the surgeon.** Tell the surgeon key facts about your medical history, including previous surgeries, diseases, medications you use, the nature of your job, and any related personal matters. Conditions such as diabetes, asthma, and heart problems need to be addressed seriously before surgery so that your surgical team can properly care for you. If you list a significant condition on your medical history, then the surgeon should ask about it. If she doesn't, that's an eyebrow raiser.

✔ **Tell all about sex, drugs, and alcohol.** These issues aren't casual. Most surgeons have no interest in your sexual orientation, but if HIV (human immunodeficiency virus) status could be an issue, you need to say so. If you use any recreational drugs, you must be honest. No one is going to call the police on you, but having surgery while you're using drugs such as cocaine can be fatal. Alcohol can be a real issue in recovery and healing, so your surgeon needs to know the truth about your drinking habits, too. Honestly discussing these issues need not prevent surgery, but it can prevent problems during surgery and recovery.

✔ **Ask for recommendations.** As surprising as this suggestion may sound, I encourage you to ask the surgeon for the names of other doctors that you should consider for your procedure. Her willingness to answer shows both confidence and professionalism. You may pose the question by saying, "I'd like to get a second opinion, so do you have someone you would recommend?"

✔ **Find out about patient education and communication.** Ask what the system is for educating and communicating with you before and after surgery. Do staff members check in on you proactively or do you have to take charge of communication about your own care? Verify that you'll receive patient education materials and that they'll help you to prepare for surgery and for recovery. The more you know, the better off you'll be.

✔ **Ask to talk to former patients.** Most practices can arrange for you to talk to one or more of their patients who've had your procedure. Cosmetic surgeons frequently operate on their office staff, and while you're in the office for your consultation, you may be able to talk to a staff member who has had your procedure. If a doctor doesn't volunteer that this conversation will be possible, ask whether it can be arranged. Most good surgeons have happy patients only too willing to talk about their positive experiences.

✔ **Get a written fee quote.** You should leave the consultation with a written fee quote that explains all the costs related to your surgery. (You can read more about this topic in Chapter 6.) You'll also want to know the costs of secondary surgeries if a complication arises or if you want a revision of your surgery.

✔ **Take the emotional temperature.** You want a great surgical result, but you also want a wonderful emotional experience. Take some time to get to know the surgeon and the staff. Do they seem like people who will be there for you after your procedure and not just while they want to get you in the door?

Watch for the dynamics among the staff. An unhappy or angry staff may be a clue that you won't get the emotional support you need should there be a complication that requires additional visits and more proactive communication from the doctor and staff.

Watch how the surgeon interacts with the staff. Is she kind and respectful or rude and abrupt? Does the staff cower in her presence or treat her as one of their own? You can be sure of this: However she treats them is how she'll treat you when the chips are down.

Evaluating before-and-after photos

Photographs are one of the most important means of evaluating a surgeon's quality. Ironically, most offices are so busy taking care of patients that they don't do a very good job of keeping their photo books up-to-date. In their defense, maintaining photos is hard to do. Many happy patients with great results don't come back for their longer-term post-op pictures, and the surgeon's real dilemma is that many happy patients, especially those with facial procedures, want privacy and won't allow their pictures to be shown.

Give extra points to the offices that provide great photo albums — they represent a level of organization and consumer understanding that says good things about the practice. If the pictures are in good order, probably a lot of other important things are well organized, too.

Evaluating each surgeon's results is a critical step and takes a "cool" eye. You need to be discerning and discriminating when you look at photos of a surgeon's work. Be sure that the surgeon shows you more than one or two examples. You want to look for flaws, but understand that in general the surgeon doesn't control the quality of the scars. The surgeon does, however, have control over all the other results.

Here are some questions to ask yourself while you're viewing photos:

- ✔ **Do the patients' results look natural?** One patient in a thousand wants to look like she's had cosmetic surgery and requests to be pulled tight so "everyone will know what I've done." Fortunately, most patients want to look like themselves — only better. Do the pictures look like a better version of the same person?

- ✔ **Do I agree with the doctor's aesthetic vision?** You and the surgeon you choose need to have the same view of what makes a good result. Ask her to show you examples of her work and to categorize the quality of the result: good (what you can reasonably expect), great, or poor. Ask her to explain her best result for your procedure and explain why she thinks it is good. Do the same for a bad result — if this were your outcome, could you be happy with it?

- ✔ **Do the results look too good to be true?** Excellent surgeons can turn out excellent results at a high rate of predictability, but even the best surgeon has average and below-average results. If all the pictures a surgeon shows you are of perfect results, then you should be concerned. Ask to see more pictures with a wider range of outcomes so you'll understand the full implications of your decision.

- ✔ **Am I sure these are the surgeon's actual patients?** When looking at a particular surgeon's photographs, confirm that you're looking at that surgeon's work, particularly if the surgeon is in a practice where photo books may show the results of several surgeons. Be direct and ask the question, "Is this your patient?"

You can use this same advice to evaluate pictures on the Internet and to familiarize yourself with what to look for and get some experience by comparing what you see. Then, when you go for your consultations, you'll feel like a seasoned pro and be better able to evaluate the surgeon's photos.

To find detailed information about what to look for in before-and-after photographs for a particular procedure, turn to the chapter where I discuss that procedure.

Talking to other patients

Many offices keep a list of patients who are willing to talk with other potential patients about their surgical outcomes and experiences. Don't hesitate to tell the physician or staff that you want to speak with someone who has had the procedure you're considering. To protect patient privacy, the staff will give your first name and phone number to the patient, who will then call you.

Sometimes patients are willing to meet you at the office or for coffee to discuss their experiences in more detail. You can find out a lot by asking the following questions:

✔ Are you happy with your surgical result?

✔ How does your surgical result rate against your expectations?

✔ Are you happy with your overall experience?

✔ If you knew then what you know now, would you have shopped differently?

✔ If you were giving advice to someone considering cosmetic surgery, what would you tell him or her?

✔ How important to you was the communication and education that you received?

✔ Did you always have to call the office or was the practice proactive about calling you?

✔ Was the staff supportive and responsive during your recovery?

✔ Did you have any complications or healing problems? If so, were you satisfied with how the matter was handled by the surgeon and staff?

✔ How has having cosmetic surgery changed your life?

Talking to staff members

When you visit an office for a consultation, talking to members of a surgeon's staff is another good way to rate a doctor and get the scoop on the procedure you're considering. Getting info from a staff member who's had the surgery you're considering is convenient — he or she is right there on the spot, so you don't have to make an extra trip anywhere or make another phone call. You also can see (and sometimes touch) the actual result, which is better than a photograph.

You can usually feel somewhat confident about choosing a surgeon whose staff trusts their doctor enough to let her perform their surgeries. These patients are generally in line for their next procedures, which is another good sign.

Taking a "test drive"

When you buy a car, you take it on a test drive. When you go shopping at the mall, you try on the shoes or dress you want to buy. When you want to move to a new house, you tour houses you're interested in. When you're planning your next vacation, you find lots of pictures or movies to help you decide. Most of life's major purchases offer you some direct means to determine in advance whether you want to go forward.

But if you're considering cosmetic surgery, it's a much more difficult issue. You may find it hard to envision what you'll really look like, thus making it hard for you to make a decision. But at your consultation, some tools do exist to facilitate communication:

- ✔ **Digital imaging:** Some surgeons have digital imaging software that can morph images of you to give you some idea of what the future holds. None of these morphing sessions absolutely represent ultimate reality, but they can give you some idea of the outcome. These systems are particularly useful in evaluating rhinoplasty, chin augmentation, eyelid surgery, liposuction, and, to a lesser extent, facial surgery. Being able to take home "before-and-after" pictures of yourself to share with family and friends can make preoperative decisions much easier. Depending upon your procedure, you may want to make this a requirement, but many good surgeons still don't offer this service. Digital imaging is not available for all procedures.

- ✔ **Breast augmentation sizing:** In the case of breast augmentation surgery, some surgeons offer sizing appointments either separately or as a part of their consultations. The goal is to give you some idea of how you would look after having your breasts enlarged. I discuss this topic in more detail in Chapter 14.

- ✔ **Before-and-after pictures:** Most surgeons offer to show you before-and-after pictures of their surgical results. If a surgeon doesn't make such an offer, move along. You can't choose a surgeon without this basic information. Check out the procedure chapters in Part III to find out what to look for in the photos.

Looking for Dr. Right

Your goal at consultation is to find a surgeon you like and trust. Trust relates to the medical side of things — the physician's training and experience and her results with patients. Liking someone relates to personal characteristics that include openness, willingness to communicate, and kindness. Your overall experience will be better if you can find both qualities in the surgeon you choose.

Evaluating the comfort level

You want to find a confident surgeon whose background and experience reassure you about the likelihood of having a positive outcome. You want your doctor and her staff to be strong and confident. What you don't need is an arrogant attitude — that sense that the surgeon and her staff are talking down to you and have no interest in getting to know you or really care about you.

To them, you're a *case* rather than a person. In most communities, you'll have so many choices that you don't need to put up with an arrogant doctor or staff.

You want to gain a level of emotional comfort with the surgeon that enables you to approach the surgical process confidently and to feel that, if anything goes wrong, she'll be there for you.

Find out during the consultation if you're comfortable with the staff as well. During your surgery, you'll probably be asleep and not talking with the surgeon. Much of your contact before and after surgery will be with the staff. If they're cold, distant, or unfriendly, you may not look back fondly on the overall experience, even if the surgical result is satisfactory.

 If in your search you find a surgeon who clearly is the best but you don't like her bedside manner, skip the "like" part and let trust be your guide by letting her operate on you anyway. Your encounters with her and her office staff will be short term, so while liking them is ideal, you can choose to make it a secondary issue because your result — which ideally will be positive and satisfying — is something that you can enjoy for the long term.

Seeking good communication

Communication is one of the most important aspects of your relationship with your surgeon and her staff. You want to use your consultation time to be sure that good communication exists. Are they listening to you or giving speeches? The kind of communication you witness at the consultations is what you'll get throughout your patient experience, so make sure you're happy with it.

I believe that the best consultation involves a conversation — a two-way approach. You share exactly what you hope to achieve (and why), and the physician describes the various surgical and treatment options available to get you there.

You need to find someone who listens, and the consultation is a great time to find this out. Suppose that you want to have your eyes done because they really bother you. The surgeon responds by saying that the *only* solution is a complete facial rejuvenation (that also includes your brow, face, and neck) and telling you she won't do just your eyes. But it's your face and your money, so if your doctor doesn't listen, find someone who does.

Understand however, that a surgeon's advice may sometimes really be the best solution, so you may want to consider what she thinks even if you ultimately decide not to take her advice. Your eyes may be the only correction you want or can afford. But if you're swayed by her advice, you may be like other patients who decide to hold off on another major purchase and spend the money on an expanded procedure instead.

Sorting though conflicting advice

Consulting with several surgeons is almost guaranteed to get you conflicting advice. Some of them will suggest the newest and latest procedures, and others will suggest procedures not even mentioned by another surgeon. Rely on your own intelligence and think with a cool head. Remember that what you want is the best *result,* not necessarily the latest procedure.

Don't necessarily choose a surgeon just because she performs the latest surgical techniques and innovations that get all the media attention. The hottest developments in cosmetic surgery may not be right for you or even be proven techniques. Just because a procedure is a hot concept doesn't mean it's the best surgical approach — even if all the celebrities are having it done. Your doctor may have very good reasons for avoiding that method and can achieve what you want by using traditional and proven approaches.

If you're struggling with conflicting advice, make arrangements to have second consults with your short list of potential surgeons. Ask them to help you sort through the various recommendations and clarify their advice. In addition to helping you make a decision, this process gives you a world of information about the surgeon's response to your particular needs. You want someone who communicates easily and shows openness and willingness to consider other options, including your ideas. Be careful if a doctor seems to take a one-size-fits-all approach.

Making the Big Decision

Now you come to the big moment and must weigh all the factors to make your decision. In a perfect world, you'll see a clear choice. The surgeon, facility, and practice each get the highest ratings on your list. You feel confident about the surgical outcome and look forward to going through the surgical experience with them. If one surgeon on your list meets these criteria, go for it.

In larger cities, you may have a number of good choices. Sometimes two surgeons you're considering both use the same surgery center and rank equally on the safety issue. If you think they have equal surgical abilities, your choice may hinge on their bedside manners or how you perceive their staffs. Perhaps the tipping point is the fact that one surgeon is always on time and another habitually runs late. That's why having the right criteria and a point system works so well.

Expanding on bumper sticker wisdom

Who knew you could find such good advice on the back of an SUV? Here are some thoughts that are particularly applicable to your cosmetic surgery search.

✔ **Don't go to a doctor whose office plants are dead.** This advice is great. Dead plants don't exactly show the attention to detail that gives you confidence in the surgeon or the organization of her office.

✔ **Cleanliness is next to godliness.** You may be surprised by the number of offices you visit that aren't clean or neat. If you're going to spend your hard-earned money somewhere, you have every right to expect a pleasant and clean environment. One patient once told me, "I chose your office because it was so clean that I knew your operating room would be clean, too."

✔ **College grad and Prowd Uv It.** Everybody makes mistakes, but if you see a lot of basic errors as you interact with a practice, you have a cause for concern. Certainly, they should learn how to spell and pronounce your name correctly.

✔ **Just say no to stupidity.** If you encounter practices with people who don't know anything, just say no. There are too many good doctors and great staffs to put up with mediocrity.

✔ **Not all who wander are lost.** You don't have to make a decision on anyone's time frame but your own. If you need more information or simply just want to wait until you're ready, then that's what you should do.

✔ **Age cures everything, but plastic surgery is quicker.** I found this quote on some cocktail napkins years ago. If you're ready and if you've found the right doctor, then go for it. Much joy and pleasure await you.

Despite your best efforts, your shopping process may not produce a clear choice. Don't force a decision if you're not sure. Sometimes the best next step is to start over. Taking time for a second look may help you clarify concerns that prevent you from making a choice.

If you can't make up your mind, go back to your list, call your top choice or choices and ask for a second consult. Most surgeons don't charge for these visits, which are often extremely valuable and may help you to clarify important issues.

Sometimes shoppers decide not to buy. If your second consults don't help, give yourself permission to delay your decision or to decide that a simple "no" is your answer. Saying no must be a viable option.

Ultimately, your final choice involves both mental and emotional factors. Analyze the results of your shopping experience and trust your intuition about the quality of the people you choose. Then make your decision and move forward confidently.

Reconstructing his life

After losing 200 pounds, Mick needed a body lift. He waited until he got close to his final desired weight loss to begin searching. He considered four surgeons and ultimately chose his doctor based on his technical expertise and "sense of caring and access." He also stressed the importance of making the patient's wishes known.

"Assuming the doctor understands what you want is a big mistake. Take time to discuss even the smallest concern or desired result — no matter how small or how much you think it is understood. Repeated visits to the doctor before the final decision are important to get that 'gut' feeling of comfort that you made the right decision."

Mick told me he's happy with the results of his body lift: "In comparison to before, I am extremely satisfied. One has to realize that plastic surgery won't make you a lean 20-year-old if you were 400 pounds and in your 40s. If you are realistic about what can be accomplished, you reduce the risk of being disappointed. Plastic surgery helped me fulfill my goal of becoming 'normal' after being obese my whole life. I feel great and look great for the first time. It was not just cosmetic surgery; it was reconstructive surgery. It reconstructed my life."

Chapter 6

Getting Ready Financially

Cosmetic surgery, like many other discretionary purchases, is expensive. There's just no other way to put it. In fact, after you hear how much it costs, you may begin to wonder if it's worth it and if you really should be doing it. If you don't like the cost, however, you can always just say no.

You don't *have* to have cosmetic surgery, and you really don't *need* to have cosmetic surgery. But you may *want* it, and if so, plan your finances carefully so that you make your decision based on not only on your finances but also on the truly important issues, such as the surgeon's training and board certification, the facility, and the anesthesia provider.

You must pay for your cosmetic surgery in advance — generally about two weeks before surgery. You can't expect any surgeon to waive this requirement, so you'll have to make a plan for paying what's due. It's just like paying for a cruise or an airline ticket or even some resort hotel rooms. You're expected to pay in advance.

Dealing with Sticker Shock

I understand that if you're thinking seriously about having cosmetic surgery, you're probably not very happy with what it costs. I'm somewhat shocked myself, and I deal with the costs daily in my own practice. One way to think about the costs is to spread them over the life of your result; for instance, if you're already getting facial fillers such as collagen or Botox, then having a facelift may actually save you money in the long run. You may also choose to postpone or waive a vacation, a newer car, a home redecorating or remodeling project, and so on in order to accommodate the costs of surgery. Table 6-1 shows you the range of fees you can expect for common procedures.

Table 6-1	Fees for Common Procedures
Procedure	**Price Range**
Botox	$200–400 per area
Collagen, Restylane, Hylaform, Sculptra	$350–800 per syringe
Artefill	$1,200–1,600
Chemical peels	$800–4,000
Laser peels	$2,000–6,000
Eyelid lifts	$3,000–6,500
Brow lift	$3,500–6,200
Facelift	$8,000–13,000
Mini facelift	$6,000–9,000
S-lift	$5,000–8,000
Midface lift	$5,000–8,000
Deep plane facelift	$8,000–13,000
Chin implant	$2,000–4,000
Facial implant	$2,000–4,000
Rhinoplasty	$4,500–8,000
Septoplasty	$4,000–6,000
Tip rhinoplasty	$3,500–6,000
Liposuction	$3,000–6,000
Abdominoplasty	$5,500–11,000
Belt lipectomy	$7,000–13,000
Thigh lift	$6,000–10,000
Buttock lift	$6,000–10,000
Lower body lift	$7,000–13,000
Brachioplasty	$5,000–9,000
Back lift	$7,000–12,000

Procedure	Price Range
Total body lift	$13,000–22,000
Breast augmentation	$4,000–7,000
Breast lift	$5,000–8,000
Breast lift and augmentation	$7,000–11,000
Breast reduction	$7,000–11,000
Breast reduction by liposuction	$3,500–6,500
Gynecomastia (male breast reduction)	$2,500–4,000

As with most things in life, a correlation exists between quality and cost. If you're planning to base your final decision for or against surgery primarily on cost, then you need to be extremely careful and be sure that you're making a wise surgical decision. Although you shouldn't just accept any fee estimates you're given without comparing them to fees from other plastic surgeons, be aware that saving money on cosmetic surgery frequently means giving up medical quality, particularly in the facility and anesthesia areas. If you can't afford the fees charged by a board-certified surgeon operating in a licensed facility, then you're better off not having surgery or waiting until you save the extra money you need to optimize the chances of a positive outcome.

Some patients try to lower the costs by leaving the country for surgery. The problem with this plan is that medical quality varies greatly, and your safety and an optimal result should be a higher priority than cost. Creative ways of paying are available, and they're better than putting yourself physically at risk if finances are a problem.

Sorting Through Fee Quotes

Chapter 4 contains more detailed information about the general process of shopping for cosmetic surgery. If you follow my advice and have three to five consultations, you're likely to end up with a range of fee quotes. Quality does cost more. But higher prices don't necessarily ensure quality. That's why being a cosmetic surgery shopper is so hard. You really have to know what you're doing. Turn to Chapter 4 for the complete details.

Comparing apples and oranges: The variables of cosmetic surgery

Cosmetic surgery involves many variables, and your role as a shopper is complex because although you get quotes for the same procedure by different surgeons, you aren't necessarily buying the same thing. If you're buying a certain model car, you can wisely decide to shop dealerships — price is the only variable. With cosmetic surgery, ways to reduce costs exist, but as I said above, if lower fees mean lower safety standards, then your best interests aren't really being considered. Make your motto "let the buyer beware."

Be sure that your fee quote describes what procedures you'll be having — ideally in layman's language so you can knowledgeably compare one quote with another.

The costs of cosmetic surgery break down like this:

✔ **Surgeon's professional fees:** Unlike internists and general practitioners, surgeons don't charge by the individual visit. Most surgeons charge you one fee for the surgery itself and include all pre- and postsurgery visits in their quotes for surgical professional fees. Be sure you know what's included in this component of quoted fees.

You're likely to find yourself in an apples-versus-oranges situation: One surgeon's fee is lower because the technique he recommends reduces surgical time and attendant costs but provides a different result. For example, a skin-only facelift is less expensive and less time-consuming to perform but doesn't last as long as a standard facelift.

✔ **Operating room fees:** Whether you have surgery in the hospital, at the surgery center, or in an office-based surgery suite, you pay a fee for using that space. Surgery at an accredited hospital or an independent ambulatory surgery center usually costs more than surgery at a certified office-based surgery suite.

Generally, uncertified office-based operating suites are the least expensive, but with good reason. To gain certification (see Chapter 3), operating room suites must have a broad range of expensive monitoring and safety equipment. They must meet costly personnel requirements and keep pricey emergency drugs on hand. If you're in a crisis situation, having a highly trained surgical team with everything it needs to handle your problem can make all the difference. I don't think saving money here can be construed as smart shopping.

✔ **Anesthesia:** Your anesthesia provider usually is determined according to where you have your surgery — by your surgeon if surgery is in his office or by the hospital or surgery center. Costs for MD anesthesiologists or certified registered nurse anesthetists (CRNAs) are about the same, and their safety records are comparable. Given the similarity in cost, I prefer MD anesthesiologists because they have more extensive education and training under their belts and because there's scientific evidence that anesthesiologists are more effective in the event of a medical crisis during surgery.

Certainly you can save money by having your surgeon or his nurse sedate you (instead of administering anesthesia), but depending on your procedure, eliminating the cost of a third-party anesthesia provider may also compromise your safety. See Chapter 3 for more on this topic.

✔ **Other charges:** Depending on the procedure you plan to have and the surgeon your quote is coming from, additional charges may be included in your quote. These may include

- Procedure-related fees: Breast augmentations include charges for implants, and liposuction procedures may include garment charges.

- Lab fees: Your surgeon may require certain preoperative lab studies that you're responsible for paying for. Some are procedure specific — many surgeons require a mammogram prior to breast surgery, for example.

- Medications: You will probably be responsible for purchasing your own medications for use during your recovery.

You can also expect to pay separately for your recovery facilities, overnight nurses, and transportation charges (if applicable). Some of these charges will be delineated on the quote itself and others in the financial policies of the practice.

Deciphering the fee quote

Fee quotes contain a great deal of vital information that you need to understand before you make your final decision. Take time to look over these quotes closely, keeping in mind your selection criteria (see Chapter 4). You may receive one of two types of fee quotes:

✔ **Global fee quote:** This quote gives you one total price that generally includes everything — the surgeon's professional fee, operating room charges, anesthesia costs, and other charges. Generally, global quotes don't show you how the surgeon arrived at the total. A global quote is more commonly used for office-based surgery where all the fees will be paid to one entity.

✔ **Standard fee estimate:** This type of quote breaks down the cost of each component of the procedure so you can see everything that goes into the total cost. Some surgeons with their own surgery centers choose to break out fees for the various components. If the surgeon uses an independent surgi-center or the hospital, you will almost always receive this kind of quote. You may even be asked to write separate checks or make separate payments to the various entities involved.

You can expect someone at the surgeon's office — generally a patient coordinator or nurse — to explain the fee quote to you. Ask any clarifying questions and don't hesitate to call back later if you need additional information. Some practices provide financial policies that explain when payments are due, what forms of payment are accepted, and so on. The fee quote or accompanying financial policies should also contain information about the practice's revisionary and secondary surgery policies.

Asking about Discounting

You may be able to negotiate some savings by asking the right questions. Make sure you ask whether the surgery practice offers any discounts. You can ask about these policies at any time during your decision-making process — at your first call, at the consultation, or before making your final choice. The following options may be available:

- ✔ **Multiple-procedure savings:** Most surgeons and some surgery centers and anesthesiologists apply special pricing or discounting when you have multiple surgical procedures at the same time. Individual procedures include extra time in the operating room beyond the actual surgical time for things — being prepped for surgery, for example. Because these costs are built into the fees, you can expect some savings when you have multiple procedures during one surgery and therefore have to be prepped for surgery only once.

- ✔ **Patient-related policies:** Depending upon the practice, you may also receive reduced surgeon's fees if you're an established patient of the practice, a medical professional, or an allied beauty or fashion industry worker.

- ✔ **Manufacturer's discounts:** Occasionally, a product manufacturer may be offering a special discount direct to the consumer on their product and the practice will pass this savings along. This is more likely to occur with facial fillers such as collagen or Botox.

- ✔ **Practice-related policies:** Occasionally patients who are scheduled for surgery must cancel at the last minute because of personal, financial, or medical clearance issues. If you're willing to step in on short notice, the practice may discount its fees. This flexibility on your part also may make it possible for you have your surgery earlier and/or to go to the surgeon who is your first choice but whom you can't afford otherwise.

When you get down to your final choice of surgeon, you may be facing a tough financial choice. If the surgeon you really want is more expensive than your second choice, take the problem to the patient coordinator of your first-choice surgeon. If she knows that you're ready to schedule surgery and the price difference is reasonable, she may be able to speak with her manager or the surgeon and adjust the fee quote to meet you in the middle so that you get your first choice. It never hurts to ask.

PERSONAL STORY

Adjusting timing to save costs

Upon losing 221 pounds after gastric bypass surgery, Theresa was left with an excessive amount of skin on her arms and breasts: "To my amazement I had lost all my breast mass and had only skin left that hung almost down to my waist. I couldn't even wear a short sleeve top, let alone a sleeveless top or bathing suit."

After losing all that weight, Theresa was down to a size 8 and yearned to wear normal clothes. So she started looking for a plastic surgeon to see how much it would cost to remove all of her extra skin. Going on a referral, she chose her surgeon after visiting the office and finding herself very impressed by his background and staff. Her research was over, but the cost of the procedure was a problem.

"Since money was an issue, they offered me a discount if I could fill a canceled surgery slot on short notice." Theresa agreed and saved money as a result. If she could afford more surgery, Theresa says she would have a lower body lift and a mini-facelift without hesitation. "I went from feeling very self-conscious about myself to being a very confident person personally, socially, and in my work as a sales designer."

Theresa says the staff made the surgery, recovery, and follow-up visits enjoyable, and she reports that her physician did a great job: "I healed fast and didn't have much pain at all. My scarring is minimal, and I'm thrilled with the results. I now wear sleeveless shirts all the time, and no one can tell that I lost more than 200 pounds."

Considering the Cost of Recovery and Additional Surgery

You can expect some costs related to recovery. Depending on the surgery you're having, costs may be minimal, but some procedures require hospitalization or a private nurse for a night or two. Extended time to recover from surgeries such as tummy tucks and lower body lifts can be an additional personal financial concern if you have a job because you may need extra time off, meaning a possible reduction in income. Turn to Chapter 18 to get the full scoop on what you can expect during recovery.

REMEMBER

Sometimes things go wrong, and you may need additional surgery, a longer hospitalization, or a longer healing period, all of which can result in extra costs. You need to be prepared financially for this potential outcome.

Most surgeons don't charge additional fees for complications or revisionary surgery within the first year after your procedure. If a surgeon has his own operating room, he may even waive facility fees under certain conditions. If your surgeon operates at a surgery center or hospital, you can expect to be charged for the facility if you need additional surgery. Generally, you can anticipate that you'll be responsible for anesthesia fees no matter where your secondary surgery takes place.

Your fee estimate or accompanying financial policies should contain the practice's policies about additional surgery — either as the result of complications during or after surgery or in case you need revisionary procedures because you're not happy with your result.

Be sure that you fully understand the costs of any potential additional surgery for complications or revisions. Get the policy in writing before you have surgery and make sure that you can afford it if it's necessary.

Paying for Cosmetic Surgery

If you decide you want cosmetic surgery, you know you're going to have to come up with some dough. Cold, hard cash is always an option. But if you don't have a stash under your mattress today, other ways of paying for cosmetic surgery are available. You need to understand the costs and formulate a plan that realistically integrates the surgery into your budget.

Many patients finally decide to schedule surgery when they receive an unexpected windfall — an inheritance, gift, severance package, or insurance settlement, for example. If you're one of the lucky ones, deciding how to pay becomes a nonissue. If not, keep reading for advice about financing. You can't imagine how creative prospective cosmetic surgery patients can be when they really want something. I've encountered many patients who use the following payment methods (and every possible combination of them).

Hoping for insurance coverage

First, let me derail the myth that your medical insurance is going to cover cosmetic surgery. Most insurance companies don't cover cosmetic surgery, and many companies don't cover additional surgery caused by the complications of cosmetic surgery. For planning purposes, you should just assume that no insurance reimbursement is available and you're on your own.

Nonetheless, it never hurts to ask. Things are changing in this area of insurance reimbursement. Maybe you're one of the rare birds who work for a great company that provides cosmetic surgery benefits. If so, you should be able to find out your benefits relatively easily from your human resources department. Even if such a benefit exists, it probably doesn't pay your surgeon's normal fee schedule. More than likely, the surgeon you want won't accept the discounted insurance payment, so you're back where you started, trying to figure out how you're going to pay for it.

Telling two sides of the inheritance story

Angela's story starts with her dad; genetics is a powerful force. "Unfortunately, I inherited heavy lids from my daddy. When he was 75, he had his lids done as did my half-brother at age 60. When my father passed away at 98, he left me some money. So I said, 'Daddy, you gave me these lids, now you're going to pay to have them lifted.'"

Angela is glad she had the surgery: "I am so pleased with the results. Someone I worked with for seven years said to me, 'Wow, you have green

eyes.' Of course she had never noticed before because my eyes were hidden by my lids." Angela is now "tickled pink" to be able to start her day doing something she always wanted to be able to do: putting on mascara and knowing it won't smear across her heavy lids. "Now I walk out of the house beginning the day on a positive note."

And her message to her father: "Thanks, Daddy. I feel great."

Starting a fix-it fund

Plan ahead for your surgery by doing your preliminary shopping, calling practices, or checking out information on the Internet. Then save your money in a fix-it fund until you have enough to proceed. You can actually sock away cash at home or in a savings account and then schedule your surgery after you've saved all the money. Or, you may want to schedule your surgery far enough in advance to give you enough time to save and a definite deadline for meeting your goal.

Prepaying your surgeon

Some patients don't want to save their money in their own account so they do the surgical equivalent of a layaway plan. They make prepayments to their surgeon until they have the amount they need to go forward. I've had a number of patients do this over the years. They've been afraid if they have access to their own money they'll spend it on something else.

If you decide to schedule way in advance and prepay your surgeon rather than keep the money yourself, be very careful. Be sure that you choose a reputable surgeon who isn't going to fold up shop and leave you holding an empty bag.

Paying with cash

If you're paying with cash, you probably can't imagine that your surgeon's practice has any issues about that payment method. You need to check with the practice you choose to find out its exact policies about payment, but you can expect to find guidelines like these:

- ✔ **Personal check:** Most practices, hospitals, and surgery centers accept personal checks but generally won't do so fewer than ten days before surgery. Otherwise, they'll want you to use a credit card or pay in cash or with a cashier's check instead.

- ✔ **Cash or cashier's check:** Depending on what you're having done, your payment for surgery may involve a payment of more than $10,000. If you're paying with cash or a cashier's check, the federal government gets involved. The practice must file a Form 8300 (Report of Cash Payments Over $10,000 Received in a Trade or Business) notifying the IRS that you have given it $10,000 or more in cash. Be ready to explain where that much cash came from.

Unlike credit cards, which always involve an expense to the practice or facility, cash or checks actually save the practice some money. If you're going to pay cash, ask whether the practice offers a discount for cash. I offer this discount in my practice, and many patients take advantage of it.

Using plastic

I can remember when using a credit card to pay for cosmetic surgery was a rare event, but doing so is common today. Like most people, you probably have three or four credit cards in your wallet. Most practices accept credit cards as do most surgery centers and hospitals. They may not accept all types of cards though, so if you're planning to use a credit card, be sure to ask.

If the credit card you plan to use doesn't offer any extra advantages, such as airline miles or cash back, you can call before you pay for cosmetic surgery and ask what benefits can be added to your card. Otherwise, you may want to apply for a card that does give added value. Why make a major purchase without getting every possible benefit?

If you encounter a surgeon or facility that wants you to pay an added charge for the privilege of using your credit card, I urge you to complain. Tell the practice that this issue may be a deal breaker. Credit card use charges are a cost of doing business, so they should be factored into your fees without additional charges. You may be able to get this policy waived and save the additional cost.

Using your home equity

Your home may be your most profitable investment. Real estate values have soared in the last few years, and low interest rates have made refinancing or home equity loans very attractive. Another added value is that money pulled out in a refinance or from an equity line of credit generally has much lower interest rates than credit cards. If you want to use your home to pay for or finance cosmetic surgery, here are two strategies:

- ✔ **Refinancing your house:** This approach works well when interest rates are dropping. You not only lower your house payment but can frequently draw out some cash for something that's important to you — like having cosmetic surgery!

- ✔ **Getting an equity line of credit:** This strategy works similarly to refinancing, but you leave your home loan in place and add a line of credit, frequently at a low interest rate. You can then write checks against the equity in your home.

Don't get carried away. You obviously don't want to use either of these strategies unless you're financially responsible. How you look and feel is important, but not that important.

Financing cosmetic surgery

You'll find several cosmetic surgery finance companies in the marketplace. Whether independent or affiliated with banks, they offer unsecured credit for financing cosmetic surgery. Many practices work with one or more companies and can refer you to one of them or actually help you apply. Please note that because this is unsecured credit, standards are high. Even so, industry-wide approvals for this form of unsecured credit are low — generally less than 20 to 25 percent of applicants are approved.

You really need to be careful if you're considering financing cosmetic surgery. Check the rates. Financing is often the most expensive form of credit. If you have any other options — saving your money, using your home equity, or using a consumer credit card — you should investigate those forms of payment first. If financing cosmetic surgery is the only option for you, try combining financing with other forms of payment. Anything you can do to reduce the amount financed saves you money in the long run.

If you need to finance all or part of your cosmetic surgery, then you really need to spend some time finding out how the world of credit works. Before you start applying for credit, find out what your credit score is. You can research this information on the Internet or call one of the major credit reporting agencies and pay a fee to find out. Be sure your credit is in as perfect order as possible *before* you start applying for credit. Then make as few applications as possible. Any denials harm your future ability to borrow.

Before you apply for financing, ask the practice or finance company what range of credit scores get approved by this particular lender and what credit history is required (often four years). If your credit score is 575 and the finance company doesn't approve anyone below 600, then don't apply to that company. If you have two years of good credit history but the company requires four years, there's no point in getting your credit dinged when you know you won't pass muster.

If you're a cosmetic surgery shopper with no approvable credit history, your only hope is to get a cosigner or a co-borrower. Even then, getting approval is fairly difficult.

If you can't qualify by yourself, try to find a financing company that allows your co-borrower with stronger credit to be first on the loan. That person's stronger credit can carry the day, and you'll have a much better chance of approval that way. You have to ask, though — not all companies allow it.

If your credit is good, you may receive offers for introductory credit cards that offer little or no interest for six months. You can create your own no-interest or low-interest financing using one of these new card offers. You can either pay off the balance in six months or transfer the remaining balance to another introductory card until you make your final payment. You do need to be disciplined financially if you choose this option.

Chapter 7

Getting Ready Physically

Cosmetic surgery sounds easy and superficial, but it's real surgery. You need to be in good enough physical condition to go through the process and heal completely. Your physical health plays a big part in your ability to withstand and recover from surgery. Taking care of your body beforehand is important. Surgery is a stress and you need to make sure you're in good shape so that you come through the surgery well and recover quickly.

If you're being treated for an illness, you may need to get medical clearance from your primary care physician, internist, or cardiologist before a cosmetic surgeon and anesthesiologist will agree to treat you.

In this chapter, I tell you about common medical problems that may require special considerations before, during, or after surgery. I also fill you in on how to assess your condition and get your body into its best presurgery state so that you'll get great results with minimal complications.

Factoring Health into Your Decision

Your surgeon and her staff need to know whether you have any medical problems that could affect your ability to handle anesthesia or could cause increased surgical complications. As part of your evaluation for surgery, your surgeon takes a medical history to find out about your past and present health. This history includes a record of any medications and supplements you take; allergies to medications, soaps, and latex; and previous surgeries.

If you have a significant medical problem that could influence your ability to have safe anesthesia or to heal normally, you need to collect as much data as possible so that your surgeon and anesthesiologist can decide whether you can safely proceed. If you have a history of heart disease, for example, you need to obtain copies of your EKGs.

You may also need to seek medical clearance before proceeding. Getting medical clearance before surgery can be expensive and can also delay surgery. The cost of obtaining clearance — usually through medical visits and tests — is your responsibility, though insurance coverage may help defray the expense. If your surgeon asks you to get medical clearance, you need to understand that it isn't a frivolous request but represents a serious concern for your safety and surgical outcome.

The following sections explain the common problems in patients considering cosmetic surgery and how they can affect surgery.

High blood pressure

If your primary care physician is treating you for high blood pressure (hypertension), then your blood pressure is probably under control with medication and your surgery can almost always proceed with no additional risk (discretion always lies with your surgeon). The exception would be if your medication doesn't successfully control your elevated blood pressure.

Control of blood pressure during the time around surgery is important because high blood pressure can cause more bleeding during and after surgery. If your pressure goes up during surgery, the surgical team can give you medication intravenously to help to control it. However, if your blood pressure is high and isn't being treated or isn't under control before surgery, your procedure may need to be delayed until the situation is more stable.

Heart disease

Many people with heart disease have cosmetic surgery safely. If you have heart disease, your anesthesiologist may request that you get clearance from your cardiologist. If you can, have your cardiologist fax copies of your electro-cardiograms (EKGs) to your surgeon's office. Although you need to inform your surgeon of your condition, you most likely will be able to undergo surgery despite heart disease. I have even safely performed a facelift on a patient following a heart transplant, demonstrating that serious problems aren't always a bar to reaching your goals.

Many times, an EKG can be interpreted as showing the possibility that you may have suffered a very recent heart attack. Anesthesiologists don't want to proceed until that possibility is clarified. If a recent heart attack has occurred and has not been treated, having an anesthetic and surgery could prompt an arrhythmia or a second attack, both of which could be fatal.

Anesthesiologists' main concern is that they not give anesthesia to someone with unstable heart disease, someone in the process of having a heart attack, or someone who may develop an arrhythmia. They certainly don't want to give anesthesia to someone who has heart failure. If you're asked to obtain cardiac clearance before surgery, don't be upset. The surgeon is making the request in the interest of your own personal safety.

Mitral valve prolapse

Mitral valve prolapse is a relatively benign heart valve problem that causes a slight "click" or murmur that your physician can hear when she listens to your heart with a stethoscope. With this condition, the mitral valve is usually a little looser than normal mitral valves, which predisposes you to developing an infection of the affected valve during the peri-operative period. If you have mitral valve prolapse, your surgeon may want take appropriate precautions by giving you antibiotics at the time of surgery. Usually, your surgeon will ask you to take oral antibiotics for a day or two before surgery, and you'll receive antibiotics intravenously during surgery.

Antibiotics prevent you from contracting *subacute bacterial endocarditis* (SBE), a very serious infection of the heart valves. Taking antibiotics almost always prevents SBE.

Smoking

Smokers have several problems that may prevent them from having cosmetic surgery. Nicotine constricts small blood vessels, so smokers have increased chances of having breathing and heart problems. Smokers also have poorer circulation in the skin, which is a special problem for patients considering such procedures as facelifts, breasts lifts, and abdominoplasties because the success of these procedures depends heavily on good or normal skin circulation. Some surgeons refuse to do facelifts on smokers.

Most surgeons make a serious attempt to get their patients to quit smoking (if only for a few weeks or months before surgery) or, if patients can't or won't quit, to at least cut back. And you can't get off easy by using nicotine substitutes such as gum and patches — they cause the same circulation problems as cigarettes.

Smoking can decrease blood flow to the surgical area, which is already stressed from the surgery, and can lead to skin loss (a small area of skin dies) at the edges of a facelift, breast lift, or tummy tuck and a much slower recovery from all surgeries. Smokers may also have increased problems with postoperative coughing and bleeding. For all these reasons, it's imperative that you're completely honest with your surgeon about your nicotine use.

Diabetes

Diabetics can have cosmetic surgery, but if you're a Type 1 diabetic, special arrangements about insulin management need to be made with the anesthesiologist before surgery. Around the time of surgery, your normal diet is disrupted, leaving you at risk of developing hypoglycemia (low blood sugar levels). Making arrangements with the anesthesiologist is the responsibility of your surgeon and her staff, but it's very important for you to be involved in these plans and arrangements. People with severe diabetes are somewhat more prone to postoperative infection, and as a diabetic you're not quite as healthy as the average person without diabetes. See Chapter 18 for more information on recovery after surgery. The increased risks of surgery are small if your diabetes is well controlled.

If, however, your diabetes is causing problems such as serious heart disease, kidney disease, or circulation problems in your feet or legs, your surgeon may decide that you're not a good candidate for surgery. You can't ignore the potential risks and must be candid with your surgeon.

Breathing problems

Asthma and chronic obstructive pulmonary disease (COPD) are diseases that interfere with the lungs' ability to deliver oxygen to the body. You must have your asthma or COPD under good control before having surgery. An asthma attack or worsening of COPD can make having anesthesia more dangerous.

If you can't walk a block on level ground or up a flight of stairs without getting severely winded, or if you need constant oxygen because of breathing problems, then you probably aren't a candidate for a major operation. You and your doctors need to carefully evaluate your medical condition before you consider having any type of cosmetic surgery.

Anemia

If you're anemic, you may need to go on iron supplements to get your blood count into a normal range before surgery. All major cosmetic operations have the potential for blood loss. If you're anemic to begin with, your "safety net" of red blood cells is already gone. What may be an easily tolerated minor or moderate blood loss in a non-anemic patient could have very different results in an anemic one; specifically, the loss of blood could make it necessary for you to have a transfusion. Almost all surgeons want to avoid giving you blood transfusions following a cosmetic surgery procedure, because the risks associated with blood transfusion (HIV, hepatitis) should not be incurred for an elective procedure.

If your anemia is severe, you may need to consult with a hematologist (blood specialist). In general, anesthesiologists don't want to administer anesthesia for elective surgery without clearance from your physician or a hematologist if your hematocrit is under 30 or your hemoglobin is under 10.

Bleeding disorders

Several bleeding disorders can make surgery somewhat risky and dangerous. If you bleed excessively following a cut or after dental work, you must report this to your surgeon. If you needed transfusions following normal operations in the past, you must report that, too. Some patients, such as those with hemophilia, lack clotting factors in their blood. These conditions mean that you may bleed excessively and not clot normally. You may still be able to have surgery safely with the assistance of a hematologist and treatment with medication or blood products. However, bleeding disorders are potentially serious problems and may require an extensive specialized workup.

Aspirin, non-steroidal anti-inflammatory agents (NSAIDS), and some herbal supplements cause increased bleeding, and you should stop taking them 7 to 10 days prior to surgery. Be sure to be completely candid with your surgeon about what medications and supplements you're taking, and don't take anything including herbal supplements without your surgeon's permission.

Some patients require the use of Coumadin (which reduces the blood's ability to clot) and other blood thinners for a variety of medical conditions. Stopping such medicines is best coordinated with the doctor who prescribed them.

Remaining physically active

Renee, a 41-year-old wife and mother of two young children, underwent cosmetic surgery for the first time in 1997, after the birth of her second child. In 2000, she then moved to, "the land of the beautiful people, a.k.a. California," and became very insecure about the loose skin and excess fat in her legs and around her hips and back. "For two years I wouldn't wear a swimsuit in public or in front of my own family in our backyard."

After additional plastic surgery (thighplasty) to address her problems, Renee reminds people that, "Surgery is not a weight-loss technique. I still go to the gym and have made changes in my diet, but the whole transformation is a process. Surgery does, however, help you with the problem spots and those last 10 to 20 pounds. If anyone is considering cosmetic surgery, my advice is, if your appearance is affecting your life in a negative way, go for it! If you have found the right physician, you won't be sorry."

Infectious diseases

Diseases such as hepatitis and HIV (AIDS) are not to be taken lightly. If your condition is stable on medications, your surgeon may agree to proceed with surgery. However, because of the increased risk of blood exposure to all members of the health-care team, you need to tell your doctor if you have one of these conditions. Obviously, active hepatitis will prevent you from having surgery because exposing an acutely ill liver to surgical stress and anesthetic agents may worsen your condition.

Some plastic surgeons are unwilling to subject themselves and their staffs to the risks of contracting human immunodeficiency virus (HIV) and therefore refuse to operate on HIV-positive patients. If questions arise about an HIV patient's current health status, clearance from their primary care physician will be needed. Severe immuno-compromise and concurrent infection at the time of surgery could lead to poor healing and wound infection.

If you have HIV but aren't "sick," then your disease shouldn't prevent you from having cosmetic surgery. If you're HIV positive, the surgeon and surgical technician will be especially careful not to stick themselves with an instrument or needle. They will take what are called universal precautions, double glove, and be exceptionally careful with the handling of all sharp objects. I believe, however, that although most plastic surgeons are willing to treat such patients, they do appreciate knowing the truth about a patient's HIV status. If you're HIV positive, I encourage you to respect the implications for your surgical team and to report that diagnosis to your physician.

Multiple sclerosis

Many people with multiple sclerosis (MS) live essentially normal lives most of the time. During the periods that you're not experiencing acute neurologic symptoms (relapses), you probably can have cosmetic surgery safely.

Undergoing any type of surgery is a stress on the body. This stress has been associated with exacerbations of multiple sclerosis, so you and your surgeon and neurologist need to confer about whether cosmetic surgery is a reasonable choice for you. If your neurologist gives her permission to proceed, most plastic surgeons will be happy to help you.

Connective tissue disorders

Lupus erythematosus, scleroderma, and rheumatoid arthritis are examples of connective tissue disorders that are chronic autoimmune medical problems. In general, such diseases don't prevent you from having cosmetic surgery unless they're in an acute phase. Although you should obviously discuss such potential surgery with your treating physician (usually a rheumatologist or internist), these diseases usually won't stop you from having cosmetic surgery.

Treatment for this group of diseases frequently includes the use of steroids. Long-term steroid usage may make your skin more fragile and decrease your ability to heal as quickly as normal. Communication between your surgeon and your treating physician will determine whether you can proceed or not.

Obesity

Being severely overweight adds some level of risk to almost any surgical procedure. Losing weight before surgery is almost always helpful. Severely obese patients have more breathing problems due to the weight of their chests or abdomens. The excess weight may also put more tension on incision lines and make wound breakdown or separation more likely.

If obesity makes it difficult for you to walk, climb stairs, and perform activities of daily living, the anesthesiologist will probably not want to give you an anesthetic except in an emergency condition. You will probably be asked to lose weight and exercise so that you can function normally prior to surgery. However, in some cases, surgeons make exceptions. For example, if you're having trouble losing weight because you have difficulty exercising, some surgeons will agree to remove the excess abdominal weight so that you're physically able to exercise and begin to lose weight. Losing weight first is safer, but it isn't always possible, and taking a small additional risk now may lessen the consequences of obesity later in life.

PERSONAL STORY

"Be at your best"

After having a breast reduction procedure, April offers the following advice to people considering cosmetic surgery: "Talk to as many friends or people who are willing to give you as much information as possible. Be sure you talk with your personal physician. Also have at least three consultations. One more thing — and this is very important — be in the best mental and physical health possible. It makes for a speedy and healthy recovery!"

If you're obese, you've probably thought of liposuction as a potential solution. Unfortunately, liposuction is not a method of weight loss. Rather, it's a method of changing your shape in localized areas. For example, if you're moderately overweight but the only area that really bothers you is your tummy, liposuction may be just what you're looking for. If, however, your abdomen, hips, thighs, knees, and back are all heavy, then liposuction probably won't solve your problems.

Alcohol and recreational drug usage

Most health experts would agree that alcohol in moderation is safe. However, drinking to excess over a long time period of time can have major effects on your body, especially on your liver, which is important for metabolizing most drugs. Most surgeons ask to you to stop drinking around the time of your surgery because it can be life threatening to mix alcohol with the pain pills that are usually prescribed after major surgeries.

If you use recreational (illegal) drugs, you must let your surgeon and anesthesiologist know and discuss the situation with them. Plastic surgeons aren't members of the International Olympic Committee or police officers — they won't report you to the authorities if they find out you're a user. But they do need to know if you use recreational drugs. You'll probably be able to proceed with surgery, but some drugs (for example, cocaine) make the heart more prone to irregular heartbeats, making anesthesia more dangerous. To avoid putting your life at risk, please be honest with your surgeon and anesthesia provider about your use of these substances.

Don't use any recreational drugs for at least a week before surgery. Following surgery, you will probably be on prescription pain pills, and you should never mix recreational and prescription drugs.

Understanding Preoperative Testing

Many surgeons request preoperative tests to verify whether it's safe to proceed with surgery. The tests that your surgeon requires for you will depend on the surgical procedure(s) you plan to have, the type of anesthesia you'll receive, your medical conditions, and your age. Some of the most common preoperative tests are:

- **Complete Blood Count (CBC):** This blood test analyzes the components that make up your blood. If you're anemic, then the test shows a low blood count (hematocrit). The CBC also measures platelets, the components in blood that assists in clotting.

- **Chemistry panel:** This test measures the concentration in your blood of various chemicals, including sodium, potassium, and glucose. Problems with the concentrations of these chemicals can make having surgery unsafe. Some medications such as diuretics (water pills) can cause electrolyte problems that need to be fixed before surgery.

- **Electrocardiogram (ECG/EKG):** An electrocardiogram measures the electrical signals from your heart. It can help determine if your heart is beating normally or if there's a problem that requires you to be evaluated before surgery. Most surgeons require ECGs on all patients over age 40.

- **Chest X-ray:** This X-ray shows the organs in the chest and can help determine whether you have pneumonia (lung infection) or congestive heart failure (water on the lungs). These conditions may cause your surgery to be postponed until they're resolved.

- **Pregnancy:** If you are or could be pregnant, be sure to inform your surgeon to avoid risk to the developing fetus. If you're of child-bearing age, many surgeons will ask you to undergo a pregnancy test immediately before surgery.

- **Mammogram:** Having a mammogram (low-dose X-ray of the breasts) prior to breast surgery is a requirement of many surgeons if you're past age 40 (sometimes 50). It's important to know that a patient doesn't have breast cancer prior to undergoing cosmetic breast surgery.

Getting Ready for Surgery

You can't just walk into surgery without preparing your body for the experience. In the time leading up to your procedure, you need to take particularly good care of yourself to make sure you're in the best possible condition for surgery. The instructions in this section are generally acceptable to most surgeons, but your doctor may have additional instructions that you should follow — or she may have different ideas altogether. Always follow your surgeon's advice.

In the days or weeks before surgery

Several factors affect your surgical outcome. Your doctor will discuss these issues with you in advance and/or give you written instructions about what to do to prepare for surgery. The general guidelines cover the following topics:

- ✔ **Stop smoking.** If you smoke, you need to stop smoking as soon as you can and for as long as possible before and after surgery. You put yourself at real risk if you don't and if you lie about this habit to your doctor. Check out the aptly titled section "Smoking" earlier in this chapter to find out why.

- ✔ **Take multivitamins.** If you don't already take multiple vitamins, your surgeon may instruct you to begin doing so. This advice is an attempt to make sure that you're at your absolute best at the time of surgery. Taking vitamins may not help, but it certainly can't hurt.

  Check the label on your vitamin bottle. Most surgeons limit your intake of vitamin E to less than 400 IU (international units) per day. Larger doses may increase the possibility of bleeding.

- ✔ **Take vitamin C.** Your surgeon will probably want you to take 1000 mg of vitamin C daily for several weeks before and after surgery because it helps promote healing. Most multivitamins don't contain this level of vitamin C.

- ✔ **Skip the supplements.** Stop taking all natural dietary supplements at least ten days before surgery. Some commonly used supplements cause prolonged bleeding and may interfere with anesthesia. Danshen, dong quai, feverfew, garlic ginkgo, and ginseng may all cause excess bleeding. Echinacea, ephedra, goldenseal, kava, St. John's wort, and valerian may cause cardiac complications, increased blood pressure, or anesthesia complications. When in doubt, ask your doctor, and, to be on the safe side, stop all supplements. You may restart your supplements ten days after surgery unless your surgeon gives you other instructions.

- ✔ **Avoid aspirin and ibuprofen.** Many over-the-counter medications and many prescription drugs contain aspirin and ibuprofen. Both products can cause excessive bleeding and need to be avoided for at least 7 to 10 days before surgery. If you need to take something for pain, take only Tylenol (acetaminophen).

- ✔ **Pass up NSAIDs.** If you have arthritis or take any nonsteroidal anti-inflammatory drugs (NSAIDs), then you should stop taking them 7 to 10 days before surgery. Like aspirin, NSAIDs cause excessive bleeding. When in doubt about your medications, ask your doctor. Your surgeon must approve all your current medications.

The night before surgery

The night before surgery should be a bit like the night before Christmas. You want to be really good and follow all the rules you've been given. This isn't a night to stay out late partying. You should do the same thing you want your surgeon to do — stay home, read or watch TV, get a good night's sleep, and arrive in the morning rested and ready for surgery.

Don't eat or drink anything (including water) after midnight or for at least eight hours before your surgery if you're having general anesthesia or being sedated. For other types of anesthesia, follow your doctor's instructions.

The reason not to eat or drink prior to anesthesia is that if you vomit while under anesthesia and inhale some of the vomit into your lungs, then very serious lung problems, pneumonia, and even death can occur.

The morning of surgery

As the big moment approaches, you have more to remember. Your surgeon may have additional suggestions for the morning of surgery, but here are the basics:

- ✔ **Food and drink:** If you're having general anesthesia or sedation, don't eat or drink anything.

- ✔ **Medications:** If you've been cleared to take your daily medicines, then take them with only a sip of water.

- ✔ **Oral hygiene:** You may brush your teeth, but don't swallow any water.

- ✔ **Make-up:** Don't put moisturizers, creams, or lotions on the area to be operated on.

✔ **Contact lenses:** Don't wear your contact lenses. You may, however, wear or bring your glasses.

✔ **Clothing:** Leave all jewelry at home and wear only loose fitting clothing that you don't have to put over your head, such as zip-up sweats or jogging outfits. I also recommend wearing slip-on shoes. Remove hairpins and wigs. Don't bring valuables with you to surgery.

✔ **Personal hygiene:** If you're having your period on the day of surgery, wear a feminine pad; don't use a tampon — you may forget about it, and no one wants to increase the possibility of toxic shock syndrome.

Part III
Exploring Your Options

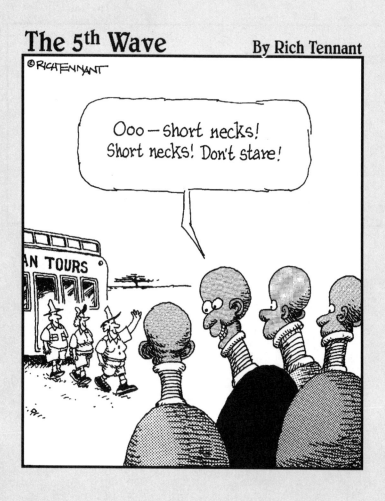

The 5th Wave   By Rich Tennant

Ooo — short necks!
Short necks! Don't stare!

In this part . . .

*W*hether you're looking to improve the shape of your nose or lift your sagging posterior, in this part you find answers to your questions about how surgeons do what they do, the risks you may encounter, and the choices you have to get the look you have in mind. I give you the lowdown on everything from where your incisions will be to how long before you're back out in the world showing off your new look.

Chapter 8

Sprucing Up Your Face without Surgery

*P*eople have searched for the fountain of youth for thousands of years. We still haven't found it, and no one can stop the ravages of time. Thanks to the marvels of modern science, however, people do have many options if they want to take a few years off their faces.

Most people want facial rejuvenation without resorting to surgery. Noninvasive treatments can and do make many people look better every day. If your skin is beginning to sag a little and looks aged, superficially wrinkled, blotchy, or discolored, some of the treatments described in this chapter may be helpful. The procedures I talk about in this chapter offer good results with very little interruption to your lifestyle. You don't have to do anything special to prepare for the procedure, and you don't have to hide out or limit your activity after the procedure.

Getting Under Your Skin: Anatomy

Your skin is a six-pound organ that acts as a protective barrier for your body: It helps maintain body temperature, transmits sensory information from the environment, and protects you from disease. Skin is composed of three layers:

- ✔ The *epidermis* is the outer layer of the skin. It sheds about every two weeks when it's healthy.

- ✔ The *dermis* is the middle layer and is made up of collagen fibers that provide structure and support, as well as elastic fibers.

- ✔ The deepest layer is subcutaneous tissue composed of fat and connective tissue with larger blood vessels.

Specialized structures in the dermis (oil glands, hair follicles, and sweat glands) are also known as *epithelial appendages.* These vary in quantity depending upon the area of the body and help heal the skin by providing new epithelial cells when it's injured. Facial skin has many more epithelial appendages when compared to neck or chest skin. For this reason, physicians can safely treat facial skin much more aggressively with deeper peels or with laser, which cause injury to the skin. The same level of treatment to the neck or chest would be more difficult to heal and could result in scarring.

Sun damage and environmental toxins, such as smoking, damage your skin and accelerate normal skin aging (see Figure 8-1). The more sun exposure you have, the worse the microscopic changes to the skin. The best treatment to prevent aging of the skin itself is avoiding the things that cause damage in the first place. But it's never too late to prevent further damage, so if you're still smoking, quit, and if you go out in the sun, protect your skin.

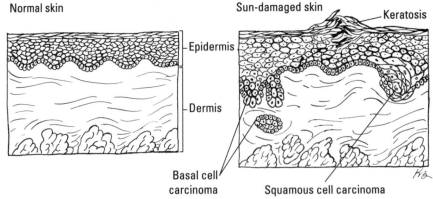

Figure 8-1: Compare the healthy skin on the left with the sun-damaged skin on the right.

Tanning your way to skin trouble

Culturally, tanned skin has strongly positive associations — with health, beauty, fashion, youth, and an upscale lifestyle. But little did medical experts know many years ago that excessive sun exposure has damaging physical effects. If you're a boomer, the importance of protecting your skin from the sun was not mainstream knowledge when you were in your teens and early 20s — and 80 percent of sun exposure usually happens before the age of 30, and perhaps before age 20. Initially, tanned skin hides the very things it later causes — a leathery appearance, lost elasticity, and sagginess. This picture isn't as depressing as it once was, however, because today you do have some control over reversing some skin damage. In the same way that you can maintain your physical health, you can maintain your skin health. You can partially reverse sun damage just as you can lose weight.

The hallmark of aging skin is a degenerative process in which collagen in the dermal layer is replaced by a thick tangled layer of elastic fibers. As skin ages, it gradually loses its dermal supporting layer and its ability to stretch and recoil. The epidermis appears disorderly and is thickened with irregular cells. The skin has an abnormal number of *melanoctyes* (pigment-producing cells) and an uneven distribution of melanin. Normal cell cycles that were six weeks are now several months, leading to increased pigmentation, wrinkles, and rough spots. Some of the cells contain excess pigment, and others contain virtually none, which explains the blotchiness of sun-damaged skin.

Smoothing Wrinkles with Botox

If you watch old movies or TV shows, you'll see the world before Botox. When actors talked, their foreheads showed lines and wrinkles, and their frowns were obvious. Look at your favorite actor or newscaster. Do you see any wrinkles? Are their frowns obvious? Is anything above their eyes in motion? You're in the land of Botox, which is the most commonly used botulism toxin product on the market at the time of this writing.

Botulism toxin is a foreign protein that binds to the nerve endings of the muscle where it's injected. Once attached, it keeps that muscle from being stimulated — it temporarily paralyzes the muscle. For example, when the muscles that attach to the skin in the area between your eyebrows contract, frown lines form (see Figure 8-2). Keeping those muscles from moving keeps frown lines from appearing. Your body eventually breaks down the botulism toxin (three to four months in most cases), and the muscles work normally again.

If a facial muscle is kept immobile with botulism toxin over a period of time (12 to 18 months), the muscle becomes weak. When muscle function is allowed to return, you should notice a definite decrease in the depth and severity of the crease or line because of the weakness in that muscle, and the interval between Botox injections may become longer. As you gradually regain strength in the muscle, you will notice an increase in the lines. The exact timing of how often you "need" Botox is variable.

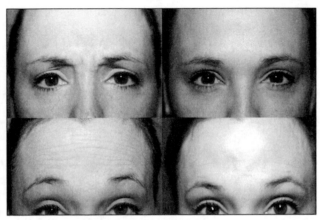

Figure 8-2:
Worry lines or frown lines can be easily and temporarily eliminated with Botox injections.

Botox is most commonly injected into the forehead, between the eyebrows, and in the area just outside the eyes (the location of so-called crow's-feet). Less common sites of injection are the upper and lower lips and chin. When injecting Botox, surgeons also can obtain a "chemical" lift of the eyebrow by carefully placing the Botox injections to result in certain muscles pulling the eyebrow up. Multiple areas may safely be injected at the same time. In some clinics, specially trained nurses inject Botox.

When Botox is injected too low on the forehead, some of the medication can migrate lower and paralyze the muscles that raise the eyelid or eyebrows. Although it looks a little unsightly, it is not dangerous and usually disappears in a month or two as the Botox starts to wear off.

Botox shows maximum effectiveness in seven days. If you feel like you have too much muscle movement at that time, you should return to the office for another injection, which many offices do at no charge or for a reduced fee.

Filling the Void with Dermal Injectables

Some of the most visible signs of facial aging are wrinkles and depressions — the lines around your mouth, wrinkles around your eyes, or frown lines between your eyes. Materials that can be injected into or under the skin to reduce or eliminate the wrinkles or depressions are called *dermal fillers,* and they work by adding bulk to the dermis. (See Figure 8-3.)

Depression in skin before collagen injection

After collagen injection

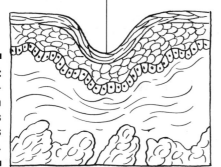
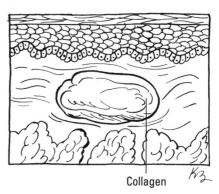

Figure 8-3: Fillers temporarily fill in depressions on the skin's surface.

Collagen

If you're bothered by creases that have resulted from smiling, laughing, frowning, squinting, or just plain old aging, dermal fillers may be a good option for you to consider. The underlying soft tissue that keeps your skin plumped up begins to thin and break down as you age. Expression lines suddenly become permanent creases and are marks of facial aging.

The areas that doctors most commonly treat with fillers are frown lines between the eyebrows, the folds between the nose or lips and cheeks *(nasolabial folds),* lines below the corners of the mouth *(marionette lines),* wrinkles in the upper or lower lips, frown lines, and smile lines at the outside of the mouth. Crow's-feet are not usually treated with fillers; the skin in those areas is thin and the wrinkles are very small, so injecting those areas frequently leads to visible beading or lumpiness no matter how much care is taken with the injections. Crow's-feet are more commonly treated with Botox.

Fillers are best used when you want only a small number of wrinkles or depressions filled; filling in a lot of wrinkles is cost prohibitive. Some type of peel (see the section "Peeling and Resurfacing Solutions," later in the chapter) or facelift (see Chapter 9) is a better solution in that case.

The results of fillers are visible immediately — just look in the mirror. You'll have some swelling in the immediate postinjection period. If you're unhappy with the results, you should return to the doctor in one to two weeks. If you leave the office and see or feel a lump in or under the skin, apply very firm pressure and attempt to smooth it out. These products can be molded with pressure. The biggest risk is that your filler has not been injected evenly on both sides. If that's the case, a return visit and some reinjection will be necessary. Virtually all injection swelling should be gone in a day or two.

When injecting fillers under the skin, a doctor can accidentally hit a small blood vessel. This problem is unusual and, if it occurs, clears up by itself in five to seven days. If dermal fillers are injected too close to the skin surface, the filler material may get into small blood vessels stopping circulation to a small area. A small area of skin can slough (die). This is very uncommon.

Trying temporary dermal fillers

As you search for products to plump up, fill in, or smooth out facial wrinkles, you'll want to consider the cost and how long the results will last. A less expensive product that gives short-term results may seem to be affordable, but when you consider the "lifetime" cost, it may actually be more expensive. However, temporary dermal fillers are a great way to give yourself a trial run to be sure that you like the results before moving to a more permanent solution. These products last up to six months, so if you don't like what you see in the mirror, you'll be back to your old self in no time. Because these fillers are temporary, they may be administered by a nurse, dermatologist, facial plastic surgeon, or plastic surgeon.

Many potential skin filler patients confuse Botox and skin fillers, discussing them as if they were the same. Botox paralyzes muscles that make wrinkles, and skin fillers actually fill up wrinkles or depressions — totally different ways of ending up in similar places.

Collagen

Collagen has been the cornerstone of facial fillers for many years. It's a good product that has made many people happy. The use of collagen products has diminished significantly, however, since the arrival of newer and somewhat longer-lasting products, such as Restylane.

Collagen is inexpensive and very convenient to use. It doesn't generally require local anesthesia for injection unless it's being placed as a filler in the lips (it actually contains some *lidocaine* — a local anesthetic). The biggest shortcoming of collagen is its short period of effectiveness. Clinical experience shows that the results last between one and six months. Unfortunately, results all too commonly last only one to three months.

Collagen is derived from bovine (brand names Zyderm and Zyplast) or human (brands Cosmoderm and Cosmoplast) dermal tissue. When using bovine-derived collagen, your doctor needs to perform a small skin test one month before injection to test for possible allergies. One or two patients per 100 may be allergic to bovine collagen. Cosmoderm and Cosmoplast don't require skin testing. These products are slightly more expensive than Zyderm or Zyplast but unfortunately don't seem to last any longer.

Approximately 50 percent of the volume of collagen injected into the skin is absorbed overnight, leaving the other 50 percent to act as the filler. Thus, the surgeon or nurse will *overfill* wrinkles or hollows when using collagen.

Hyaluronic acid

Hyaluronic acid is a natural complex sugar substance that comes as a clear gel that tends to attract water. This tendency helps maintain its volume over time within the skin. Hyaluronic acid is relatively inexpensive and will last from three to six months (sometimes longer) depending on the site of injection.

Hyaluronic acid injections are more painful than injections of collagen products, and local anesthesia is frequently used before injection, especially if hyaluronic acid is being used to augment lips.

Two products currently on the market — Restylane (see Figure 8-4) and Hylaform — use hyaluronic acid as the filler material. Each has received FDA approval for the treatment of smile lines but is being used for other facial wrinkles as well.

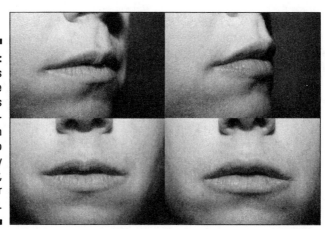

Figure 8-4:
Restylane is one of the many fillers on the market that can be used to temporarily create fuller, smoother lips.

Trying semipermanent solutions

If you're seeking a longer-lasting effect, then you can move up to the products that produce results for 6 to 18 months. If you're one of the lucky ones, you may even experience positive results for two years or longer.

Poly-L-lactic acid

Poly-L-lactic acid, which has the brand name Sculptra, is a recently released product that has been used in Europe (sold there as New-Fill) for several years and was recently approved by the FDA for use in the United States. This product contains microspheres (small particles) of poly-L-lactic acid, a synthetic polymer that has been used for years in absorbable sutures.

The FDA approved Sculptra for use in depressions in cheeks caused by loss of fatty tissue in patients with AIDS but is being used off label as a cosmetic dermal filler. Early clinical experience appears to show that Sculptra lasts approximately six to twelve months when used as a dermal filler.

Sculptra costs more than collagen or Restylane. It's relatively easy to inject but may require multiple injection sessions spaced several weeks apart. The main advantage of Sculptra is that it seems to last up to one year or more in certain people. Patients don't need a skin test before injection.

Calcium hydroxyapatite

Radiesse (formerly Radiance) is a synthetic implant composed of smooth bone-like microspheres suspended in a watery gel. These consistently shaped and sized particles have proven safe and are well tolerated in the body. Radiesse costs two to three times more than Restylane. It doesn't require any local anesthesia unless it's being injected into the lips. Its main advantage is that it can last one to two years depending on the person. Radiesse has FDA approval for use as filler for vocal cord defects. It has not been approved as a cosmetic skin filler to treat wrinkles.

Radiesse's main disadvantage is that it's white and, when injected too superficially, can be visible through the skin and mucosa (the lining of the inner surface of the lip). When put in the lips, it tends to dislocate and clump. I don't recommend injecting this into the lips, and I use it only cautiously in the rest of the face.

Harvesting your body's own fat farm

Autologous fat is fat that has been harvested from your own body. This procedure costs more than using collagen or Restylane because the fat has to be removed from your body (a small liposuction procedure) and prepared for injection. This step requires a local anesthetic and, in some cases, additional sedation or even general anesthesia. After the fat is harvested (usually from those areas where you think you can spare it — the abdomen, hips, or thighs), doctors can inject the fat into all parts of the face. Usually, at least local anesthesia is required for injection.

One disadvantage of this procedure is that your body reabsorbs a lot of the fat. In order for fat transfer to be permanent, the injected fat has to develop blood vessel connections. This does occur some of the time to some of the fat, but when it doesn't, the fat dies and is absorbed by the body. As a result, autologous fat falls somewhere between the categories of semipermanent and permanent solutions. This procedure works well for filling larger defects or hollows (in which case some of the injected fat probably will become permanent) but not so well for filling small wrinkles.

Studies and physicians have varying opinions about how long autologous fat that has been harvested from your body can be stored for future injections. Three months is the general rule.

Taking the plunge: Investing in a permanent solution

Judging from experience with over 250,000 patients treated in Canada and Europe, Artecoll is the only dermal filler that appears to be permanent. Although Artecoll isn't available in the United States, a second-generation product, Artefill, has preliminary FDA approval and is expected to be released in the United States in mid-2005.

Artefill consists of microscopic beads made from a synthetic polymer and suspended in ultrapurified U.S. bovine collagen. The beads in Artefill are slightly smaller and more highly polished than the beads in Artecoll. The permanent microspheres stimulate your body to produce its own collagen to encapsulate each microsphere individually. The end result is that approximately 80 percent of the permanent filler volume is made up of your own collagen. Side effects have been reported to be extremely low (1 in 10,000 patients), but can result in a delayed reaction that causes a lump at the site of injection. If the lump is permanent, it can be treated with steroid injections or it can be excised.

The cost of Artefill is uncertain at this point, but it'll probably be slightly more expensive than collagen and hyaluronic acid. If not injected properly, Artefill may have some tendency to forms lumps in the lips. If you get good results from collagen or hyaluronic acid injections, however, Artefill may turn out to be the permanent solution everyone has been waiting for.

Because this product is permanent, I recommend that only a plastic surgeon, facial plastic surgeon, or dermatologist inject Artefill.

Peeling and Resurfacing Solutions

Facial peels and resurfacing procedures are performed to make the surface of the skin look smoother, younger, more evenly pigmented, and somewhat tighter. These can be excellent procedures for younger patients with reasonably tight skin who have surface scarring or pigment problems. Chemical or laser peels also remove precancerous lesions and some very superficial cancers, so these procedures have some medical benefit in addition to the cosmetic benefit. Various lasers are available to treat isolated dark (hyperpigmented) spots, but if the overall quality of your skin is damaged, a total facial peel may be much better.

A good general rule is that the level of correction is related to the level or depth of skin damage (from sun, smoking, acne, and so on). The greater the skin damage, the more extensive the correction (and the injury to your skin). In turn, the deeper the injury, the longer the healing time. A lunchtime peel gives you a fresher look (and quick recovery) but not much correction. A series of these lighter peels can be beneficial, however, when done in conjunction with a therapeutic cream.

No matter what method of resurfacing you chose, you must protect and take care of your skin following that treatment.

Using a chemical approach to better skin

A chemical peel is a water-based solution of chemicals that's painted on the face, and it works by killing a layer or more of tissue that gradually peels off. How deep the peel goes depends upon a number of factors such as which chemical is used, the concentration used, how long it's left on the skin, and whether it's covered after being applied. Lighter peels damage the surface to a shallower depth and heal within one to five days. In deeper peels, the skin surface heals in seven to fourteen days.

The risk of peeling deep enough to get a perfect result is that you might end up with some superficial scarring. I judge the depth of the peel (as it is being performed) by certain changes I see in the skin. Facial skin isn't of uniform thickness, so the depth of the peel has to be adjusted in different areas to prevent scarring.

Alpha hydroxy acid

Alpha hydroxy acid peels, which use products such as lactic, glycolic, and fruit acid, give you smoother and more radiant skin. They don't require any local anesthesia, and you can return to your normal daily activities immediately following the peel.

When done in a series and used in combination with Retin-A, vitamin C, and hydroquinone, these peels can help improve the surface of your skin. Very few risks are associated with this type of peel. However, you can't expect these very light peels to solve major skin surface problems, such as deep surface wrinkles or severe pigment changes.

Saying goodbye to Pippi Longstocking

A freckle-face ever since she can remember, Melissa despised her "sun kisses" (as her relatives lovingly referred to them) and tried everything she could to cover them up. "I bought bleach creams, heavy costume makeup, and anything new on the market that promised clean, flawless skin." Hours spent at the beach trying to get the rest of her skin to match her freckles only seemed to make things worse. "I can't even begin to add up all the money I spent on dark self-tanners in the hopes of turning myself into one big freckle."

Melissa had come to terms with the fact that she would have freckles all of her adult life until she found out that a TCA chemical peel could improve pigmentation. "I didn't think twice about having the procedure done. If there was any chance of my getting a 'clean palette,' I was ready to go."

"For me, the process was rather simple and completely painless. The worst part was trying not to pick my peeling skin to help things along. As I watched all the sun damage come to the surface and peel away, I saw my first glimpse of perfectly smooth, pink, new skin underneath . . . with no freckles in sight!

"I'm now one of those people who can go without makeup whenever I want to. I can honestly say it's changed the way I look at myself and boosted my self-confidence — and it's cut my getting-ready time in half!"

And does she still bask in the sun? "I feel I've been given a second chance to take care of my skin, so I'm very good about putting on SPF every day. I still go to the beach, but I'm much more careful than I was before and aware of what the sun can do to people with fair skin like mine."

Jessner's peel

Jessner's solution is made up of lactic acid (an alpha hydroxy acid), salicylic acid (a beta hydroxy acid), and resorcinol. This solution, for light to medium depth peels, can be used to lighten areas that have dark pigment and to treat sun-damaged skin. The solution can be used on the face, neck, and chest but should be used with some caution when peeling skin off the face. You will peel and flake for about a week and then the new skin surface will appear. You can undergo a second peel in about four weeks if further improvement is desired. As with all skin peels, you should protect your skin after the peel with sunscreens and clothing when possible.

Trichloracetic acid

Trichloracetic acid (TCA) peels are the next most aggressive level of peels. The primary benefit is a more uniform color to your skin. Check out the results in Figure 8-5. In addition, you should notice some reduction in fine lines and wrinkles, as well as some restoration of skin elasticity. This peel also removes some precancerous lesions.

Your doctor can perform TCA peels with or without anesthesia. If the concentration of the acid is over 15 percent (TCA peel solutions are available for clinical use in concentrations from 5 percent to 40 percent), I recommend sedation and local anesthesia with monitoring of your vital signs. Your doctor probably will prescribe antibiotic and antiviral medications that you'll start the day before the peel and continue until you're healed.

Your skin will need from three to ten days to completely peel, depending upon the depth of the peel. Most often these peels are done as medium to deep peels, so peeling will not be complete for seven to ten days. After the peel, you'll have very little discomfort. Here are a couple tips on how to care for your skin after the peel:

- ✔ Do not assist in the peeling process by pulling off the loose flakes or sheets of skin.
- ✔ Use mild washes and a moisturizer.

After your skin is completely peeled, it will appear slightly red or pink, and you'll be able to apply makeup. Your risks depend to a large extent upon your skin type. The darker the skin, the greater the immediate risk of postinflammatory hyperpigmentation (dark blotches). You can decrease this risk by starting on a prepeel regimen or using an aggressive postpeel regimen, which starts the day you're healed. A pretreatment regimen that includes glycolic acid, hydroquinone, and Retin-A helps control your pigment-producing cells before the peel to minimize postpeel hyperpigmentation.

Loss of pigment is unusual after a TCA peel. The possibility of superficial scarring is a risk for any peel but low for this type of peel.

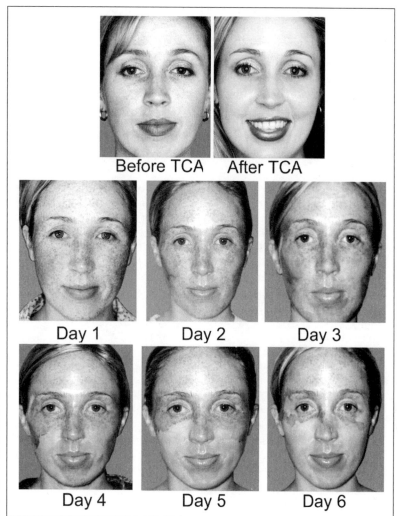

Before TCA   After TCA

Day 1   Day 2   Day 3

Day 4   Day 5   Day 6

Figure 8-5:
This patient
eliminated
years of sun
damage and
removed her
freckles with
a TCA peel.

Croton oil peel

Croton oil peels are the most aggressive of the chemical peels. Croton oil has always been a component of phenol peels, but doctors previously thought that phenol was the most active peeling agent in phenol peels. More recent evidence has shown that croton oil is more effective. Phenol peels worked extremely well in removing wrinkles but took most of the color out of the skin. In addition, they were painful and almost always healed with severe crusting of the skin surface. Croton oil peels can achieve aggressive deep surface changes with less bleaching of the skin than occurred with phenol peels. Most plastic surgeons no longer use phenol peels.

Today you can still get some of the wonderful benefits of phenol peels — without the loss of skin pigment — by having croton oil, or modified phenol, peels. Here are some of the primary benefits you can expect from these peels:

✔ Reduction of both the number and depth of the lines in your skin

✔ Restoration of elasticity

✔ An increase in the tightness of your skin

✔ A more even appearance to irregular pigment blotching

✔ Removal of precancerous and cancerous lesions

This type of peel requires an anesthetic; I recommend local anesthesia with sedation and monitoring of your vital signs. Your doctor probably will prescribe antibiotic and antiviral medications that you'll start the day before the peel and continue until you're healed. Expect healing from this peel to take five to ten days. You'll need to apply a series of moisturizers in the immediate postpeel period, until you're completely healed. Most patients also require some sort of pain medication after the peel. Figure 8-6 shows you an example of the healing process.

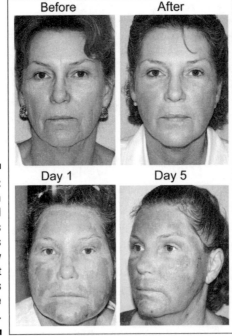

Figure 8-6: The croton oil peel process isn't always a pretty sight, but the results can be incredible.

You should expect to be red to pink for up to six months. Your risk of doing this peel depends to a large part on your skin type. The darker the skin, the greater the immediate risk of developing dark blotches. You can decrease this risk by starting on a pretreatment regimen that includes glycolic acid, hydroquinone, and Retin-A to help control your pigment-producing cells and minimize postpeel hyperpigmentation (dark skin color). Loss of pigment is unusual, and the blotchiness present posttreatment goes away. Superficial scarring is a risk for any peel, but it's uncommon. Antibiotics and antiviral medications will be started before the peel and continued after the peel in order to reduce bacterial and viral infections (herpes simplex, cold sores).

Body peeling

Body peeling is becoming more common, but it has limitations: Deep peels can't be used because the skin of the body isn't as forgiving as that of the face. I use a thin layer of glycolic acid augmented with trichloracetic acid to peel the neck, chest/back, and upper and lower extremities. For the best results, a series of peels is necessary. You can expect reduction in irregular pigment and some decrease in depth of fine lines and wrinkles.

Using a skin resurfacing approach

Skin resurfacing usually refers to a surgical procedure that physically removes layers from the surface of the skin. Rather than killing a layer that gradually peels, this procedure removes the tissue layer at the time of surgery. Laser resurfacing and dermabrasion are the two types of skin resurfacing available. Laser treatment destroys the epithelial surface to an even depth. Dermabrasion mechanically (wire brush or rough wheel) grinds down the surface of skin until the surgeon sees the changes he wants.

Laser resurfacing

Cosmetic surgeons and dermatologists use two types of lasers today for laser resurfacing: the carbon dioxide (CO_2) and the erbium YAG lasers. They have slight differences that are topics of debate among physicians. Many surgeons feel that the CO_2 laser gives more reduction in facial wrinkles, but it usually results in more residual redness following treatment, as well as some increase in potential pigment loss. Figure 8-7 shows you the results of a CO_2 laser treatment.

The erbium YAG laser doesn't give you quite as good a correction of your wrinkles, but you won't have red or pink skin for as long, and your chance of pigment loss is significantly lower. Combination (CO_2 and erbium YAG) lasers that are now on the market have been somewhat successful at combining the benefits of both.

Figure 8-7:
A CO$_2$ laser treatment gave this patient her youthful skin back, along with a second chance to take care of it.

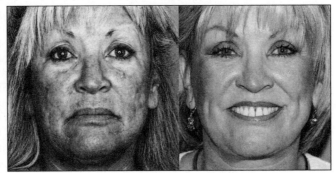

A laser peel can offer the following benefits:

✔ A reduction in the number and depth of the lines of your face

✔ Restoration of elasticity

✔ An increase in the tightness of your skin

✔ Reduction in unwanted pigmentation

Laser peels can be done under general anesthesia or monitored local anesthesia with some sedation. Your doctor probably will prescribe antibiotic and antiviral medications that you'll start the day before the peel and continue until you're healed. You'll be healed from your peel and able to wear makeup seven to ten days after the procedure. Postpeel care involves the application of moisturizers until you've healed. Your doctor also will prescribe pain medication. You can expect your skin surface to be red to pink for several months following laser resurfacing. Redness following dermabrasion is usually gone within a month.

Your greatest risk with a laser peel is temporary hyperpigmentation in the short term and permanent loss of pigment in the long term. This result may not be evident for up to one year. Physicians are especially cautious when doing aggressive peels on dark or olive-skinned individuals, as any potential pigment differences between peeled and nonpeeled normal skin will stand out and can be permanent and difficult to hide. Immediate problems with hyperpigmentation can be decreased by a pretreatment regimen that includes glycolic acid, hydroquinone, and Retin-A; this pretreatment helps control your pigment-producing cells before the peel to minimize postpeel hyperpigmentation.

If you have darker skin and need or want laser resurfacing, try and find a physician with an erbium laser, because the risks of pigment loss are significantly reduced with that type.

PERSONAL STORY

Finishing touches

Although the first thing that prompted Loretta to pursue cosmetic surgery was upper eyelids that touched her lower lashes, she also wanted to do something about the texture of her skin. Although surgical removal of excess skin would certainly give her a more youthful look, she wanted to do the finishing touches that would improve the surface of her skin. After discussions with both her husband and her plastic surgeon, Loretta opted for complete facial rejuvenation: facelift, eyelid lift, neck and brow lift, chin augmentation, and a full face laser resurfacing.

Speaking six months after the procedures, she says that her results continue to improve and she is very happy with the outcome, "Last week I approached a fellow employee who used to work with me. I asked her, 'How are you?' She looked at me for a few minutes and finally said, 'Loretta, I didn't know it was you until I looked at your name badge. I can't believe it's you! You look 15 to 20 years younger. What did you do?' I just smiled and said, 'Thank you!'"

Microdermabrasion

Microdermabrasion is an excellent way of smoothing out surface irregularities with little if any downtime. This process involves gentle abrasion of the skin by a machine that blows fine crystals of aluminum oxide, baking soda salt, or corn cob granules through a handpiece onto the skin surface. The shallowest layer of the epithelium is abraded off. The depth of injury to the skin surface is always very shallow and is controlled by the operator, who is usually an aesthetician or nurse. You may find microdermabrasion an appealing option for the following reasons:

- ✔ It's performed with no sedation or anesthetic.
- ✔ The operator can target certain areas of the face, such as acne scars or crow's-feet, which can be softened over time without the risks associated with other procedures.
- ✔ It has been demonstrated to stimulate new cells and collagen formation.
- ✔ It's appropriate for all skin types.
- ✔ It gives the skin a healthy glow.
- ✔ You can resume normal activities immediately.

Be aware, however, that microdermabrasion requires multiple sessions to achieve the desired result. This method can help fine surface irregularities, but it won't significantly help deeper wrinkles.

Mechanical dermabrasion

Mechanical dermabrasion is most commonly used today to treat deep vertical lip lines and acne scarring on the face. Physicians use rotary wire brushes or rough-surfaced wheels to grind down the surface of the skin. Surgeons and dermatologists usually perform this procedure.

The problem with mechanical dermabrasion is that the deeper the skin is dermabraded, the more likely the possibility of pigment loss and color change (hypopigmentation or hyperpigmentation).

Healing takes approximately one week, and patients have only minor chances of prolonged redness. When used for acne scarring, dermabrasion softens the appearance of acne scars but does very little for the depth of the scars. If you have an isolated area of wrinkle lines (radial lip lines), dermabrasion can give you an excellent result. Dermabrasion is also known to stimulate collagen formation and new surface cells.

Evolving technologies

Newer technical innovations come to the marketplace all the time. Some don't stand the test of time, but others do. The following three technologies show real promise and are important enough for you to consider as you look for ways to improve the quality or tightness of your skin.

Thermage and Titan skin treatment systems

Nonablative skin tightening, being used in both the Thermage and Titan skin treatment systems, is the latest technology to be evolving in cosmetic surgery. The term *nonablative* means that the superficial layer of skin is left intact. These noninvasive methods are purported to promote healthy skin by doing the following:

- Reducing redness in some cases
- Decreasing pore size
- Decreasing laxity
- Improving skin tone

The presumption of this technology is that the deeper tissues can be stimulated to produce more connective tissue without injuring the more superficial layers. Each of these systems provides uniform heating of the deep tissues, which causes contraction of the collagen layer while protecting the superficial layer with intense cooling. The Thermage system uses a radio frequency, and the Titan system uses a laser to heat the dermis, which is believed to make the collagen contract on a permanent or semipermanent basis. The end result is tighter skin.

The advantage of these procedures is that patients have minimal or no downtime associated with the procedure, and skin tightening is a significant part of the treatment benefit. The procedures take between 30 and 90 minutes, depending upon the area being treated.

These procedures have two main disadvantages:

✔ Doctors have no good way to judge the effectiveness of the treatment while it's being done.

✔ A certain percentage of patients will have no visible response at all.

In addition, the patients who respond can expect only a small improvement when comparing the results to standard procedures (such as facelifts).

Those who may be good candidates are patients who shouldn't have surgery, those whose skin is losing its elasticity, and those who have previously had surgery and want to maintain the tightening achieved. Recent interviews with patients who have had Thermage treatments indicate that they had an initial good result that diminished or disappeared after three months. The technology is interesting, and some patients have benefited longer term, but many patients report extreme disappointment.

Intense pulse light (IPL) therapy

Intense pulse light (IPL) therapy has proven effective at treating a number of skin irregularities. Unlike a laser, which has a single wavelength of light, an IPL delivers a multitude of wavelengths simultaneously through a treatment tip that is gradually applied across the area being treated on the face, neck, or chest. Either small areas or the entire surface may be treated. Generally, several (three to six) treatment sessions are required and are performed at one to four week intervals. IPL does the following:

✔ Reduces diffuse redness

✔ Improves the appearance of freckles, age spots, spider veins, birthmarks and other discolorations

✔ Causes gentle heating of the dermis for collagen regeneration

✔ Decreases pore size

✔ Can remove unwanted hair

✔ Improves skin tone and texture

Fraxel laser

A new laser potentially combines the best of both worlds — a safe, no-downtime procedure that is effective in rejuvenating the skin surface. A very small laser spot (so small that it cannot be seen without magnification) is moved randomly across the skin surface by a computer in the treatment tip that contacts the facial skin.

In one treatment session, only about 20 percent of the skin surface area is treated, and generally this causes only temporary redness for a few days. Multiple treatment sessions are needed and usually performed at weekly intervals. Although the Fraxel laser is new technology, it appears to be very promising for the treatment of uneven red or brown pigment, rough texture, and fine wrinkle lines as well as tissue laxity.

Combining Facial Treatment Options

You're more likely to get the best result in nonsurgical facial treatment if you have several different procedures. Combining different treatments isn't dangerous and can in fact provide additive benefits. Each procedure complements the other, and you usually have little associated downtime unless you're having a full face peel. Here are some possible combinations:

- **Combining Botox with dermal fillers:** Two of the most common procedures that I combine in my practice are the use of Botox and dermal fillers. Botox can't completely remove an established line or crease, and a filler is temporary at best at improving the crease. But by combining these two procedures, you can have an immediate improvement in contour and make the filler last longer because it's muscle action that helps cause breakdown of the filler.

- **Combining Botox and skin peels:** Lines that occur near your eyes, known as crow's-feet, can be minimized with Botox. These lines can also be reduced with the use of chemical or laser peels, either as an isolated peel or in conjunction with a full face peel. The peel decreases the visibility of the lines, and Botox keeps them from returning.

- **Combining fillers with other procedures:** Cosmetic surgeons frequently inject dermal fillers into frown lines or nasolabial folds after they have completed a facelift. The only requirement is that you and your surgeon have a preoperative understanding about what your goals really are.

- **Combining skin peels and surgery:** Skin peels are often combined with surgical rejuvenation of the face. After the gravitational aging has been addressed with a facelift, eyelid lift, or brow lift, a customized peel helps improve the quality of the skin and "polishes" the result of the surgery. It's usually performed a few days later after normal healing is assured.

- **Designer combinations:** You may be able to combine these treatments in some other way. All of them complement each other to some degree, improving some aspect of the skin's appearance and of the aging face. Discuss the possibilities with your surgeon.

If you wish to combine different kinds of skin treatments, you need to discuss timing with your doctor so that you can achieve the maximum improvement that your skin and the various treatments will allow.

Identifying Pre- and Posttreatment Considerations

Knowing what to expect *after* your skin has been treated is just as important as knowing what to do and expect prior to treatment. You get the best possible result when you're fully informed and prepared for what lies ahead.

Finding the best doctor for the job

Experience is the number one attribute a physician should have when doing any of the procedures explained in this chapter. The more experience a physician has with a procedure, the more predictable the result will be. For best results, consider the following tips when shopping for your surgeon:

- ✔ Stick to the three types of specialists trained for these procedures — plastic surgeons, facial plastic surgeons, and dermatologists. Not all these physicians will have interest in or experience with all the treatment options in this chapter. In general, plastic surgeons and facial plastic surgeons have great experience with CO_2 and erbium lasers and dermabrasion for wrinkle removal; cosmetic dermatologists usually have a wider range of lasers available for treating all the other skin problems.

- ✔ Seek out a physician who has all the different tools on hand to give you the approach most appropriate for you. There are usually several different ways to treat a single skin issue, some being more aggressive than others, and you want a physician who adapts his treatment to your particular skin type and problem.

- ✔ Look for a medical setting where a physician can provide local anesthesia if you need it. Chapter 3 tells you more about anesthesia.

- ✔ Make certain that your doctor is board certified in plastic surgery, facial plastic surgery, or dermatology.

- ✔ Hold out for someone who has experience. Ask the doctor how often he performs the procedure you're considering.

- ✔ Ask about the technology and why the doctor recommends particular procedures. You want to avoid treatment based on old technology that has been superceded by newer, better equipment. On the other hand, you don't want the latest and greatest if it hasn't shown its worth in real practice.

Considering age and health

Your health is more important than your age when considering cosmetic procedures. The benefit of nonsurgical procedures is that you have minimal downtime and minimal risk. You can have all the procedures in this chapter with no anesthesia or local anesthesia with some sedation.

A standard battery of blood tests and EKG (heart tracing) is done when you undergo any sedation procedure. Your doctor also will take a standard medical history and do a physical exam. Your doctor will perform additional blood tests if any factors in your history or physical make them necessary.

Taking a test drive

Software programs are available to simulate peel results, but I don't feel that the simulated results are very informative. In addition, predicting the absolute response of your skin to different peeling solutions is difficult. The best way to reassure yourself that the procedure you're considering will work is to see or talk to other patients. Ask the physician or his office staff to arrange a meeting or phone call.

Avoiding the magic wand syndrome

All cosmetic procedures, including nonsurgical ones, have trade-offs and limitations. As a consumer, you must have realistic expectations and understand the limitations of the procedures you're considering. You and your doctor need to assess the risk of potential scarring, loss of pigmentation, temporary hyperpigmentation, prolonged redness, and immediate or prolonged downtime after the procedure before proceeding.

Not all the effects of skin aging can be reversed or eliminated. If you have deep-seated pigment irregularities, you may need a series of peels or several different peels to give you the most reduction in pigment possible. Some of the pigment irregularities may still exist after all these procedures. Deep creases in the skin may be significantly reduced but can never be totally eliminated. Are you willing to wear makeup for months after a skin peel in order to significantly reduce the visibility of posttreatment redness or pinkness? Nonablative therapies such as Thermage have shown results in many patients (though the results may be short-lived), but ten percent of patients get no improvement at all. Are you willing to take the risk?

All the procedures I discuss in this chapter work equally well in men and women. I do have a word of caution for men undergoing a deep skin peel: Men don't commonly wear makeup, so the redness that results from the peel will be visible without makeup for a period of time.

Getting ready for — and recovering from — skin peels

Preparation for a skin peel depends mainly on the type of skin you have and will ultimately be decided by your doctor. I don't feel that fair-skinned people need to be treated before peeling. If you have skin of color, however, then you're at increased risk of developing dark spots following your peel. In this case, a pretreatment regimen including glycolic acid, hydroquinone, and Retin-A (retinoic acid) is frequently suggested to help minimize the possibility of post-operative hyperpigmentation, make your peel more uniform, and decrease your downtime. As a general rule, you should follow the pretreatment regimen for three to four weeks.

After your treatment, most surgeons will give you prescriptions for antiviral medications and antibiotics. I prefer the use of the antiviral drug Valtrex because you can take it once or twice a day. Physicians vary from practice to practice on what topical creams and ointments they prescribe to reduce pain and inflammation. Your physician will determine your specific postpeel regimen.

Here's what you should know about your recovery from a peel:

✔ You need to be prepared for your appearance more than anything else. You'll look worse than you feel, but your appearance will improve very rapidly in the first week after your procedure.

✔ You'll swell to some degree, but swelling will diminish fairly rapidly in the first few days. Having some one around to help with activities such as dressing changes and meal preparations is a good idea.

✔ Any discomfort you experience will be short-lived but can be significant for the first few days.

✔ You'll see your physician either daily or every other day for the first week to have your wound assessed.

✔ You'll probably want transportation to the office for the first few visits. You may be very swollen, and discomfort may interfere with driving ability.

✔ Peels can be uncomfortable for a few days, and the peeled area may look unsightly. Some patients want to hide the peeled area.

Getting through the pain

In general, anyone who undergoes a TCA peel will have a relatively painless posttreatment course. The injured skin stays on the wound and acts as a dressing. This skin doesn't peel off until the underlying skin is healed. Your skin will feel tight and you will feel like you can't apply enough moisturizer. Pain, however, isn't the major symptom.

Laser peels and croton oil peels are deeper than most other peels, and for a few days, you'll experience discomfort from the open wound created by the peel. You'll receive pain medication and detailed dressing instructions to follow until you're healed. I prefer the use of topical anesthetics in the immediate posttreatment period to help alleviate the discomfort. You'll also start taking an anti-inflammatory medication before the peel and continue it until you've healed. If pain becomes intolerable, call your doctor's office.

Taking it easy

After a skin peel, you need to stop all vigorous physical activity. If you're taking any pain medication, you won't be able to drive because the medication may slow your reaction time or make you drowsy. You'll be swollen as well, so if you have trouble opening your eyes, you shouldn't drive. In addition, you should avoid any activity or environment that causes you to sweat because sweating will make your ointment or cream runny and more likely to get into your eyes, causing irritation and blurriness.

Laying low or hiding out

Moderate and deep skin peels do have associated downtimes. You'll want to hide out for seven to ten days, depending on the depth of the peel, because you'll have excessive peeling during this time or the need to apply heavy coats of petroleum jelly to keep the wound moist. After your wound has completely *epithelialized* (grown new skin), you can apply coverup makeup and resume normal life activities.

Knowing what's normal

Deep skin peels, either with the laser or chemicals, require more labor-intensive care than other peels in the first few days (see the section "Croton oil peel," earlier in the chapter). You'll experience irregular healing based upon skin thickness, and the wound won't look good to you. You'll need reassurance from your surgeon that your appearance is normal. Somewhere between two and seven days, you'll probably wonder if it was all worth it. Be reassured, however, that you're experiencing normal healing.

Judging the result

Deep skin peels, either laser or chemical, take several months to heal. Redness means that your skin is still inflamed and still generating collagen. The final result won't be evident until the redness is gone. The timing of a second peel, if you need one, is up to your doctor. At a minimum, you have to wait until you're completely healed from the previous procedure, which in most cases takes several months. I don't even consider doing a second peel for six to nine months.

Taking better care of your skin

The nicest thing about skin care is that it's something positive that you can do daily no matter what surgical procedures or noninvasive treatments you're considering or have had. If you're going to invest in your face, an accompanying skin care program makes a lot of sense and can definitely further improve or help you maintain your results for a longer period of time.

A skin care specialist can tailor a skin care program specifically for your needs. I recommend that you seek the advice of a skin care specialist who works in conjunction with a physician because more products are available to you through a physician's office, and you can be more certain of the therapeutic benefit of those products.

In my practice I suggest that patients use a combination of products that include glycolic acid, hydroquinone, vitamin C, and the cyclical use of retinoic acid, which I discuss later in this section. I recommend using Retin-A for a three-month cycle, preferably in the cooler months when the sun is not an issue. After patients complete a course of Retin-A, I switch them to a vitamin C–based system. Correction of your skin doesn't happen overnight, so you need to be on a program that you can comply with over a period of time. Eventually, you'll notice that your skin is getting better. Pore size will decrease, irregular areas of pigment will fade, fine lines and wrinkles will lessen, and you'll no longer feel like you always need to apply moisturizers.

Most over-the-counter cosmetics that you can buy in a department store contain low levels of the active ingredients that are known to work. These products cover up age-related changes in the skin while providing very little if any correction. Therapeutic creams (which can only be prescribed by a physician) not only make your skin feel and look better, but they also can reverse some of the sun-related changes in your skin. Therapeutic creams generally have higher percentages or levels of the "active" ingredient. Many therapeutic skin care products actually help make the surface of the skin look younger to the eye and under the microscope.

New products enter the market almost daily. The research behind some of these products is limited and in some cases amounts only to the experience of the person who formulated the product. You probably won't hurt yourself, but you do risk getting ripped off if you invest in these untested products.

The following products have stood the test of time and have been found beneficial by numerous patients.

- ✔ **Alpha hydroxy acids** work by breaking the bond between epidermal cells. After the bond is broken, the superficial layer is sloughed off, and the cells below this are forced to the surface for replacement. These cells sometimes contain excess pigment so that repeated peeling will tend to lighten the skin and sun spots. Your skin will feel smoother, pore size will decrease, and your skin will appear healthier. Note however, that no skin "correction" or permanent healing has occurred, so your skin goes back to its preexisting state as soon as you stop using the product.

- ✔ **Hydroquinone** is a skin bleach that stops the production of the skin pigment melanin by blocking an enzyme in cells that produce it. When used by itself, hydroquinone lightens the skin only very slowly because the melanin that has already been produced is cleared through cell cycles. The cell cycles in sun-damaged skin take longer to complete, so dark spots may not be cleared for several months.

- ✔ **Glycolic acid** is found in most products that contain hydroquinone. The hydroquinone works to turn off the production of melanin, and the glycolic acid forces quicker turnover of the cells, causing the irregular pigmentation depositions to clear quicker.

- ✔ **Retinoic acid (Retin-A)** stimulates the cells at the basement membrane to begin dividing. This process causes peeling of the superficial layer of skin as the damaged cells are pushed or sloughed off. In addition, it causes an increase in blood flow to the skin. Retin-A is the only product I know of that improves skin surface quality by reprogramming the epidermal cells to divide at normal six-week intervals and to reset the melanoctyes to produce normal amounts of pigment.

Retinoic acid also causes your skin to produce new collagen for a period of time. Because of the increase in blood vessels in your skin, retinoic acid makes you both heat sensitive and sun sensitive. While using Retin-A, protect your skin with sunscreens and appropriate clothing.

- ✔ **Vitamin C** creams and serum contain either vitamin C or the ester of vitamin C. Use a cream that has a vitamin C concentration not less than ten percent. Vitamin C helps block the chemical reactions that cause sun damage. Don't confuse vitamin C with a sunblock, which blocks the sun's rays from hitting your skin. Vitamin C works *after* the fact to neutralize the free radicals that have been caused by sunlight.

Vitamin C stimulates collagen production and restores some of the normal immune function to skin that has been damaged by the sun's ultraviolet rays. Sunscreens should always be applied in addition to vitamin C because vitamin C isn't a sunblocking agent.

Chapter 9

Finding Out about Facial Cosmetic Surgery

*Y*ou're living a longer and more active life than your parents and grand-parents did, so someday you may find yourself looking in the mirror and wondering who that old or tired-looking person looking back at you is. Perhaps you're starting to see your parents in yourself, but you realize that that you don't *feel* like the person you see in the mirror. These are the moments when many people start thinking about cosmetic surgery.

Patients get younger and younger

Many people visiting plastic surgeons today are younger than they used to be. Patients now begin noticing the effects of the aging process and seeking help when they're in their 30s and 40s. They no longer wait until they're in their 50s and 60s. Thirty or more years ago, plastic surgeons turned down patients who wanted procedures on their faces in their late 30s and 40s. They frequently told their patients to come back in 10 to 15 years. Now, younger people know what they want, and many more plastic surgeons are willing to help. I think that virtually all plastic surgeons (and others doing facial surgery) feel that younger patients have the right to look better if they wish. An advantage to operating on younger patients is that they look younger and better after healing!

In this chapter, I discuss the many surgical alternatives for your face — eyelid lifts, mini facelifts, facelifts, neck lifts, forehead lifts, and more. It can seem like a jungle out there, with everyone offering a patented cure for the aging face, but it doesn't have to be that complicated.

Understanding Facial Aging

Despite the fact that all of us are unique individuals, our faces change in predictable ways as we age. Aging and gravity are powerful forces, and the changes that you're seeing happen to everyone, sooner or later. These changes start at different ages in different people, often determined by genetics, environment, activity, and general health. Most people start seeing the very first changes sometime in their early 40s.

Losing structural support

Your skin sags, your cheeks start to fall, your chin droops, the skin under your neck stretches. What's happening? You're losing structural support. The fine connective tissue framework of your face is loosening and stretching due to gravity and years of changing facial expression. You'll hear descriptions such as "turkey neck" or "jowls" used to refer to these changes.

If you think your face reflects loss of structural support and you don't want to have surgery, then you have to learn to live with whatever is bothering you. Noninvasive facial treatments, such as those described in Chapter 8, do little to solve the problems of loss of structural support.

Losing skin quality

You see lines and wrinkles (called *rhytids* in plastic surgery parlance) where your skin used to be smooth. The surface of the skin looks older, and you may notice discolorations and blotchiness. What you see is damage done by aging, which decreases the elasticity in your skin. Exposure to the sun accelerates aging, and if you were or are a smoker you probably have additional wrinkles because nicotine damages the skin.

The effects of sun damage and cigarette smoking are often very difficult to treat with total satisfaction. Surgery helps the skin surface to some degree by stretching it. I discuss tightening your aging skin with facial surgery in the sections under the "Putting On a Happy Face: Getting a Lift" section, later in this chapter.

More and more men get into the act

Approximately 20 percent of all facelifts are performed on men. In a recent week, however, I did three male facelifts in a row, so either the trend or my practice is changing.

Cosmetic facial procedures for men work just as well as for women. Many surgeons use a slightly different incision for men because they usually can't cover the incision lines with long hair.

Quite commonly, a couple has some type of facial surgery in tandem and go through the healing process together.

If the damage is minor, non-surgical techniques such as microdermabrasion, photofacials, and superficial chemical peels can sometimes correct it. Nurses and aestheticians — not surgeons — usually perform these procedures. Surgeons perform resurfacing procedures designed to tighten the skin, including laser peels, deeper chemical peels, and dermabrasion.

Dealing with the effects of dynamic aging

Many muscles in the face have an attachment into the skin. These muscle attachments make it possible for people to have many different facial expressions. These expressions, repeated many thousands of times, eventually cause permanent wrinkles in the skin. A good example is the wrinkles between the eyes known as frown lines. When you frown, you create a temporary fold or wrinkle. Over the years, the temporary folds become permanent.

These permanent wrinkles can be improved with botulism toxin (Botox) or with one of the injectable skin fillers described in the section "Checking out injectables," later in this chapter. The surgical solution, a brow lift, is a skin-tightening operation that reduces the activity of the corrugator muscles, which are the culprits behind frown lines, by partially excising them. The corrugator muscles can also be partially excised through eyelid or eyebrow incisions.

Losing facial volume

Another change that you may see as you age is the loss of fat and volume around your lips and cheeks and the areas around your eyes. The loss of fat and muscle leads to a hollow or sunken appearance that is often associated with aging or ill health.

The solutions to muscle and fat loss are twofold — surgical and noninvasive. I discuss the surgical options, fat grafting and facelift procedures, in the section "Correcting Lost Facial Volume," later in this chapter, and the noninvasive solutions, facial peels, in Chapter 8.

The Eyes Have It: Procedures for Your Brows and Lids

If the eyes really are the windows to the soul, you may be wondering why yours look so much older than you feel. What makes your eyelids look tired or old is excess skin, bulging fat deposits, or a combination of both.

The eyelids are very complex structures that provide coverage and protection to the eye itself. One set of muscles closes the lids, and another raises the upper lids. The tear ducts are in both the upper and lower lids.

Normal-appearing lids contain fat that doesn't bulge. As people get older, however, the fat appears to grow and bulges outwardly, causing so-called fat pockets. In the lower lids, the bulges cause shadows when the light is overhead. You may think that your lower eyelid skin has turned dark when, in fact, what you're seeing are those shadows. Look in the mirror and pull your lower lid skin gently to the side. See if the discolored skin doesn't disappear. Excess fat in the upper lids also is usually visible as a bulge, but fat in that area doesn't cast a shadow. Figure 9-1 shows you the procedure for an upper and lower eyelid lift.

Lifting your upper eyelids

With advancing age — and sometimes for congenital reasons when you're young (25 to 35) — you may develop redundant skin and excess fat in the upper eyelids, creating a tired look and a heavy feel to the lids. As a result, you may find it harder to keep your lids open as the day progresses. You may even find yourself straining your brow upward to keep the upper eyelids off your eyelashes. And if you wear eye makeup, you know how annoying it is when it smears and smudges right after you apply it.

An upper eyelid lift, known as an upper lid *blepharoplasty,* is the surgical solution to these issues. The surgeon marks the excess skin to be removed above the fold in your upper lid. The shape of the excision is a semiellipse. The scar will be in the normal lid fold but will extend, in most cases, to the side of the lid for a centimeter or so. See Figure 9-2.

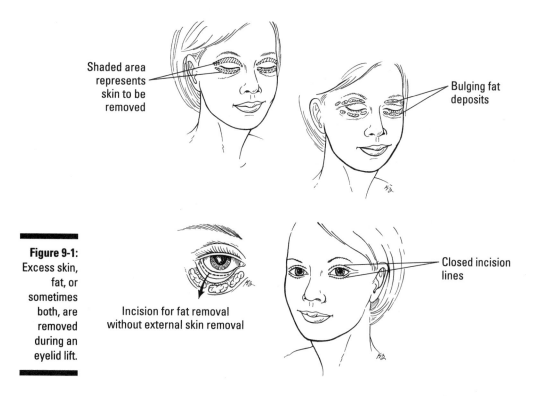

Shaded area represents skin to be removed

Bulging fat deposits

Closed incision lines

Incision for fat removal without external skin removal

Figure 9-1:
Excess skin, fat, or sometimes both, are removed during an eyelid lift.

The surgeon removes the excess skin and underlying muscle, revealing the fat pads. If the fat pads are prominent —which they almost always are in older patients — the surgeon reduces them. After removal of all the extra tissue, the surgeon closes the incision with very tiny sutures. The incision almost always heals with a thin, barely detectable scar.

Figure 9-2:
This woman had her upper and lower eyes done along with laser resurfacing under her eyes and a brow, face, and neck lift.

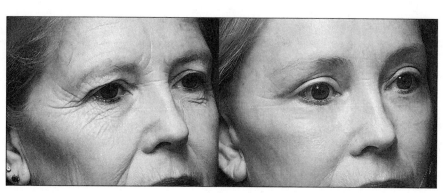

If you're Asian or have Oriental ancestry, the anatomy of your upper eyelid is slightly different from Caucasian lids. You don't have a well-defined upper eyelid crease, but you may decide to have a "western fold" created with a special suture technique. You can have a blepharoplasty just to create a western fold or as you have your lids lifted. If you have extra upper lid skin and don't want a western fold, your blepharoplasty can be done in the standard way.

Not all surgeons are well versed in this operation, which is a little trickier than standard blepharoplasty techniques. Make sure your surgeon discusses the difference between Oriental and Occidental (western) eyelid surgery with you in detail. Ask to see pictures of Asian patients who have had this type of surgery.

Resolving lower eyelid issues

The most common complaint I hear about the lower eyelid is, "Doctor, my friends ask me if I got a good night's rest — even after I've slept perfectly." The puffiness that makes you look sleepy is due to three distinct fat pads sitting under the lower eyelid muscle and bulging outward. Usually this area also has extra skin that is frequently wrinkled.

Surgeons use two different approaches to reduce the fat pads in the lower eyelids, and the method your surgeon uses depends on her own preference.

- ✔ In the traditional approach, an incision is made through the skin and muscle one millimeter below the eyelashes, and the fat pads are then exposed and can be reduced. The excess skin is removed and the incision closed. This incision almost always heals nearly without a trace.

- ✔ In the transconjunctival approach, the fat pads are removed through incisions made on the inside of the eyelid. If you're young and have no extra skin, removal of fat through those incisions may be all you need to make your lower lids look normal. If you also have extra skin, you may need an external excision as well, to trim the excess. The surgeon makes this incision a millimeter or two under the eyelash line.

Some surgeons believe that rearranging the lower eyelid fat pads, rather than removing them, gives a more natural result.

Addressing tiny wrinkles

If your only problem in the eye area is little, fine crisscross wrinkles under the eyelids and you don't have significant bulging and puffiness, you may benefit from lower eyelid skin resurfacing, or tightening the skin without surgical incisions. This can be achieved with a chemical peel, but is more commonly accomplished using laser resurfacing. Turn to Chapter 8 for the full scoop on laser resurfacing and chemical peels.

Occasionally, skin resurfacing is combined with skin excision. This approach can be very helpful when surface eyelid wrinkles are prominent enough that excising the excess skin will not smooth the skin out.

Dealing with drooping brows

If your friends tell you look tired or angry, your problem may be a drooping or sagging forehead (brow). A sagging forehead positions your eyebrows too low and contributes to saggy upper eyelids. A brow lift is the best solution for a drooping brow and that angry look. A brow lift (see Figure 9-3) raises the forehead skin to a more normal position, but also partially removes the muscles that cause frowning (corrugator muscles) so that your ability to frown is reduced.

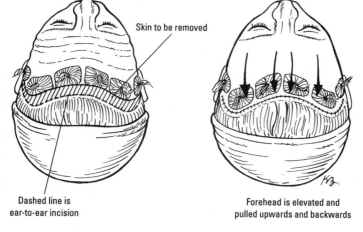

Figure 9-3: Incision lines for a brow lift run from ear to ear.

Skin to be removed

Dashed line is ear-to-ear incision

Forehead is elevated and pulled upwards and backwards

Stand in front of the mirror and lift your entire forehead upward. If moving your skin like this opens your eyes and makes you look more happy and relaxed, you could probably use a brow lift.

Figure 9-4 shows you the results of a brow lift.

The coronal brow lift

The traditional approach to brow lifting is a coronal (or open) brow lift, in which the surgeon makes an incision across your scalp that is hidden within your hairline. Your surgeon then lifts your scalp and forehead tissues and partially removes your corrugator muscle and excess scalp. She then closes the incision and your forehead is repositioned (lifted) into a more normal and younger position.

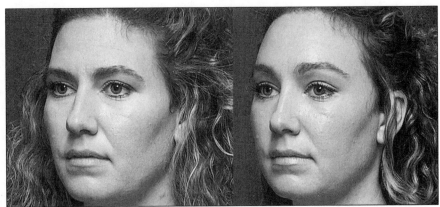

Figure 9-4: A brow lift gave this patient more youthful-appearing upper eyelids and a smoother forehead.

This operation is easy to combine with a facelift because your surgeon joins your facelift and brow incisions within the hairline above your ears. The advantage of a coronal brow lift is that it's completely reliable: The result obtained during surgery is what you will see later. The disadvantages of this technique are that the scar across the scalp is longer than the one you'd get from an endoscopic browlift, and you may have more problems with prolonged numbness of the scalp.

The endoscopic brow lift

A newer technique for forehead lifting involves the use of specialized surgical equipment — a skinny television probe called an *endoscope*. Surgeons need special training to use the endoscopic equipment for this procedure.

With this technique, no scalp tissue is removed in order to lift the forehead, and instead of one continuous incision across the top of your head (coronal brow lift), your surgeon makes multiple — most commonly three to five — incisions within the hairline. Guided by the endoscope, the surgeon separates your forehead and scalp tissue and partially excises the corrugator muscles. The entire scalp is pushed upwards to the desired position and fixed into position with a permanent, dissolvable, or removable device. No tissue is removed (except for the corrugator muscles), but the scalp is repositioned at the desired location. The forehead tissues scar down to the bone in the new elevated position, providing a permanent forehead lift.

Fixing up for the fab 50s

Although Julia says she inherited the family hooded eyelids and sagging "turkey chin," it took her 20 years after she first thought about cosmetic surgery to finally pick up the phone and call. She wanted to look great for her 50th birthday, and after speaking with a girlfriend who had already had a facelift done, she signed up for the procedure with confidence.

Julia said that although the first three days after the surgery weren't much fun, "It was over quickly, and my doctor did such a great job that after four weeks, when I had a family emergency, no one could see the scars or notice anything except that I looked really rested." She doesn't mind looking in the mirror now, and people tell her she looks great. "Just last week, I saw a high school friend that I haven't seen in 20 years, and she said I looked younger than I did 20 years ago and asked if I was ever going to age. I said 'No, not as long as my doctor is still practicing.'"

The advantages of the endoscopic lift are that the scars are shorter and you probably won't have as much numbness as you would from a coronal brow lift. The disadvantages are that the short scars may sit closer to the hairline and end up more visible than the scars from a coronal lift, and the lift may not be as long-lasting or as symmetrical as a coronal brow lift.

If you have a high forehead and don't want your hairline to go even higher, your surgeon may place the central coronal incision in front of the hairline and then run the incision behind the hairline in the area above the ears. You'll have a scar that's visible if you pull your hair back, but your hairline actually will be lower. Many women with high foreheads are used to wearing bangs to hide a look they don't like, and the bangs will hide the scar as well.

Putting On a Happy Face: Getting a Lift

You can choose from among many types of facelifts, and you, along with your plastic surgeon, have to determine which type is right for you.

One of the often unexpected side effects of a facelift is that you may need to make some adjustments to your hairstyle. Making the incisions through which the facelift is performed and then tightening and removing the excess skin can pull back and pull upward the hairline in front of and above your ear. Behind your ear, your normal lower hairline will probably develop a notched or indented appearance because of the excision of your extra neck skin. Your hair stylist can be invaluable in helping you choose a new do.

Standard facelift

The modern standard facelift addresses the changes from aging that occur from the eyes down to the base of the neck. A facelift can correct problems such as sagging cheeks, the deepening fold between the cheek and lip (the *nasolabial fold*), the sagging skin along the jaw line, and the extra skin and fat in the neck. This procedure takes two to four hours and is usually performed under general anesthesia.

The incisions for a standard facelift vary from surgeon to surgeon and from patient to patient. But as a rule, the incision will begin two to four inches above the ear and then curve gently around the front of the ear (usually inside the little cartilage bump you feel in front of the ear canal, the *tragus*), around the earlobe into the crease behind the ear, and into or along the hairline behind the ear. Check it out in Figure 9-5. The surgeon often makes a separate incision in a crease under the chin, through which the muscles are tightened. These scars usually heal beautifully and, if they're placed well, are barely detectable.

Scars take 9 to 18 months to fully mature (become smoother and fade from purplish or pink to whitish skin color). So the way they look at one month after surgery isn't the way they'll eventually mature. Figure 9-6 shows you the process of healing from facial surgery.

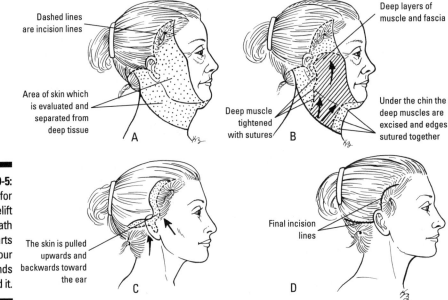

Dashed lines are incision lines

Area of skin which is evaluated and separated from deep tissue

Deep muscle tightened with sutures

A

Deep layers of muscle and fascia

Under the chin the deep muscles are excised and edges sutured together

B

Figure 9-5: Incisions for a facelift follow a path that starts above your ear and ends behind it.

The skin is pulled upwards and backwards toward the ear

C

Final incision lines

D

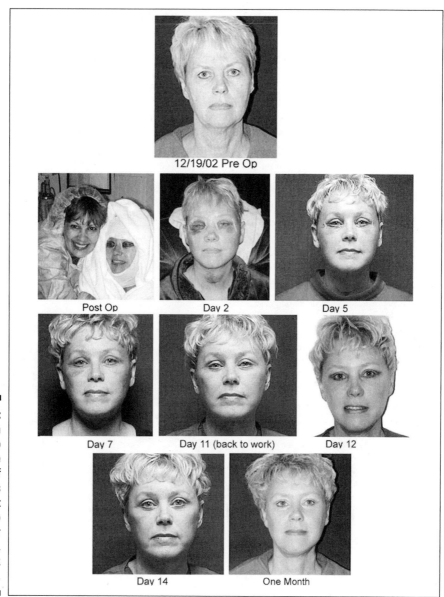

12/19/02 Pre Op

Post Op

Day 2

Day 5

Day 7

Day 11 (back to work)

Day 12

Day 14

One Month

Figure 9-6:
Along with a facelift to combat the signs of aging, this patient decided to have her eyes, brow, and neck lifted.

After making the incisions, your surgeon lifts and separates the skin and fat from the underlying muscles and their covering layer, known as fascia. How much of the skin is lifted varies, but it's lifted enough so the skin, when tightened, will redrape without creases or folds. The skin in the neck will generally be lifted nearly down to the collarbone and across your entire neck. After all the skin dissection is done, most surgeons also tighten the next deeper layer in a procedure known as submusculoaponeurotic system (SMAS). The SMAS makes a facelift last longer than facelifts that lift only the skin and keeps the smooth neck from disappearing as quickly.

The way the SMAS procedure is done is also variable, but in all cases, the muscles of the neck and the connective tissue of the cheek are tightened. Some surgeons also use suspension sutures to anchor tissues they want lifted or repositioned. Next, the excess skin is trimmed and the incisions closed.

Most surgeons leave a little drainage tube under the skin on each side to evacuate the blood and fluid that invariably collect under the skin. This drain is usually removed a day or two after surgery. At the end of surgery, your hair is usually washed, and any residual blood left from surgery is removed. Finally, most surgeons apply a big bulky football helmet–type dressing, and you're ready to go to the recovery unit and wake up. Figure 9-7 shows you the results of a facelift.

Figure 9-7:
Along with a neck lift to give her a more defined jawline, this patient underwent a facelift, brow lift, eyelid lift, rhinoplasty, chin implant, and laser skin resurfacing.

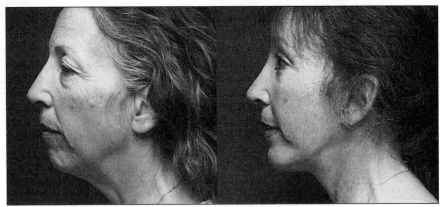

Mini facelift

The definition of a mini facelift isn't set in stone, but generally it means anything less than a standard facelift. It's usually performed in patients who need only a little correction along the jaw line or cheek. Mini facelifts may also be useful if you've had a standard facelift but are now becoming a little saggy and need your skin tightened. Usually the mini facelift involves much less work in the neck than a standard facelift and limited, if any, muscle work. The incisions are also shorter, not going far above the ear and usually not as far behind the ear.

Be aware that this operation gives limited results, so don't expect it to substitute for a standard facelift. Mini facelifts may or may not require drains and usually have a shorter recovery. Be sure you ask your surgeon exactly what she means by a mini facelift and what you can expect in the way of results and duration of results.

In my practice, mini facelifts are an excellent choice for younger patients who don't have bands or cords (folds of skin and underlying muscle that hang from under the chin down toward your clavicles), or severe sagginess in the neck. If the only problems in the face and neck are caused by excess skin (no cords or bands), a mini-lift can be a perfect solution. Figure 9-8 shows you an example of a mini facelift.

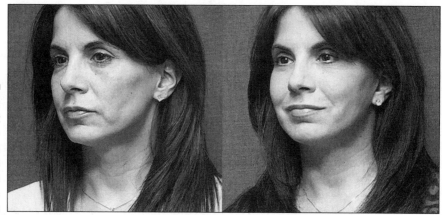

Figure 9-8:
This patient had a mini-lift and is shown here 14 days post-op.

S-lift

The S-lift uses a short S-shaped incision beginning slightly in front of and above the ear, extending down around the earlobe and up behind the ear. Good results can be obtained, but logic suggests that the shorter the scar, the less skin that can be removed. Consider the S-lift to be a variant of the mini-lift. If your surgeon suggests an S-lift, compare the cost to a standard facelift by the same surgeon. If the cost is the same, go elsewhere. On average, a surgeon can perform the S-lift, which includes muscle tightening, in one-third less time than she needs to perform a standard facelift. If you have minor facial and neck skin sagginess, the S-lift may be an ideal procedure.

Midface lift

Midface lifts focus on improving the area from your cheekbone down to your upper lip. You lose the youthful fullness of your cheeks as you age, and that skin and the underlying fat begin to sag down from the lower eyelids. Surgeons frequently perform the midface lift in conjunction with a standard facelift, but it can be done as a stand-alone procedure.

The surgical incisions for a midface lift are either in the temporal hairline or in the lower eyelid skin. All of the soft tissue of the cheek is separated from the cheekbone, at the level of the bone surface. Depending on the surgeon's preference, the lifted tissues are anchored to bone, *periosteum* (the covering of bone), or *fascia* (the covering of muscle).

A secondary benefit if this procedure may be some decrease in the depth of the *nasolabial folds* (the creases extending from the side of the nose toward the corners of the mouth).

If your surgeon suggests this procedure, make sure you ask to see pictures of patients who have had it done and also ask about complications. Although the results from a midface lift can be dramatic, the complications can be quite serious and difficult to correct. These include sagging of the lower eyelids, injury to nerves that supply some of the facial muscles, and prolonged swelling.

Deep plane and subperiosteal facelifts

In the past ten years, surgeons have become more aggressive in searching for different and better surgical methods of performing facelifts. Two methods, deep plane and subperiosteal facelifts, have arisen in response to that movement. The theory behind both operations is that lifting the full thickness of the soft tissues in the face (not just the surface skin, fascia, and muscle) will lead to a more natural-looking result.

The deep plane facelift has largely fallen out of favor because of prolonged swelling after surgery and because of higher risks of nerve injury.

Surgeons who perform these procedures operate in somewhat more dangerous territories. Some of the dissection is performed "blindly" (meaning that the surgeon dissects by feel). An injury to the nerves can cause a partial facial paralysis, which may be either temporary or permanent. Although these nerve injuries are possible with the standard facelift as well, the chance of them occurring is much lower.

Subperiosteal lifts aren't as likely to cause nerve injury as deep plane lifts, but they don't elevate the facial tissues as much. A subperiosteal lift is best suited for a younger patient who has some early sagging along the jawline and upper cheek area. The potential downside is that moving all the layers of tissue up and back can make the face look somewhat less natural.

Before you commit to one of these procedures, ask your surgeon about the possible complications and how common are they are. You also may want to talk to some patients who've had this procedure to find out whether the pain of waiting is worth the benefit of the result.

If your surgeon suggests a deep plane or subperiosteal facelift, find out how many of these procedures she does per year. Some surgeons perform many facelifts and use one of these procedures as their primary technique. I would discourage you from having this procedure performed by anyone who does fewer than 40 or 50 of them per year.

Having a tiny-incision facelift

Many patients want the outcomes of facial surgery without actually having a big operation — they're looking for magical procedures that can remove excess skin without larger or longer incisions. And plenty of nonsurgeons are rushing in to fulfill this fantasy. Remember the adage "If it sounds too good to be true, it probably is!"

Facelifts with tiny incisions are commonly performed by dermatologists with little surgical experience or training. They usually involve microliposuction of excess fat in the neck as well as tightening of the neck muscle through a short incision under the chin. When combined with facial peels, good results can be obtained. If, however, you have a marked excess of neck skin, these less-invasive procedures need to be combined with a neck lift (skin excision and tightening) in order to achieve an optimum result.

Limited surgery means limited results. Frequently, disappointed minimal-surgery patients who got nowhere near the result they expected or were promised end up coming to plastic surgeons for help.

To determine whether these less-invasive procedures are right for you, ask your physician about the traditional facelift procedures and whether she performs those as well and has privileges to perform them at the hospital. Remember that any doctor who tries to sell you on a minimal or limited surgical procedure may be doing so only because she isn't competent or qualified to perform other procedures.

If a physician suggests that you undergo one of these limited alternatives, ask to see pictures of patients who had standard facelifts. If she doesn't have any such pictures, she probably isn't qualified to perform standard facelifts.

Noninvasive facial procedures

Two other types of facial tightening procedures are now available. Thermage (see Chapter 8) helps tighten collagen within the skin. A newer method, developed in Russia, is called the Feather Lift or Aptos Lift. It's a nonsurgical method using barbed sutures placed through the skin of the cheeks that are suspended from the fascia above and in front of your ear to tighten your cheek skin.

The Feather Lift may be useful in correcting cheek sagginess, but it will never replace traditional facelifts. I haven't performed this procedure but have friends who have used it in Canada and Mexico who say it's a good technique for certain patients.

Correcting Lost Facial Volume

If your cheeks have taken on a hollow look and the skin under your eyes is seemingly sinking into your bones, you're experiencing what doctors call a loss of facial volume. A typical side effect of aging, loss of facial volume means that the fat and muscle in your cheeks have atrophied. Plastic surgeons can address this problem by filling the depressions and hollowness with implants, implantables, or injectables. Fat transfer is probably the most commonly used method of augmenting cheeks.

Understanding implants

Implants are usually used to augment or enhance bony structures, such as a weak chin (see Figure 9-9) or flat cheekbones. Cheek implants, chin implants, and even lip implants can be used to help replace tissue lost to the aging process. These implants are made of alloplastic material, meaning that they aren't biological in origin. After the surgeon inserts them, they stay intact and don't get absorbed into the body.

Chin implants are usually inserted through an incision inside the lower lip or under the chin. Cheek implants are placed through an incision under the eyelashes of the lower eyelid or through an incision in the mouth, but they can also be placed through a browlift-type incision.

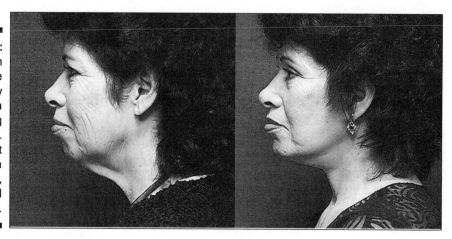

Figure 9-9:
Chin implants are a good way to combat a receding chin line. This patient also had a face, neck, and eyelid lift.

Investigating implantables

Implantables are called implants as well but are softer than cheek or chin implants. These substances are used to fill out soft tissue volume loss, such as in thin lips or in furrows such as the cheek folds.

Usually these implantables are quite soft and can be placed through small incisions and then threaded or pulled to where they're needed. Implantables can be either synthetic and permanent, such as Gore-Tex, or biological, like AlloDerm, which is derived from human skin. The latter often have a softer feel, but unfortunately, they're not permanent.

AlloDerm can be used to augment lips or can be placed under wrinkles or depressions. It's very well tolerated, but it lasts a limited period of time, ranging from several months up to two years or more. AlloDerm is human dermis (the undersurface of skin) that has been harvested from healthy cadavers. All the cellular structures have been removed (so no one is allergic to AlloDerm), leaving only the framework of connective tissue.

The biggest benefit of this product is that it feels extremely natural after it's implanted. The biggest disappointment with the product is that it sometimes largely disappears in six to nine months (although it occasionally lasts for several years).

ePTFE (Gore-Tex) is a synthetic implant that's available in threads or sheets and can be used in ways similar to AlloDerm. Gore-Tex appears to be well tolerated in the body. If you have an infection or tissue reaction, Gore-Tex is relatively easy to remove. In recent years, Gore-Tex has been used most commonly for lip augmentation by providing a more defined lip border.

Combining facial procedures with other surgery

The impact of aging affects all areas of your face: Your brow droops, your eyelids get heavier, your neck sags, and so on. So when you visit a surgeon for a consultation, she'll most likely discuss all possible "problem" areas that she sees but also, more importantly, pay attention to what bothers you. If you have more than one area of concern, addressing all areas in the same operation is a reasonable and logical approach. In fact, cosmetic surgeons typically perform multiple facial procedures simultaneously.

Almost everyone has seen *Extreme Makeover* or one of many similar television programs that show patients having more than one type of surgery. Probably because of such shows, surgeons are getting more and more inquiries about combining facial rejuvenation procedures with other cosmetic surgeries. In many cases, combining, say, a facelift with a tummy tuck or a breast lift is fine, provided you're in good health and have a clear understanding of risks and recovery time.

Checking out injectables

Safe injectable skin fillers, which are used to address loss of volume, have been available for years and include collagen products and, more recently, hyaluronic acid. All these products last a relatively short time, but they work well and have made many patients very happy. Longer-term (one to two years or more) injectables are now also available. Fat (from your own body) has been used as an injectable for many years. For more detailed information about these noninvasive solutions, turn to Chapter 8.

Facing Up to Cosmetic Surgery

More cosmetic facial surgery is being performed at this time than at any time in the past. Part of the reason for this is that the techniques are better and the results are more predictable. In addition, anesthesia has become dramatically safer. There are also more plastic surgeons and a larger population that wishes to look better and younger.

Although facial cosmetic procedures are very reliable, not every patient has a "fantasy" result. Some patients hug their surgeons because the result is so good. Others complain that their jowls aren't quite tight enough. Reality is in the middle somewhere, with most patients showing significant improvement, but not perfection. The results depend on a number of factors, including the quality of the patient's skin, the amount of fat in the face and neck, the age of the patient, the surgeon's skill and the patient's ability to heal.

I believe that every person over the age of 40 or 45 will look better following facial surgery (provided quality surgery is performed and healing falls in the normal range). Does that mean everyone over 40 should rush into the plastic surgeon's office? The answer is obviously a resounding NO!

Understanding cultural issues

One reason for the increase in facial cosmetic surgery is that people's attitudes have been shifting toward acceptance of these procedures. Societal changes now make cosmetic surgery something to brag about rather than an event to hide from friends and neighbors. Reality television shows such as *Extreme Makeover* and *The Swan* are giving even more people "permission" to consider updating or improving their appearances.

In cultures that respect and revere age (such as the Chinese culture), the demand for older people to look younger is probably smaller. The U.S. culture is youth oriented, however, so people who look older may find themselves being excluded or ignored to some degree. Thus, many people feel true cultural pressure to look younger. In many circles, women are almost expected to have a facelift when they start to look saggy. It may be an indictment of our society, but it's reality.

Considering your health

Facial cosmetic surgery is superficial, blood loss is minimal, no body cavities are entered, and you're not confined to bed rest after the surgery is over. Consequently, almost everyone who doesn't have serious health problems can have facial surgery. Even patients who do have some ongoing medical conditions are frequently able to have this surgery.

Don't take chances with your health. If you're older than 45 or 50 and preparing for facial surgery and the surgeon or her staff doesn't really look into your health and fitness, go somewhere else. If, on the other hand, your surgeon and her staff request tests by your cardiologist or clearance from your internist, they have a reason to do so, and the reason is to protect you. Follow their advice.

If you have a health issue but are willing to cooperate with the health screening process, you'll probably be able to have surgery. In my own experience, almost all the patients canceled for health reasons were unwilling to be completely evaluated. When patients were evaluated and the patient, the consulting physician, the anesthesiologist, and the surgeon discussed the problems, probably 95 out of 100 were able to proceed.

Staying in the game

John, a 60-year-old salesman, hired a nationally renowned executive coach to help him take his career to the next level. Surprisingly, he told John to get a facelift! John recalls, "At first, I was shocked. I expected assistance in marketing and presenting my qualifications to senior management, but I didn't anticipate being told that I looked old and tired or how my droopy eyes and sagging neck were hurting my chances to succeed." Important factors playing into his decision were cost and bottom-line return on his investment. The surgeon's staff also was extremely important in his decision: "Their professionalism exceeded my expectations by an order of magnitude. The way they ran their business told me that they were accountable and committed to serving the customer." So John decided to have facial rejuvenation (facelift, necklift, eyelid lift) to help his career advancement.

"Although competing against people without my experience and love of the craft is no problem," John said, "getting the chance to get into the game is tougher when the person doing the hiring sees you as older than you feel and far more tired than you'll ever be. Looking tired, worn out, and unenthusiastic is a death knell to a career in sales! The cosmetic work I underwent aligned my face with the person inside. I have recovered the costs of my cosmetic surgery many times over in opportunities seized and commissions earned!"

Smoking causes particular dangers for facial surgery. Some surgeons will not perform facelifts on smokers because of the extreme healing problems that nicotine can cause. Nicotine decreases the flow of blood through the skin by constricting the small blood vessels in the skin. Nicotine patches and pills have the same effect on the skin as cigarettes.

Factoring age into your decision

One of the most common questions facial plastic surgeons get from patients interested in facial rejuvenation is "Doctor, am I too young/old to have a facelift?" I usually answer that your physiological health matters more than your chronological age. I've known 78-year-old patients in excellent health who sailed through their procedures. I've also seen patients in their 30s whom I've advised to avoid elective surgery because of their multiple serious health problems.

Most plastic surgeons agree, however, that a better, more natural, and longer lasting result is possible if patients are in their 30s, 40s, or 50s because they have better, more elastic skin. I estimate that half of my patients who have cosmetic facial procedures are between the ages of 42 and 52. People on the young side of that range probably don't want a full facelift, but they're frequently excellent candidates for a mini-lift, midface lift, brow lift, blepharoplasty, or some combination.

Finding the right surgeon

With all the baby boomers and others interested in plastic surgery, a whole industry has grown up around this specialized surgical field. You only have to pick up a copy of your local newspaper or upscale suburban magazine or turn on the television or radio to be bombarded by advertisements for plastic surgery clinics, plastic surgeons, facial plastic surgeons, cosmetic dermatologists, ophthalmologists, and others — all vying for the chance to improve your looks.

I give you all the information you need to find the right surgeon and the right clinic in Chapters 4 and 5. As you're looking, keep in mind the following additional guidelines.

Evaluating before-and-after photos

Ask to see pictures of previous patients. Almost all plastic surgeons have albums of before-and-after pictures. Study these photos in detail, but be aware that surgeons are probably showing you their *best* results. When looking at the postoperative pictures, evaluate whether or not you think the people look better and "normal."

Look very carefully at the necks. If you see residual wrinkles or folds under or near the chin, think about going elsewhere. Look also at the earlobes, and if you see a fold of skin that's not smooth or if the earlobe is pulled too low, find another surgeon. Ask about the surgeon's complications as well. If no pictures of complications are available to show you, get a verbal description of what went wrong and why. If the surgeon says she has no complications, get up and leave. She either has no experience or is lying. Most of all, protect yourself, be careful, and make rational, not hopeful, observations.

Taking a test drive

The easiest way to see what a facelift may do for you is to look in the mirror and pull your facial skin slightly upward, but mostly backward. Understand that a facelift will be the equivalent of a light or moderate pull. If you pull enough to distort the corners of your mouth, you're pulling too hard.

Imaging (digital photography and digital manipulation of the photos) of the face can sometimes be performed, but it's clumsy and doesn't really show the potential result as well as pulling your facial skin in front of the mirror.

Considering anesthesia

Sedation with local anesthesia and general anesthesia are the two methods commonly used for facial surgery. Both are equally safe if the same monitoring equipment is used. The main advantage of sedation and local anesthesia is that you have less chance of postoperative nausea. The advantages of general anesthesia are that you feel nothing and there's less movement by the patient during surgery to distract the surgeon. More than 90 percent of facelifts are performed under general anesthesia.

Avoiding the magic wand syndrome

Facial surgery is real surgery. You can expect scars, swelling, bruising, puffy eyelids, discomfort, and small complications that can delay your good result. You need to take a realistic approach and be willing to take a little bad with the good along the healing road.

Be happy with a very good outcome. Perfection is seldom achieved. Most plastic surgeons want you to end up looking like yourself — only better and younger.

Assessing the Risks

Facial cosmetic surgery is generally very safe, and thousands of patients successfully have this surgery every year. Nevertheless, every operation has certain risks associated with it, and facelifts are no exception. Your doctor should discuss these fully with you before surgery so that you don't have any surprises afterward. She should also discuss what to expect during a normal recovery, which includes the following:

- ✔ **Bleeding:** Bleeding is probably the most common risk and complication following a facelift. Bleeding can cause problems that range from excessive bruising, which is really more of a nuisance, to a marked swelling under the skin (hematoma) that may require another operation. Moderate lumps or swelling under the skin caused by a small hematoma can usually be suctioned out with a needle or small cannula (suction tube). Usually, small hematomas have no long-term implications but can delay complete healing and smooth contours for a month or more.

- ✔ **Infection:** Infection is unusual in facial surgery because of the excellent blood supply to the face, but it can happen if you're unlucky or if synthetic implants are placed. If an implant becomes severely infected, the surgeon may have to remove it. If you wish to have it replaced, you'll need to wait for several months. Otherwise, your risk of infection is higher.

- ✔ **Wound healing problems:** Sometimes incisions don't heal as expected, but time usually solves this problem. Prominent scars can develop if a wound heals slowly. The most feared wound healing problem is the death of an area of skin due to poor circulation. This complication occurs more commonly in smokers, but it can occur in nonsmokers as well due to skin tension or poor circulation.

✔ **Nerve damage:** Damage to the branches of the facial nerve, leading to partial facial paralysis, is probably the most distressing complication. Fortunately, this complication is rare, and in most cases, the nerve is merely bruised or stretched and recovers on its own over the course of weeks or months. All experienced plastic surgeons know where the facial nerve branches are located, so they're able to avoid them during surgery.

✔ **Asymmetry:** If you notice after your facelift that one side looks slightly different than the other, the cause is probably local swelling. Another possibility is that your face was slightly asymmetrical before surgery but you weren't aware of it. Occasionally, one side is pulled or tightened differently or pulled more than the other side during surgery. Should this be the case, the looser side can be redraped with a secondary surgery.

Recovering from Facial Surgery

In general, facial surgery heals quickly enough that you should be able to rejoin society within 10 to 20 days, with 14 days being the average time after a facelift. If you have eyelid surgery only, you should be out and about sooner. Some patients go to the store within a day or two, while others don't show their faces for three weeks. Do whatever is comfortable for you.

Getting through the pain

Pain isn't usually an issue after facial surgery. If you hurt, take the pain pills prescribed. Because of swelling and tightness, you won't be able to turn your neck fully. As you heal, your neck will turn more and more easily with time. You probably will feel discomfort, heaviness, and swelling and some numbness in the areas that have been operated on.

Taking it easy

Don't do anything aerobic or strenuous for at least ten days after facial surgery. As far as other activities, let your body tell you what you can do (and not do). When you feel you can drive, drive. You may find that gentle sex is therapeutic. You may eat what you wish, but avoid alcohol for approximately one week because alcohol increases the likelihood of postoperative bleeding.

Knowing what's normal

After surgery, you'll probably have areas of numbness, and your face will feel swollen, tight, and uncomfortable. These are all normal reactions. If you have severe pain, however, something is probably wrong, and you should call your doctor. A low-grade fever is normal for a day or two, but higher fevers aren't normal and should be reported.

Your emotions may ride a roller coaster after surgery. Facial plastic surgery patients typically feel a little depressed a few days after surgery. Your routines have been disrupted, and you're probably isolated from your friends and work, so feeling a little sorry for yourself is understandable. In addition, you're swollen and bruised. Pamper yourself, and these emotions will pass.

Judging the result

Don't judge the results until the swelling is essentially gone (which takes at least two to three months), unless you have some obvious wrinkle or fold that clearly is not disappearing with time. If you chose your surgeon wisely (which I'm sure you did if you followed the information in this book), give her the benefit of the doubt. If she says you'll have a good result, believe her.

Your scars won't look "normal" (meaning that they've faded but may still be somewhat visible) for six months or more. In the interim, they'll be reddish or pinkish. If, after four to six months, you don't like how you look, have a frank talk with your surgeon. If something is wrong and can be fixed, she'll almost certainly do so. For more information on dealing with less-than-satisfactory results, see Chapter 19.

Chapter 10

Winning by a Nose: Rhinoplasty

*R*hinoplasty (also known as a nose job or nasal reshaping) is an operation that changes the external shape of your nose, with the goal of making it more attractive. Of all the many cosmetic procedures that exist, rhinoplasty procedures are probably the most complex, most difficult to understand, and most difficult to master.

I advise against changing your nose on a whim. After your nose has been altered, getting your old nose back is difficult. One of the best surgical results I ever obtained ended up making the patient very unhappy. When her family saw her new nose, they said she no longer looked Greek. She then wanted to reverse her operation, but doing so was essentially impossible.

Understanding the Anatomy of the Nose

For such a small structure, your nose is very complicated. The framework or support of your nose is made up of nasal bones (which are not moveable and which you can feel between your lower eyelids) and of cartilage (which is moveable and makes up the support of the end of your nose). The space inside your nose is divided into two passages by your nasal septum. Your nasal cavities are lined with nasal mucous membrane, except for the areas just inside your nostrils, which are lined with skin. The vertical structure between the two nostrils that attaches your nasal tip to your upper lip is called the *columella*. The attachments of your nostrils on each side to your cheeks are called the *alae*.

If your nasal septum is crooked or deviated because it grew that way, or because you suffered a severe nasal injury with a fracture of your nose and septum, then the outside shape of your nose may be crooked in the same way. A crooked nasal septum can also restrict breathing on one side or both sides of your nose. Sometimes, correcting a crooked nose not only enables you to breathe better but also reduces snoring.

A surgeon changes the shape of your nose by modifying or reducing the size or shape of nasal cartilages and bones. Cartilage may be harvested from your nasal septum, your ear, or a rib if you need extra cartilage to replace or augment an injured or depressed area. Cartilage may be useful in improving the shape of your nasal tip.

In general, the surgeon makes no incisions on the outside of your nose except in the case of open rhinoplasty, which involves an incision on your columella (see the "Open rhinoplasty" section, later in this chapter), or Weir excisions, which narrow your nostril bases (see the "Weir excisions" section, later in this chapter). Wide nasal tips aren't reduced by removing nasal tip skin, nor are noses narrowed by removing skin from the top of your nose. They are narrowed by excising cartilage, placing retention sutures, or both. All the changes in your nasal shape are accomplished by operating inside the nose, with the exception of the open rhinoplasty incision and the possible incisions from Weir excisions.

Sniffing Out Motivations for Rhinoplasty

Exploring the possibilities of rhinoplasty for yourself or someone you care about requires doing your homework. This decision is an important undertaking, so seriously weigh the pros and cons of the actual procedure. Then get really clear on why you'd like to alter your nose.

If you're healthy, you don't like the shape of your nose, and you aren't motivated by a whim, you're probably a good candidate — provided that a qualified nasal surgeon sees the same problem that you do and feels that he can improve it surgically. If you've become obsessed with a minor flaw in your nose, however, don't be surprised if the nasal surgeon declines to operate. You may be seeing something that just isn't visible to anyone else, including a potential surgeon.

Rebuilding confidence

A childhood sports injury initially prompted Terri to have her nose done: "My nose was severely fractured in a softball game when I was 12 years old. A ground ball popped up and struck me right between the eyes, breaking my nose. I had surgery to correct the damage, but was unhappy with the results."

After enduring constant harassment and teasing throughout junior and senior high school, Terri found that her confidence was shot. "I did not think I was pretty and believed that people only saw a girl with a big, deformed nose. Cosmetic surgery was always in the back of my mind, but at the time it was not as common as it is today, and I thought it would be too expensive."

When she turned 30, Terri moved to Southern California, which she describes as "practically the capital of the world when it comes to cosmetic surgery. I began to research the benefits, risks, and costs of having surgery — particularly for rhinoplasty. I wanted to be knowledgeable about the process and procedure in order to make an informed decision. Once I decided to proceed with surgery, I began to search for a reputable doctor." After much research for an experienced physician and many discussions with her family, she decided to have surgery.

She found that the first few days following the procedure were the most difficult, but she was able to return to work about five days after surgery. Of her outcome Terri says, "I can honestly say I am very happy with the results. I did not expect to look like a movie star after surgery; I just wanted to have a normal-looking nose. I especially like looking at my profile — wow, what an incredible difference! I believe my self-image has significantly improved."

Although Terri says her confidence is higher now, she points out that "cosmetic surgery does not solve problems. It is a step toward rebuilding self-esteem and confidence."

You may be envious of a nose you've seen in a film or magazine and want it for yourself. Creating an exact duplicate of a nose from a magazine picture is almost always impossible, but this doesn't mean the surgeon won't be willing to operate. However, most surgeons aren't eager to operate on a patient with unrealistic expectations.

Various physical issues can prompt you to consider cosmetic nasal surgery. Most of them fall into one of three categories:

- **Congenital problems:** If you're like most people wanting a nose job, you probably inherited your problem from your family. Hopefully you also got some good traits as well.

- **Post-traumatic problems:** If you broke your nose in the past, you may have developed a post-traumatic nasal hump. Or if you fractured your nasal bones and your nasal septum, your nose may now be crooked.

Insurance coverage may be available for the correction of post-traumatic nasal deformities, so check with your insurance company.

✔ **Ethnic considerations:** In a perfect world, people could live with their differences and be content. But ours is not a perfect world, and noses that would look perfect in other countries may be embarrassing to their owner in the United States.

If you think of nasal abnormalities on a scale of 1 to 5 (with 5 being the worst), you can probably change a 5 problem to a 3, or a 4 problem to a 2, but changing a 5 to a 1 is extremely difficult and probably impossible. Accepting real improvement rather than obsessing about perfection is the key to a satisfactory outcome.

Nasal tip asymmetry

Your nasal tip may look a little different from one side to the other. One side may be lower or higher or slightly twisted or have a protrusion not present on the other side. Because the external shape of the nasal tip follows the shape of the underlying cartilages, your nasal tip shape can be improved if the cartilages can be straightened or made more symmetrical. This problem is probably congenital but may also be the result of an injury.

Crooked nasal tips are almost always improved or corrected via the open rhinoplasty approach (see the "Open rhinoplasty" section later in this chapter). Cartilage grafts, tip grafts, or even very small implants may be required in order to obtain maximum correction.

Crookedness

Crooked noses occur when your nasal bones or your nasal septum (or both) do not sit symmetrically in the midline of your face. This condition can occur if you inherited it from your family, suffered a small birth injury, or broke your nose or septum in a later injury. You usually need to straighten your crooked septum as well as your nasal bones to obtain permanent correction. Doing only a rhinoplasty — without correcting the deviated septum — almost always results in some persistent crookedness.

Excessive nasal tip projection

Nasal tip projection is the distance that your nasal tip protrudes out from your face. If your tip projection is abnormally large, your entire nose will look too big. If you have this problem, you inherited it. This problem doesn't develop after injury.

Fixing this problem is an area of controversy among nasal surgeons. Some surgeons reduce nasal tip projection via an open rhinoplasty approach (see Figure 10-1). Others camouflage excessive tip projection by raising your *nasal profile* (bridge of your nose) to match the current tip height.

Figure 10-1:
Nasal "humps" or extended tip projection can be reduced and reshaped through open rhinoplasty.

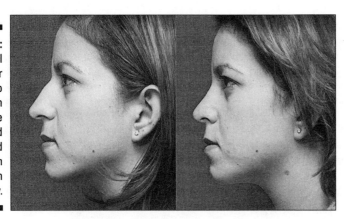

These two ways of improving your nasal appearance can both work very well. Some surgeons know both methods, but some do not. At the end of your consultation, you want to have a clear understanding of what the surgeon has recommended for you. You must make a decision as to whether you want to leave your nasal tip the same height or whether you want it smaller.

Excessive width

If you think your nose looks good in profile but you don't like the thickness or width of your nose, you may wish to have it thinned. If the skin on your nose is thicker than average, your surgeon may not be able to thin it as much as you hope. If the extra width is due to wide nasal bones, your surgeon can probably make a significant improvement. Wide nasal bones can usually be surgically fractured inward. They can also be narrowed by rasping (filing) your bone. Remember, however, that very wide nasal bones can never be made very thin; they can only be made *thinner*.

Having thick nasal skin significantly reduces your chance of getting a sculpted, modeled nose with good definition. Surgeons are unable to reduce the thickness of your skin. The overall size and shape of your nose can be changed, but after you've healed, you may still think your nose is too wide or too thick. In this circumstance, you must be willing to accept a result that is less than your fantasy.

Overall size

If your nose is too big or too small to fit your face, you may find a surgical solution that gives you the proportions you have in mind.

Too big

Some noses are just too large in all dimensions and are out of proportion to the face (see Figure 10-2). Very large noses can be reduced to a moderate size — but not to a very small size. There are real limitations to the changes that can be made. The surgeon can narrow the tip, reduce overall nasal width, lower the nasal profile, narrow the nostril base width, reduce the size of the nostrils, reduce the projection of the nasal tip, and shorten the overall length of the nose by rotating the nasal tip higher so the tip doesn't hang too low toward the upper lip. Not all patients need to have all these surgical steps performed to correct a large nose, but all are available if needed.

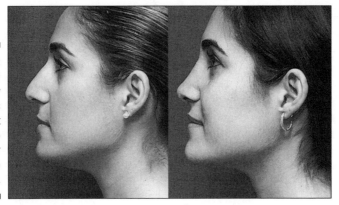

Figure 10-2:
A standard rhinoplasty gave this patient at nose to match her delicate features.

Too small

Maybe it's not a smaller nose you're after but a larger one. For example, you may want a larger nose if an accident has crushed in the bridge of your nose or if you're an Asian with a very low nasal profile. Whether you're looking to correct an injury or improve on what nature gave you, your surgeon has various techniques and materials that he can use to make these corrections.

The materials available fall into two groups:

- ✔ **Tissue taken from your own body** *(autologous tissue):* Your own cartilage can be harvested from your nasal septum, your ear, or one of your ribs. Bone can be taken from your hip. The advantage of using your own tissue is that you'll never reject it. Occasional disadvantages are that it can reabsorb or twist.

> ✔ **Various types of implants:** Implants are made out of silicone rubber or other bonelike materials and are preformed into the commonly needed shapes for nasal augmentation. They don't absorb or twist, but they may shift position and occasionally get infected.

Length

If you have an excessively long nose or an overhanging nasal tip (where the tip of your nose hangs over your upper lip), you probably inherited it. Rhinoplasty surgeons measure the angle between the upper lip and columella; this measurement is called the *nasolabial angle*. The ideal angle in women is approximately 100 degrees and in men is about 90 degrees.

In general, long noses are totally correctable problems, and surgeons use a combination of techniques to fix them. Surgeons can shorten noses by reducing the length of support cartilages within the nose, by shortening the nasal septum, by occasionally anchoring (suturing) the columella to the end of the septum, and by excising skin within the *nasal vestibule* (the area inside the nostrils). Except under unusual circumstances, noses are almost never made smaller or shorter by removing external nasal skin.

Bumps

You can be born with a nasal bump or develop one after an injury. A nasal bump or hump is caused by enlargement of your nasal bones. You may have a hump in combination with any of the other nasal problems discussed in this chapter. If a nasal hump is your only problem, the success rate of surgery is extremely high when performed by a good nasal surgeon.

If your only problem is a nasal hump, most rhinoplasty surgeons use the closed rhinoplasty approach, which I discuss later in this chapter. The open approach, however, is the choice of many excellent rhinoplasty surgeons for all nasal surgery, including surgery to correct bumps.

Tip size

If the tip of your nose is too rounded, too bulbous, or too broad, you can blame your parents and grandparents because these problems are usually congenital. Surgeons can achieve dramatic improvements in the external tip shape by modifying the tip cartilages. Making your round nose as thin as you want may not be possible. Improvement — not perfection — should be your goal. Sometimes, the culprit in thick nasal tips is thick skin, and if that's the case, improvement is much harder to obtain.

Doing something for herself

Some people spend the majority of their time giving to others and neglect their own needs. Such is the case for Jennifer, a nurse: "I work in a very giving profession, and it was time to do something I've wanted to do for a very long time. Ever since I was in my teens, I have been very self-conscious about my nose. My profile was what bothered me the most. I was very self-conscious of how I positioned myself in photos, and it just seemed to be the prominent feature on my face."

After hearing about a doctor through a recommendation and personally seeing the results of other patients, not just the photos, Jennifer chose her physician and signed up for a nose job. Since the procedure, she says, "I think I feel a greater confidence about myself. I've always been fairly happy with my appearance, but I think we all have something about ourselves that is our own personal nemesis. Others may not see it, but I don't think that really matters; it's all about what's best for you personally. Could I have lived without the surgery and been happy? Yes, no doubt. But I had the means to do it, so I did, and I'm happy I did."

Before the procedure many people told Jennifer they didn't think she needed it, but she said she wasn't interested in what others thought. "The greatest thing about my surgery was that it wasn't this drastic procedure; I just look like a better me. People who haven't seen me for a long time don't realize what is different. They just say I look younger and I look great. My nose is very natural and just fits me! Why not do something for yourself?"

Most, but not all, nasal surgeons improve tips via an open rhinoplasty approach, which I describe in a section by that name later in this chapter.

Nostril width

You may find that the base of your nose is wider than you would like. This occurs more commonly among some ethnic groups such as Latinos, African Americans, or Asians. Your surgeon can remove a wedge of tissue at your *nostril bases* (the area where your nostrils attack to your cheeks) in a procedure called a Weir excision, which you can read about in its own section later in this chapter. This technique can narrow your nostril bases, reduce the length of your nostril sidewalls, and make your nostrils smaller, depending on the design of the wedge excisions.

Checking Out the Rhinoplasty Options

Whether you're looking to correct an injury or improve what nature gave you, your surgeon has various techniques to get the result you want.

Before you make an appointment with your rhinoplasty surgeon, look at your nose very carefully and have some real ideas about the changes that you want to make. Your surgeon may show you some options you haven't considered, but always come prepared with some of your own thoughts as a starting point for your discussion.

Rhinoplasty operations can last from 45 minutes to several hours, depending on the complexity of your problems and the operating speed of your surgeon.

Augmentation rhinoplasty

Augmentation rhinoplasty is an operation that adds size to an area of your nose. You may want a higher nasal bridge or a different nasal tip, or some area of the nose may be depressed or deficient. Depending on what needs correction, the surgeon can perform the operation by using a standard rhinoplasty approach or an open rhinoplasty approach.

As part of the same operation, cartilage is harvested from your nasal septum, your ear, or one of your ribs and used as a graft for reconstruction or as augmentation material. Implants available are made from silicone rubber, polyethylene (Medpor), human dermis (AlloDerm), and Gore-Tex (Gore S.A.M., made of ePTFE).

Closed rhinoplasty

Closed rhinoplasty means that all the incisions are inside the nostrils. Closed, or standard, rhinoplasty was the surgical approach used for essentially all rhinoplasties until the open technique was introduced 20 or more years ago. Many up-to-date rhinoplasty surgeons use this approach when the nasal tip is not excessively projecting, excessively wide, or deformed. If a nasal hump or excessive width of your *nasal vault* (the part of the nose above the nasal tip) is the only problem, closed rhinoplasty works extremely well, without placing an external scar on your columella. Adequate exposure to perform meticulous surgery is available through intranasal (inside the nose) incisions. Surgeons can trim or reshape cartilage, rasp, or fracture the nasal bones, and remove excess soft tissue.

Some sophisticated rhinoplasty surgeons do all their rhinoplasties by using the closed approach and obtain superb results. However, the technique your physician uses is not as important as the results he or she obtains.

Open rhinoplasty

Open rhinoplasty is a relatively new technique — it's been around for about 20 years now — in which the surgeon makes an incision across the lower or mid columella. The initial incision is connected to other unseen incisions inside the margins of your nostrils. This approach enables your surgeon to lift all the skin over your nasal tip upward, allowing complete exposure of the cartilages that make up the nasal tip and providing your surgeon with direct vision of your nasal bones, septum, and upper nasal cartilages.

If you come to me because you don't like something about your nasal tip — it is very bulbous, sticks out, or projects too far or if the tip is twisted or slumping (see the section "Nasal tip asymmetry," earlier in this chapter) — I always suggest using an open rhinoplasty approach (see Figure 10-3). The small scar on the columella is essentially invisible after complete healing has occurred, and the extra exposure in this procedure provides a much better chance of correcting your tip problem.

Figure 10-3:
Incision
lines
typically
used in
open
rhinoplasty
procedures.

Dashed lines represent incisions made for open rhinoplasty

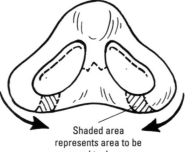

Shaded area represents area to be removed to decrease nostril size

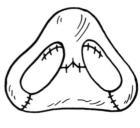

Closed incision lines

Septoplasty

Septoplasty is performed either through the open rhinoplasty exposure of the columella or through a separate incision deeper inside the nostril (nasal vestibule). Both approaches work well. If you have a crooked nose and a crooked septum, you need to correct both problems in order for your nose to stay straight. If you have nasal obstruction due to a crooked septum, straightening your septum usually enables you to breathe easier because the mechanical blockage has been removed. The septum can be straightened by removing deviated cartilage and bone, fracturing the deviated cartilage and bone back to a normal position, or releasing the septal attachments and replacing the cartilage in the midline.

If you want to correct a crooked nose, you should probably avoid any surgeon whose operative plan does not include a discussion of your septum.

Weir excisions

If your nostril bases are wider than ideal, excisions of a wedge of tissue at the nostril base, a procedure known as *Weir excisions,* can narrow the nostril base width. If you have an exceptionally protruding nasal tip and your tip projection is reduced surgically, the rims of your nostrils may appear too large and buckle outwards. Weir excisions can solve this problem, and they can also be used to make oversized nostrils smaller (see Figure 10-4).

The scars from Weir excisions sit in the normal skin fold at the side of your nostril bases and are almost always virtually invisible. In any case, the benefit of the excisions outweigh any negatives of any slightly visible scars.

Figure 10-4:
Weir
excisions
have
reduced the
size of this
patient's
nostrils.

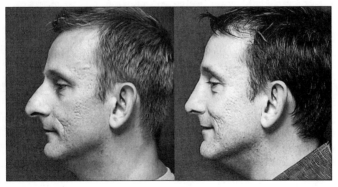

Tip rhinoplasty

Occasionally, a tip rhinoplasty (see Figure 10-5) is an alternative to a full rhinoplasty. In a tip rhinoplasty, the scope of the operation is limited to the nasal tip only, so the operating time and cost are reduced. Tip rhinoplasties can be done by using either a closed or open approach, depending on the problem with your tip. In general, your surgeon will use an open approach for more complicated tip problems.

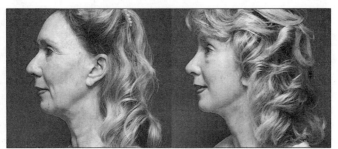

Nosing Into Important Considerations

You have a few issues to consider before you decide to pursue rhinoplasty. You want to be sure that you choose an experienced surgeon and that you communicate clearly about your potential results. Rhinoplasty can easily be combined with other procedures but it does affect your anesthesia choices.

Factoring your age into your decision

You can have cosmetic nasal surgery after age 13 or 14. In reality, most people who have rhinoplasty do so during high school or college. During this time, the desire to be accepted and appreciated by peer groups and the opposite sex is enormous. Some, however, must wait and have nasal surgery after they've worked long enough to be able to afford the procedure. There's no real age cap for having rhinoplasty.

I once did a rhinoplasty on a 75-year-old woman who had wanted her nose done since she was a teen, but her mother had always discouraged her from doing so. When her mother died, family resistance disappeared, and she was able to fulfill a lifetime dream.

Combining rhinoplasty with other operations

When patients combine rhinoplasty with another surgery, a chin augmentation is frequently requested. For many people with large noses and small or receding chins, the combination of these procedures creates a much more balanced facial appearance. Modification of chin projection can be accomplished with chin implants or with sliding genioplasties (procedures in which surgeons move the chin bone forward).

Many patients wish multiple procedures at the same time as a way of saving both recovery time and money. My rule is that I'll do a combination of procedures if they take no longer than six hours, providing blood loss isn't an issue and you're healthy. Examples of such combinations include a facelift and rhinoplasty or a tummy tuck and rhinoplasty.

Avoiding the magic wand syndrome

Great surgeons frequently make wonderful things happen for patients, but they don't do it by waving a magic wand. Rhinoplasty isn't a painless, perfect, instant fix for your problem. If you understand that scarring, swelling, and pain management are all part of the healing process (check out the upcoming section, "Recovering from Rhinoplasty"), you're more likely to be a satisfied consumer and a wiser decision maker.

Your chances of getting the exact results are slim to begin with — nothing in life is perfect — and they're even slimmer if the modification you're after is complex. You need to discuss specific procedure limitations with your rhinoplasty surgeon and make certain that you're prepared to live with and accept improvement rather than perfection.

Making sure your surgeon is a pro

Probably no other cosmetic surgery procedure requires as much care in your choice of a surgeon as does a rhinoplasty. Any rhinoplasty procedure affects not just the way your nose looks but the way it functions, so be sure you consult with an experienced and qualified doctor before considering rhinoplasty. Of all the different operations that plastic surgeons or head and neck surgeons learn during their residencies, rhinoplasty is almost universally considered the most challenging. Because rhinoplasties are so difficult, many surgeons perform very few of them. You want to find an expert, which means finding a surgeon who regularly does this surgery and produces consistent results that you like.

Some plastic surgeons initially were trained in otolaryngology (head and neck surgery) rather than general surgery, and these "double-boarded" plastic surgeons (see Chapter 3) are probably the best-trained nasal surgeons and your best choice because both specialties include training in rhinoplasty.

Rhinoplasty is considered to be a major procedure, so you should have the procedure performed at a hospital, in a certified surgery center, or in an office-based certified surgery suite.

Asking the right questions

Because nasal surgery is so complex, be sure that you ask the right questions at the time of your consultation (see Chapter 5 for more details on consultations). Use your in-office time wisely. Ask the following questions of every potential surgeon:

- **How many rhinoplasties do you perform per year?** If the number is under 25 or 30, be careful! More experience usually means better results. However, the best surgeon in your community may still be the newest physician out of residency who has both skill and passion. Experience is just one part of the equation.

- **May I see before-and-after photos of your work?** I tell you how to evaluate these photographs in the upcoming section, "Evaluating before-and-after photos."

- **Do you have a system of showing me potential results for my nose?** The most common way is to produce an image of your nose by using digital photography and special imaging software. I tell you about this and other options in the upcoming section, "Picking your new nose."

- **How do you handle redos?** Because of the uncertainty of the healing process, rhinoplasty surgery probably has the highest rate of revision procedures, also called touch-up or secondary procedures. You want to know upfront what your position will be if you need such surgery. Ask what secondary surgery will cost you and how long you'll need to wait to have the surgery (probably 6 to 12 months).

You need to be a discriminating shopper and accept realistic goals. Don't be intimidated by the surgeon, and ask enough questions so that you can form an intelligent decision about whether you want the surgeon to operate on you.

Evaluating before-and-after photos

Evaluating pre- and postoperative photos is your best opportunity to see what a surgeon can accomplish. If a surgeon is unable to show you before-and-after photos, go elsewhere. If he can only show you one or two results, he probably does very few noses. If he tells you that showing photos is a patient privacy issue, go elsewhere, because clearly he's giving you excuses.

When looking at before-and-after images, be critical. If you see a lot of results that you don't like and none that you do, consider seeking another surgeon. For nasal surgery, you may want to take your show on the road and travel to another city to see a super-specialist.

Making a very large nose small or an extremely bulbous tip narrow is difficult, if not impossible. What you need to evaluate is improvement: Do the postoperative noses look better?

To help you analyze what you see, ask yourself the following questions:

- ✔ Does the nose really look better after surgery than it did before?
- ✔ If the nose was crooked, is it now straight?
- ✔ If the tip was too big or too wide, is it now smaller and narrower?
- ✔ If the nose was too big, does it look smaller?
- ✔ Does the nose fit the patient's face?
- ✔ If the patient is a woman, do you think her nose is feminine enough?
- ✔ If the patient is a man, does he still look masculine?

Although these questions seem basic and intuitive, many patients, under the possible anxiety of the consultation, don't get these questions answered in their own minds. If you don't trust your ability to judge your responses while in the stressful environment of the consultation, take a friend or relative with you. If none of the noses that you look at would make you personally happy, move on to the next surgeon. If, however, all the noses look extremely good, you've probably found your surgeon.

Most offices can arrange for you to talk to a postoperative rhinoplasty patient who is happy with her result. Talking to a patient can be one of the best ways of obtaining firsthand information about your potential surgeon and the entire surgical experience.

Picking your new nose

Imagine asking a friend to pick up some biscuits for a party you're throwing, but he brings dog biscuits. Errors in communication are all too common in life, and when you're planning to change your body, you can't rely on words alone. To make sure you're communicating well, surgeons use imaging.

Imaging is a system comprised of digital photography and a software program that allows the images to be manipulated. In my opinion, the best use of imaging in cosmetic surgery is in planning for rhinoplasty.

Because your nose can be changed in so many ways and you can choose from so many looks, you need to have some idea of the result you want before going to see your nasal surgeon. Look at your nose in the mirror; better yet, look at it with two mirrors so that you can see yourself from the side and really think about how you want your nose to look.

Imaging and other visual methods of choosing a new nasal shape provide an opportunity for you to choose a shape that would make you happy. They also give your surgeon an opportunity to show you what can potentially be achieved. If there is a difference between what you want and what he thinks he can do, then a new image can be created and agreed upon. You need to understand that the image you choose is only a guideline. Your surgeon will make every attempt to achieve a result that is exactly like the imaging, but in reality, results that exactly match the imaging very seldom occur.

You're likely to be offered the following types of imaging:

- **Digital photography and imaging software:** You, your family, and your surgeon can all sit in front of the computer screen while the options for changing your nose are manipulated, stored, saved, and printed. Imaging allows you to show the doctor what would and would not please you. The surgeon can show you minute changes in the position of your nasal tip or in the contour of your nasal bridge. You and your family can go home with before-and-after images to evaluate and compare.

- **Transparencies:** Some physicians take black-and-white photos and draw on an overlay transparent sheet. This process isn't as high tech as digital imaging, but it works well, and you shouldn't be deterred from using a surgeon who uses this method. He may not be a computer whiz, but he still may be your best choice for a surgeon.

- **Photographs:** Some surgeons draw directly on photographs taken of your nose. Unless the photographs are life-sized, this method is the least sophisticated and may indicate that the surgeon doesn't specialize in nasal surgery. It could be a reason to consider moving on.

During your consultation, if the surgeon is unable to perform imaging (by any method), be careful. If the surgeon says something like "I understand exactly what you want. Trust me," you probably don't want to work with this surgeon. Chances are this surgeon doesn't do many rhinoplasties and can't afford or won't take the effort to learn any imaging system. I advise you not to proceed without some form of a mutually agreed upon visual goal.

You and your surgeon must reach a clearly understood goal. Imaging is a guideline and not a promise. You must understand that imaging and the subsequent choosing of an image don't guarantee your surgical result.

Some surgeons won't image noses for fear that patients will consider the process a guarantee. No nasal surgeon in the world can produce noses exactly like the imaging provides 100 percent of the time. I like to use imaging for its value as a communication tool, but I accept its limitations — and encourage patients to do likewise.

Considering anesthesia

You have some anesthesia options when you're having a rhinoplasty by itself. For more information on anesthesia, see Chapter 3.

✔ **Local anesthesia with intramuscular (IM) or intravenous (IV) sedation:** In this method, sometimes called twilight sleep, you're sedated with intramuscular or intravenous medications, local anesthetic is infiltrated into your nose, and the operation proceeds. The level of sedation determines whether you won't feel the injections at all or whether you will feel them minimally. Your nose is easy to make numb, and this method works very well. One advantage of this method is that you'll probably bleed a little bit less during the surgery, making it slightly easier for your surgeon to operate. The only potential drawback is that you may be slightly aware that you're having surgery. Pain during surgery is almost never a problem.

✔ **General anesthesia:** Many patients wish to hear or feel nothing during surgery, and for them, general anesthesia is the method of choice. The disadvantage is that there's a slight potential increase in postoperative nausea. When you combine rhinoplasty with other procedures, you and your surgeon will probably decide on general anesthesia.

Understanding the Risks

Rhinoplasty operations have their own specific risks.

✔ **Unhappy result:** An outcome that leaves you unhappy is the biggest risk. But before you proceed with surgery, you need to accept that rhinoplasty operations have the highest revision rate (secondary procedures to correct minor flaws after healing) — 20 percent or more.

✔ **Bleeding:** The mucosa (nasal lining) may be cut during rhinoplasty, and suturing the cut edges may be impossible because of the location and small spaces. Bleeding can occur after surgery, but it can usually be controlled with pressure and nasal sprays. If the bleeding is severe, some type of nasal packing may be required. Bleeding problems are uncommon, however, as most nasal surgeons now close all the intranasal incisions. If mucosal tears are known to exist, surgeons may place nasal packing for a day or more at the time of surgery.

✔ **Infection:** Infection following rhinoplasty is rare and is more likely to occur if the surgeon uses cartilage grafts or implants. Oral antibiotics usually heal the infection quickly, but in the worst-case scenario, the surgeon may need to remove an implant or a graft in order for the infection to clear up.

✔ **Absorption or twisting of cartilage grafts:** If cartilage grafts have been placed, later absorption or twisting can occur in spite of your surgeon's best efforts. If the problem is severe, you may need revisional surgery.

✔ **Abnormal scarring:** Unusually thick or wide scars can occur from the open rhinoplasty incision on the columella or from Weir excisions at the alar bases. If this occurs, excising the scars and resuturing them usually solves the problem.

Rhinoplasty also has serious but rare risks — including heart attack, blood clots, and pulmonary emboli — that are inherent in all major surgical procedures. For more info on the risks, see Chapter 17.

Recovering from Rhinoplasty

If you're like most patients, you worry that your entire upper face will be black and blue and that you'll have a lot of pain. Yes, you'll likely have some bruising and pain, but the reality is that rhinoplasty is a relatively easy procedure from which to recover.

In most cases, you should look presentable within a week. Keep in mind, however, that *all* the postoperative swelling and postoperative changes in shape don't go away for approximately one year.

Getting through the pain

You can expect to have some pain after the anesthetic has worn off. By the following day, your pain level should be much reduced. Oral pain medication prescribed by your surgeon and ice packs control most postoperative discomfort with little difficulty. For a week or two after surgery, your nose will be tender to the touch.

Rhinoplasty is more uncomfortable if your nose is filled with gauze packing after the operation. If your surgeon uses packing to reduce postoperative bleeding and swelling, you'll experience postoperative pain and discomfort until the packing is removed. Your postoperative pain is reduced by approximately 80 percent if nasal packing isn't used. Surgeons who don't use nasal packing close or suture all the incisions inside the nose, thereby reducing to near zero the possibility of bleeding. Very good rhinoplasty surgeons may use either method.

If your septum is being straightened at the same time, you may have septal splints sutured across the septum to hold the septum in the midline during healing. The splints reduce your airway slightly and are usually removed in about a week, making it easier to breathe.

Taking it easy

You can be up and about after the anesthetic or sedation wears off. Don't do anything strenuous, but if you look and feel good enough, you may go to the movies, out to dinner, or even shopping. If your surgeon doesn't use nasal packing (see the preceding section, "Getting through the pain"), rhinoplasty is one of the easiest cosmetic surgery procedures from which to recover.

Knowing what's normal

Some swelling and bruising are normal following rhinoplasty, but extreme swelling and bruising are not. Persistent bleeding is also abnormal. Call your surgeon's office if something feels wrong.

Judging the result

Healing after rhinoplasty takes a long time. Probably 80 percent of the swelling is gone within the first 30 days, but the last 20 percent may take six months to a year or even longer. You need to be patient and understanding during this process.

If your nose doesn't turn out close enough to the projected goal, your surgeon may want to do a small secondary procedure to make both you and him happier. Your surgeon probably won't be willing to reoperate until at least six months to a year after the original surgery.

Dealing with Disappointment

Rhinoplasty has a higher than average revision rate because healing isn't always predictable. Most revisions are relatively small and simple and should lead to good patient satisfaction.

If you feel that your nose has turned out terrible after the first or second procedure, you need to sit down with your surgeon and discuss your feelings and your options. You should probably get second or even third opinions from physicians your surgeon recommends or from your second or third choices gathered when you were evaluating surgeons.

Sitting down with the surgeon and discussing all the issues involved can frequently smooth out some difficult bumps in the road. Surgeons sometimes realize that the result hasn't turned out as anticipated, and they're unclear on how to make it better. Some surgeons would rather refer you to a colleague for further attempts at correction.

Chapter 11

Getting the Skinny on Liposuction

. . . .

In This Chapter

▶ Looking at fat cells

▶ Figuring out whether you want liposuction

▶ Weighing the risks

▶ Covering all the presurgery bases

▶ Planning your recovery

. . . .

*O*nce upon a time the perfect female figure was a 36-24-36. No more. Today's cultural definition of the perfect body is more like 38-22-34. In an attempt to achieve that "perfect" shape, many women are turning to liposuction. Many other women (and men) seek liposuction so that they can just look more proportional and fit into the clothes they wish to wear. Men typically want liposuction on their abdomens, flanks ("love handles"), and chests (breasts).

Lipoplasty (another name for liposuction) is the most popular cosmetic surgery in the United States, with more than 300,000 procedures performed in 2003, according to the American Society for Aesthetic Plastic Surgery.

Understanding Body Fat

Even if you've dieted and exercised as much as possible and are pretty much within normal weight ranges, you may have unwanted fat deposits in different areas of your body. Even some of your thin friends have extra fat in certain places. These pesky bulges remain even in people who are marathon runners. The reason is genetics.

Subcutaneous fatty tissue, which exists above muscle and under skin, is a well-defined layer that creates softness and hides the angularity of the bones of the body. When excess fatty tissue is deposited in certain areas (including the abdomen, hips, buttocks, thighs, knees, and chin), a person looks overweight or less than perfect according to today's standards of beauty. Liposuction is an excellent technique to help sculpture the body by removing these unwanted fat deposits.

The fat cells can be removed with their accumulated fat, leaving behind the connective tissue, the blood vessels, and the nerves. The space left after the fat cells are removed is obliterated with small amounts of scar tissue. As long as the skin is elastic enough to contract, a pleasing, smaller contour can be achieved. Some elasticity of the skin is present in most people under 50 so that when the total volume of the abdomen or hip is reduced, the remaining skin contracts and still looks normal. This might not occur to the same extent if you're 65 or older. More than 95 percent of liposuctions, however, are performed on people under 50 years of age.

Every person is born with a certain number of fat cells — okay, billions of them, if you must know. When you gain weight, you don't grow new fat cells (unless you become morbidly obese), but rather the fat cells you have fill up with fat and become larger. If fat cells are removed with liposuction, they don't regenerate. Suppose that you have liposuction and achieve a better contour but subsequently gain weight and look fat. If you lose that weight again, you should look the same as you did after liposuction. Liposuction causes a permanent change in your shape. Even if you subsequently gain weight, you can anticipate doing so in your new profile.

Checking Out Your Options

The location of your fat cells dictates your shape; heredity and gender influence the location of those cells. You can change your size through weight reduction, but shape stays relatively the same. Liposuction can improve both your size and shape.

Defining liposuction

Liposuction, also known as lipoplasty, suction-assisted lipectomy (SAL), or liposculpture, is a procedure in which your surgeon sculpts your body by removing unwanted fat deposits in specific areas (see Figure 11-1). *Cannulae,* or suction tubes, are used to extract fat. Liposuction removes the fat cells while sparing nerves, blood vessels, and connective tissue. Liposuction can permanently change the shape of your body.

The amount of fat removed varies. If your body build is average but you have way too much fat, the maximum amount of fat and fluid that is considered safe to be removed (at one operation) is 5,000 cubic centimeters (cc), or approximately 1½ gallons. If you're a smaller person, your surgeon may not wish to remove more than 3,000 or 4,000cc at one operation.

Returning for a second procedure in three to six months is much safer for you than attempting to remove 7,000 or 8,000cc at one time. Unfortunately, a second procedure costs extra, but your safety is worth it.

Liposuction never removes all the fat cells in any area. Some fat cells are always left behind and are necessary to provide normal contours.

Taking a look at the procedures

Over the past 20-plus years, significant improvements in liposuction have occurred. The method a surgeon employs to perform liposuction is largely dependent on personal preference. Equally good results can be obtained with any method.

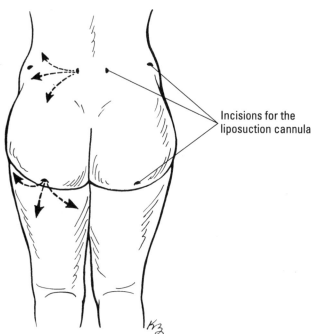

Figure 11-1: Liposuction can eliminate unwanted or difficult-to-get-rid-of fat deposits.

Incisions for the liposuction cannula

Arrows represent liposuctioned areas

The type of technique employed is less important than the skill of the operator. The fact that a surgeon uses the latest $75,000 laser liposuction machine doesn't guarantee a better result. Your surgeon may have bought it because it may save a little time and she hopes that it may result in slightly less blood loss. But in the end, the surgeon's judgment is what's important.

Suction-assisted lipoplasty (SAL), or liposuction, is how liposuction began and is basically how it is still performed today. The cannulae, connected to suction, are inserted under the skin and fat is suctioned. In this traditional method of liposuction, the surgeon guides the device in order to suction unwanted fat.

Liposuction is an inherently safe procedure, if performed carefully using safe guidelines. Serious complications occur when too much local anesthetic agent is infiltrated, when too much fluid is injected, when too much fat and/or blood is removed, when the cannulae are inserted into the abdomen or chest cavity (instead of under the skin), and when non-trained nurses or physicians attempt this operation.

Syringe technique

Using this system, cannulae attached to a large syringe are inserted, the barrel is withdrawn and locked (creating suction), and liposuction is performed until the syringe is filled. In this manner, liposuction is done 60cc at a time. This technique is elegant and requires less physical "work" (because there is no weight of the suction tubing).

Ultrasonic liposuction, or ultrasound-assisted lipoplasty

Ultrasonic liposuction, also called ultrasound-assisted lipoplasty (UAL), has many adherents. Ultrasonic energy is directed from the tip of the cannulae to "liquefy" the fat. The "melted" fat is then suctioned out by the ultrasonic cannula or by a second cannula. One potential problem with ultrasonic liposuction is a slightly increased occurrence of fluid collections under the skin postoperatively. Another potential problem is the occurrence of burns to the skin. Fortunately, neither of these problems is common.

External ultrasound-assisted lipoplasty

External ultrasound-assisted lipoplasty (E-UAL) uses external ultrasound waves (transmitted through the skin) to liquefy subcutaneous fat cells. Fluid containing local anesthetic is injected into the area of concern, and ultrasonic energy is transmitted to liquefy the fat before removing it. I tried this method extensively but found that it wasn't very helpful. Frequently, suctioning the fat after the application of the external ultrasound was no easier than if no ultrasound had been applied.

VASER-assisted lipoplasty

VASER-assisted lipoplasty (VAL) is a variant of UAL that uses slightly different technology in which either continuous or intermitted bursts of ultrasonic waves break up fat cells before removal by suction.

Power-assisted lipoplasty

Power-assisted lipoplasty (PAL) uses a motor in a handle to which the cannula is attached. The motor either moves the cannula forward and backward or rotates the cannula back and forth in a circular manner. The rotary type of PAL is the method of choice in my office. It removes fat easily and quickly, and blood loss is minimal.

Microliposuction

This technique uses suction cannulae that are the size of injection needles or slightly larger. Fat can be removed in small quantities through tubes that are very small in diameter. This technique can be quite useful in treating fatty bulges in the neck and on the face. In such areas, the removal of as little as 5 to 10cc can make a significant difference.

Microliposuction requires special equipment. The use of regular liposuction cannulae, even if they're small, doesn't seem to work as well, in my opinion, as microliposuction equipment. If you think you would benefit from this procedure, ask your surgeon some pointed questions, such as "Do you have the correct equipment?" and "Is it a procedure you perform frequently?"

Understanding tumescent liposuction

The name "tumescent liposuction" was coined by dermatologists doing liposuction under local anesthesia with sedation. Plastic surgeons never liked the term, but the general public uses it. *Tumescent liposuction* has come to mean a procedure in which all the areas to be suctioned are filled with fluid before treatment, no matter what type of anesthesia is being used.

Physiologic saline with a dilute amount of adrenaline (a natural substance that constricts blood vessels and reduces bleeding), known as tumescent solution, is injected into the fat.

A volume of solution two to three times the estimated amount of fat to be removed is injected under the skin into the fatty layer if the procedure is being performed under local anesthesia. This fluid makes the fat easier to remove and helps reduce blood loss and bruising. If you're having liposuction under general anesthesia by a plastic surgeon, the amount of solution injected into the fat is approximately equal to the amount of fat to be removed.

Deciding Whether Liposuction Is for You

You may have exercised hours each day and watched your calories but still don't look the way you want in your dress or bikini. Or perhaps you just want to be your best and have decided to give yourself a present. You've decided that liposuction may be just what you want. A careful preconsultation evaluation of your own body and the goals you want to reach will make your consultation and decision-making process easier.

Considering cultural ideals

Liposuction is one of the most popular cosmetic procedures for both men and woman. For many people, the inability to have an attractive, youthful shape creates great stress, particularly for those who have tried to improve their figure through diet and exercise programs. A focal point of discontent for many men and women is the isolated fat deposit (see Figure 11-2). The knowledge that liposuction can reduce those disproportionate localized accumulations of fat and help improve body contour irregularities often brings great relief to many people.

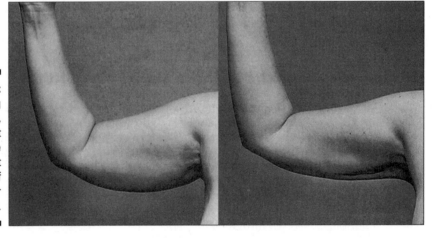

Figure 11-2: After having liposuction, this patient feels more confident showing off her upper arms.

Some young women aren't successful socially because they believe that their bodies are not attractive. In a different society or era, women may not have those feelings, but modern society does place a lot of emphasis on shapely bodies. Making those bodies closer to what society perceives as normal occasionally causes social miracles, something I see in my own practice.

Sizing up your health and body

If you're considering liposuction, you're an ideal candidate if you're healthy, in good physical condition, and have tight, smooth skin (no cellulite or surface waviness). If you don't fit this ideal model and still want to consider liposuction, don't worry. Although the ideal patient can achieve an excellent result, you can achieve a very good or good result if you don't fit the ideal criteria. One of the happiest patients I ever had was a woman with extremely wrinkled thigh skin who had never fit into a pair of jeans. After liposuction, her skin quality was unchanged, but she slid into her jeans with ease.

Dramatic changes can be achieved if you have localized areas of bulging caused by fat under the skin. For example, if you have very large hips and/or large outer thighs but otherwise have a normal shape, you're a good candidate for liposuction (see Figure 11-3). These areas respond extremely well to liposuction, and you can have a normal shape the rest of your life.

Liposuction can't help with generalized obesity, intra-abdominal fat, or excess loose skin. Some people with bulging tummies hope that liposuction can help but find out that almost all of the excess fat is "inside" the abdomen, wrapped around the intestines. Liposuction can't help in that instance.

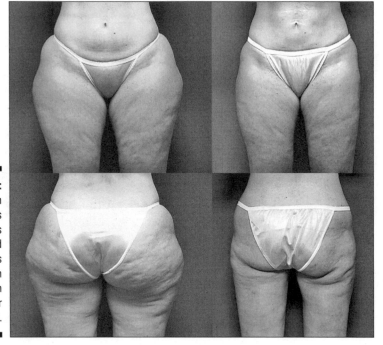

Figure 11-3: Liposuction enabled this patient's hips and thighs to be in proportion with her small waist.

People who are moderately overweight can benefit from liposuction, and there are no absolute age limits. However, older patients usually have diminished skin elasticity and therefore may not receive an optimal result.

I discuss the general health issues related to surgery in Chapter 7. If you have a bleeding disorder or take anticoagulants, you're probably not a good candidate for surgery in general and for liposuction in particular. If you have heart disease, pulmonary disease, or diabetes or are excessively overweight, you'll have a slightly higher chance of complications with all surgery. If your surgeon or her staff asks you for clearance from your physician or cardiologist before surgery, don't be upset. Those requests let your surgeon know that you can withstand the surgery safely.

What liposuction can (and can't) do

You have dieted and exercised and are stuck with a body that's still slightly too full in several areas. In women, the areas are usually the abdomen, hips, thighs, inner knees, and sometimes the upper arms and back. In men, the areas are usually the abdomen, flanks, and chest or breasts. The other areas of your body are normal, or at least as normal as you can get them. Liposuction can help you solve these problems (see Figure 11-4).

Figure 11-4: Although she went to the gym regularly, this patient could reduce the size of her outer thighs only through liposuction.

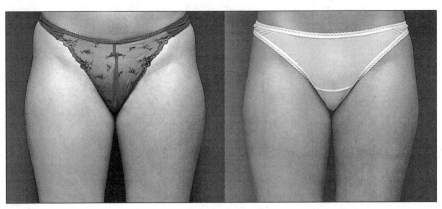

After 25 years of liposuction, surgeons have found that additional areas, such as knees, ankles, the face, and areas around the breasts and armpits, can also undergo liposuction with wonderful improvement. If you have localized excess fat essentially anywhere on the body surface (except perhaps the upper and lower eyelids), it can be liposuctioned. In my experience, the ankles and calves are difficult areas to treat but get great results. Many patients want their backs liposuctioned and end up slightly unhappy that they don't see greater changes. The reason is that the skin on the back is very thick and loose and the thick skin is frequently confused with excess fat.

Liposuction of fatty chests or breasts works extremely well on men. The procedure is also a good alternative to breast reduction surgery for men and in some women with very large breasts (see Chapter 16).

Avoiding the magic wand syndrome

Your goal for liposuction should be to improve body contour, understanding that it will not change the way your skin looks. Liposuction removes persistent fat not responsive to diet and exercise and establishes more normal proportions between areas of the body. It also improves your appearance both in and out of clothing.

Eliminating the curse of the pear

Karen, a 40-year-old female interior designer, began pondering the idea of liposuction in 1984, but it wasn't until 16 years later that she got serious about things. She's 5-foot-2, and no matter how much she dieted or exercised, she always carried too much weight on her thighs and bottom. With the encouragement of her husband, who knew how much the extra bulk bothered her, she made the decision to move forward with surgery.

She never regretted having the procedure done and even though the surgery itself went smoothly, it was painful for her. But she was so excited with the results that she felt better as each day passed, and within a couple weeks, she was feeling like herself again. One of the best emotional changes according to Karen is she "just enjoys everything more, including sex. My husband never, ever complained about my figure, but he still giggles now after 15 years of marriage that he feels like he has a new wife! If

that's not a reason to get a little help from a cosmetic surgeon, I don't know what is!"

Though it's a bit more of an effort for her to keep her weight down than she had expected, she still manages to do it. Karen says that her body wants to maintain a certain weight no matter what. The good news is that if she happens to put on a few pounds it goes all over, not back to the old pear spots. Now that she's motivated, though, when she gains weight, she says she just buckles down and gets it off.

So was it worth it? Karen says, "I'm wearing clothes I never could look at before, and I'm so much more confident. My figure was upside down for my height. Now I dress with attention to my figure, instead of covering it up. By ridding myself of the excessive fat in the lower region of my body, I feel tidier, sexier, and prettier. Now I enjoy my figure and get a bit of attention, too. I enjoy life more, and it shows."

You must be aware that the usual goal is improvement, not perfection. Having realistic expectations can make the entire experience much more satisfying and reduce your chances of disappointment. If you start the process with tight, hard skin, you will probably end up the same way, but with better contours. If your skin surface is wavy, dimpled, or wrinkled to start, your contours will improve, but the surface may stay the same.

Some patients, in spite of receiving all this information, still believe in some recess of their brain that liposuction will make them perfect. When they realize that surgery hasn't made them perfect, they end up disappointed, even if they have a wonderful result. Matching expectations with reality is why your surgeon gives you so much information before surgery.

Assessing the Risks

Performed properly, with good anesthesia in an accredited surgery center, liposuction is almost always safe. It is, however, major surgery, and people do sometimes die after the operation. Think through your decision to have or not have liposuction with a clear mind.

Patient deaths after liposuction virtually all occur because of technical errors of one kind or another. These errors include passing the cannula into the bowel or lung (instead of keeping the cannula under the skin), giving the patient too much fluid, or taking too much fat and fluid out. Another error is overdosing the patient with too much local anesthetic. Your best protection against these and other mishaps is to have a board-certified (see Chapter 3) liposuction expert perform this surgery in a certified operating room with an upper limit of 5,000cc being removed in an average-sized patient. If you follow this advice, I believe liposuction is as safe as any other major surgery.

Patients always have some blood loss after liposuction, but the amount is much less now than it was in the early years of this procedure, before the use of tumescent solutions and smaller cannulae. Nevertheless, on occasion, the trauma of the cannula suctioning the fat under the skin causes prolonged oozing of blood after the operation is over. On rare occasions, patients need blood transfusions.

Other risks are less serious than blood loss and can include the following:

- ✔ Temporary discoloration
- ✔ Swelling

> ✔ Discomfort such as pain or sensitivity
>
> ✔ Numbness
>
> ✔ Lumps or irregularities

More permanent complications include the following:

> ✔ Scars
>
> ✔ Waviness seen as surface irregularities
>
> ✔ Asymmetry
>
> ✔ Pigmentation changes (which occur only rarely)

Many of these problems, if they occur, are only temporary. The final contouring may not be complete for four to six months. Check out Chapter 17 to find out more about the risks associated with surgery.

Getting Set for Surgery

Liposuction is an elective, invasive procedure, so you need to be in good health before surgery. Making sure that you're eating right and exercising can help you stay healthy. Your doctor may ask you to attempt to lose some weight before liposuction. The best contours can be achieved if you're nearer to an ideal body weight.

Because of the bleeding issues with liposuction, you can't take aspirin or non-steroidal anti-inflammatory agents within a week or 10 days before surgery.

Making sure your doctor is a pro

Many medical practitioners represent themselves as qualified to do this procedure. Some are, but many are not. You're probably better off if you stick to a specialist who's been specifically trained to do liposuction, such as a board-certified plastic surgeon or a dermatologist. Facial plastic surgeons (who are ear, nose, and throat trained), general surgeons, obstetricians, and family practitioners usually have very limited training relative to liposuction and essentially learn on the job.

You really need to make an informed choice, so follow some simple rules when considering liposuction.

Asking the right questions

When choosing a surgeon, ask all candidates whether they were trained to do liposuction in their formal training or whether they learned it in a weekend course. Plastic surgeons and dermatologists receive liposuction training in their residencies and fellowships, so that fact should probably count heavily as you decide on a surgeon.

Ask surgeons you're considering whether they're board certified in plastic surgery or dermatology (see Chapter 3 for more information). Dermatologists performing liposuction under local anesthesia have excellent safety records.

Evaluating before-and-after photos

Pre- and postoperative photos may help give you an idea about the results you can expect from your surgeon. When evaluating photos, look for symmetry. Even if the skin quality is poor (both before and after liposuction), you're looking at a good result if both sides look improved and symmetrical. Also look at contours. For example, if the suctioned area looks hollowed out and the surrounding areas are normally rounded, you're looking at a bad result. The bottom line is, are you looking at a result you'd like for yourself?

Checking out the images

In order to envision the changes that may occur, a surgeon can perform imaging on the computer, giving you some approximation of the results you're trying to achieve. Imaging doesn't give you a very good sense of the quality of your skin surface after liposuction. Your skin quality won't change; the volume of the area being treated and contours will.

Choosing the facility

Most liposuction procedures are performed in an outpatient setting because the costs are much lower than in a hospital. However, you still want to be sure that the surgery suite is certified and that your doctor has privileges to perform lipoplasty in an accredited hospital.

In an accredited outpatient facility, the risks are about the same as in a hospital. Turn to Chapter 3 to find out more about safety and certification for outpatient facilities.

Considering anesthesia

Depending upon the technique used, your anesthesia choices vary. You need to discuss your anesthesia options — local anesthesia with sedation or general anesthesia — with your surgeon. Your choice relates in part to the amount of fat being removed and the specialty of the doctor you're choosing.

Traditionally, plastic surgeons perform liposuction by using the tumescent technique under general anesthesia. A board-certified anesthesiologist or nurse anesthetist administers general anesthesia, allowing the surgeon to focus on your surgery. Because you're fully asleep, your surgeon can also remove greater volumes of fat over larger areas in a rapid fashion.

Dermatologists tend to perform liposuction under local anesthesia, with or without mild sedation. This technique can also be very effective. However, they can't remove as much fat as a surgeon can under general anesthesia, and the patient may have a greater level of discomfort due to the local anesthetic injections or attempts to suction slightly beyond the areas of anesthesia. When performed skillfully, this method works extremely well.

Telling the whole truth — and nothing but

Be honest with your surgeon and anesthesiologist about any underlying medical conditions that you may have. Also tell them about any drugs (recreational and prescription) you use and your family medical history. Share with your operating team any special conditions that you may have, such as neck stiffness or back pain, so that the surgical team doesn't aggravate your condition when they position you on the operating table. Your anesthesiologist is your best ally for helping you avoid postoperative nausea. Let everyone know about your special concerns.

Recovering from Liposuction

After your surgery is over, follow the doctor's instructions. You can really compromise your results by inattention to your postoperative instructions.

Depending upon the type of anesthesia and the amount of fat removed, your doctor will give you instructions about whether you need to have someone stay with you overnight. If you have general anesthesia, your surgeon will require you to have someone stay with you the first night. Even with a local anesthetic, having a caregiver the first night is a good idea.

Your caregiver must be able to assist you safely into your home, help you get settled, and monitor you until you can fend for yourself. After liposuction, these duties generally involve offering assistance to the bathroom, giving you your medications, and helping change dressings beneath your support garment as needed. Caretakers also see that you get fluids and light meals.

If you have an emergency or even just a simple question for your doctor, you need a caretaker who can effectively describe your concerns to the doctor over the phone. If you need to see your physician, you need someone who is willing and able to drive you to that appointment.

After surgery, you'll have to restrict your activities for a few days and wear a support garment. The support garment gives you a little circumferential compression and provides the feeling that you're being "held together." Initially, you'll have dressings beneath the garment. The incisions that have been well hidden in skin folds or stretch marks may be loosely sutured and will have some bloody leakage for about 12 to 24 hours or more.

Within 24 to 48 hours, you may shower and then return to normal activity in just a week or more. Patients usually have minimal restriction placed on their activity after liposuction. Swelling can exist for up to three weeks, and the final result becomes fully apparent between four and six months after surgery.

Getting through the pain

Most physicians advise you to let pain be your guide when it comes to how active you can be. If it hurts, don't do it. For most patients, liposuction is uncomfortable but not very painful, and a few pain pills take care of the problem.

Naturally, liposuction patients run the full spectrum as far as pain is concerned. Some say they never have pain, and others say it hurts terribly. Most patients however, are somewhere in the middle. The average patient feels as if the muscles in the treated area are recovering from an extreme workout. Most patients, if they wish or need to, can return to work within a few days to a week.

Taking it easy

In general, most physicians let postoperative liposuction patients do what doesn't hurt. You shouldn't run or exercise strenuously for the first week or longer. You may, without risk, go to the store, dinner, or a movie whenever you feel comfortable doing so. If, however, you feel weak or woozy, you may have some temporary anemia. Discuss these symptoms with your doctor.

Ask your doctor how soon after your surgery it is safe to drive, and remember never to lift anything heavier than a few pounds in the early postoperative period. You don't want to do anything that can cause bleeding. While recovering, be careful around your pets and children, who can be overly active or rambunctious and cause a great deal of soreness if they jump on you or bump into your freshly operated areas.

Knowing what's normal

Physically, you can anticipate some bruising, swelling, and altered areas of sensation after liposuction. The asymmetry, lumps, surface irregularities, discomfort, and discoloration dissipate nicely over a few weeks. Your scars should be minimal and short (less than ½ inch). Increased skin pigmentation over the treated areas is very rare. Most people have some evidence of surface irregularities or waviness, particularly in areas that had preexisting laxity of skin.

Emotionally, you may find that you're on an initial downer — you don't feel that you've had any improvement or that the changes are taking place more slowly than you'd like. Please discuss these concerns with your surgeon and the nurses. Take consolation in the fact that postoperative photos, taken several months after surgery, will enable you to see for yourself the tremendous improvement when compared to your pre-op pictures.

Judging the result

When judging the result, keep in mind that all the swelling won't disappear for approximately four to six months, so that's when you can expect to see optimal skin shrinkage over the new contours. A possibility for disappointment exists when a patient has excessive intra-abdominal fat or preoperative loose skin. Intra-abdominal fat responds only to weight loss. Also remember that subsequent alterations of body contour will occur as a result of continued aging, weight gain, weight loss, and pregnancy.

Generally speaking, you have no guarantee as to the results after your cosmetic surgery. You and your surgeon can usually expect good results, but occasionally, surgical revision may be indicated following the original liposuction procedure. A surgeon can easily touch up a bulge remaining after liposuction with additional liposculpture. However, a postoperative depression or divot is much more difficult to treat. Occasionally, liposuction around the edges of a depression can improve the situation. Another possible solution, but one that's less likely to result in improvement, is fat grafting (fat transfer) into the divot or depression.

Chapter 12

Dejunking Your Trunk: Body Contouring Procedures

*I*f diet and exercise could solve all the problems that bother people about their bodies, the body contouring procedures described in this chapter wouldn't exist. If you see loose skin or loose skin and excess fat when you look in the mirror, this chapter is for you. If you've lost massive amounts of weight and you have very large amounts of excess skin, then the surgical procedures described in this chapter can be modified (see Chapter 13). If excess fatty deposits are your only problem, then you'll want to read Chapter 11 about liposuction.

I focus in this chapter on the surgical procedures that enable your surgeon to recontour your torso and upper thighs — tummy tucks, arm lifts, and buttock and thigh lifts. Procedures for the breast are discussed in detail in Chapters 14 through 16.

Checking Out Body Contouring Options

Body lift and body contouring procedures remove loosened skin, resize and reshape the body envelope, correct both vertical and horizontal laxity, and also use liposuction to improve bulging contours. The procedures can also tighten abdominal muscles.

Body contouring procedures aren't for the faint of heart. They involve large surgical incisions with significant recovery issues, but they solve loose skin problems that can't be resolved in any other way.

Body contouring procedures can be life-changing — physically and emotionally. Tummies can be tucked, hips can be smoothed, arms made smaller, and thighs and buttocks lifted. You must understand and accept realistic goals as part of the planning process. Surgical removal of loose skin can lead to dramatic results, but in order to achieve such results, you need to accept that you'll have long scars. You can usually hide your scars under clothing, but they may take almost a year to fade from pink to skin color.

Tucking your tummy

A tummy tuck *(abdominoplasty)* is the most commonly performed body contouring procedure. If you have excess abdominal skin, a saggy tummy, or bulging of your abdomen, some type of abdominoplasty will probably be necessary to achieve your goal. Your abdominal muscles can become lax through inactivity or stretched and separated because of pregnancy. You may have been born with a tendency toward lax abdominal skin, and both weight fluctuations and pregnancies can stretch the skin to the point that it will no longer contract.

Plastic surgeons have a number of different abdominoplasty techniques, depending on the severity of the skin laxity. In general, tummy tuck procedures contour your protruding abdomen by tightening your abdominal wall (your *rectus abdominus* muscles) and removing excess skin and fat from the area. Figure 12-1 shows you the procedure doctors use. Your surgeon's challenge is to keep the scars hidden inside underwear areas and to leave skin that conforms nicely to your body.

Standard abdominoplasty

A standard abdominoplasty is an excellent operation for women (or men) who have loose skin above and below the belly button that does not go away with weight loss or exercise.

Prior to surgery, your surgeon marks your incisions with a skin-marking pen. Before your surgeon marks you, be sure to tell him about any special clothing goals you have. If you want your scars to be hidden beneath a bikini or a favorite style of panties, then you need to let your surgeon know that. If this is important to you, you can bring the garments with you at marking time.

During an abdominoplasty, here's what happens, step by step:

1. The surgeon makes an incision encircling the edge of your belly button (umbilicus) and another curved incision from hip to hip along the top of your pubic hairline.

2. Your surgeon separates your skin from the abdominal muscle underneath, leaving your belly button and its umbilical stalk attached to the abdominal wall.

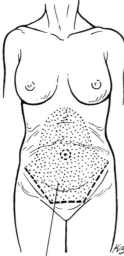 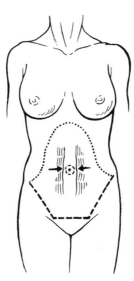 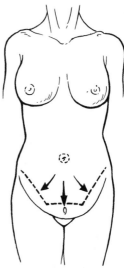

Figure 12-1:
In an abdomino-plasty, excess skin is separated from the underlying muscles and excised.

1. Area where skin is separated from the underlying muscles

2. Tightening of the underlying muscles. Arrows indicate the direction in which muscles are pulled and sutured

3. The elevated skin is pulled down and the excess is removed

3. He tightens your rectus muscles with large sutures. The rectus muscles run parallel to each other from the rib cage to the pubic bone (on either side of the vertical midline of your abdomen).

4. He measures, marks, and removes your excess skin.

5. He makes a new opening for your belly button, which is pulled through and sutured in place.

6. He places suction drains under your skin and then closes your abdominoplasty incision. The drains expedite your recovery by helping remove excess fluids. They remain in place for at least several days and perhaps for a week or more.

You can see the result of a standard tummy tuck in Figure 12-2.

Mini-abdominoplasty

If your skin laxity and muscle weakness problems are limited to the area below the belly button, you may be a good candidate for a mini–tummy tuck. This is a smaller operation than a standard abdominoplasty, with a shorter scar, and the belly button is not released or moved. Scars created by the incision are permanent but are deftly placed to be hidden by the type of bathing suit or undergarment you usually wear. Figure 12-3 shows you the results of a mini-abdominoplasty.

Figure 12-2:
If you have
a
substantial
amount of
excess skin
to be
removed,
you may be
a good
candidate
for a
standard
tummy tuck.

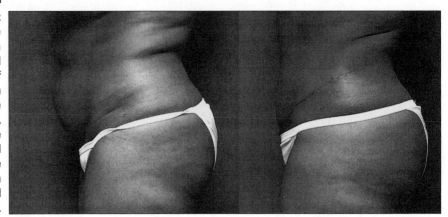

Mini-abdominoplasty procedures solve excess skin and bulging problems of the lower abdomen. They're usually performed in younger women who develop a permanent skin excess or bulging problem after pregnancy and delivery. Many women wanting mini-abdominoplasties want the operation with only a three- or four-inch scar. Unfortunately, it doesn't work that way. The scar has to be long enough to remove the excess skin.

Figure 12-3:
Many
women are
still able to
wear bikini
bottoms
after a
mini–tummy
tuck
because the
incision is
relatively
easy to hide.

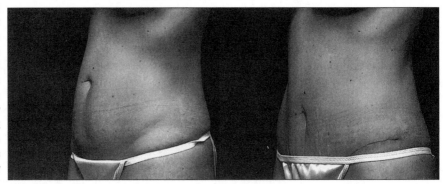

Extended abdominoplasty

This operation is similar to a standard abdominoplasty, but the incision is extended to include excision of skin and fat from the hip areas and lower back. The scar can extend to near the posterior midline or can cross the midline to encompass a total buttock lift (belt lipectomy, see next section). The longer incision enables your surgeon to deal with excess skin and bulging of areas of your hips and back that aren't addressed in a standard abdominoplasty technique. Figure 12-4 shows the results of an extended abdominoplasty.

Figure 12-4: An extended tummy tuck is generally the only answer to remove the excess skin resulting from more than one pregnancy or substantial weight loss.

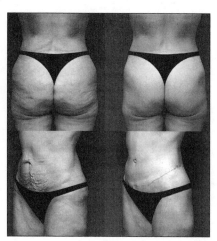

If you require tightening of skin over your hips or your buttocks, you will have longer incisions that are strategically placed within underwear or swimsuit lines. This procedure takes longer to perform and generally requires an assistant surgeon to expedite the operation. Because the surgery is more extensive, you also have a have a slightly higher chance of complications.

Belt lipectomy

If you have excess skin and fat involving not only the abdomen but also the hip and lower back areas, with some sagginess of your buttocks, you're likely to be a candidate for a belt lipectomy. Belt lipectomy removes skin from your abdomen, your hips, and lower back (and also tightens your buttocks and outer thighs to a significant degree). Another way to think of this operation is to consider it a combination of a standard abdominoplasty and a buttock lift.

Belt lipectomy is similar to an extended abdominoplasty, but the scars go completely around the body (see Figure 12-5) instead of stopping near the midline of the back. A belt lipectomy allows more dramatic lifting of the buttocks and the central back. Figure 12-6 shows you the results of a belt lipectomy.

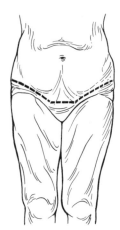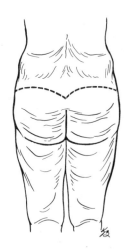

Figure 12-5:
True to its name, the belt lipectomy leaves patients with a permanent incision, much like a belt.

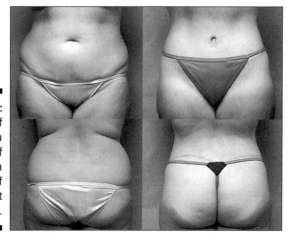

Figure 12-6:
Removal of this extra "belt" of skin is a major relief to most patients.

Modified abdominoplasty

You may be one of a few people who want an abdominoplasty and also have a very highly placed belly button and minimal excess skin above the belly button. If you're one of these few patients, your surgeon can move your belly button lower without having to make any incision around the belly button as is typical in standard abdominoplasty procedures. He'll separate your belly button from its connection to your abdomen and leave it attached to your skin. When he pulls your abdominal skin down, he reattaches your umbilical stalk to your abdominal wall in its new location.

Considering thigh and buttock lifts

If you have loose skin on your thighs that doesn't respond to exercise, you may want to consider some type of thigh lift. If your buttocks are saggy, a buttock lift may be the answer. There are times when both are appropriate at the same time.

Thigh lifts

You may want to consider a thigh lift if you have lax or loose skin in your thighs. The most common thigh lift is the inner (medial) thigh lift or thighplasty.

The incision for this procedure begins somewhere in the front groin and proceeds around your inner thigh onto your buttocks. If your inner thigh skin sagginess is excessive, a vertical wedge of skin can also be removed along the inner thigh, thus allowing horizontal as well as vertical skin tightening. The vertical excision also leaves a vertical scar extending from the inner groin down toward the inner knee. The vertical wedge excision is an infrequently performed part of thigh lifts.

If you want or need a thigh lift, you must understand that the scars end up in very personal and intimate areas. The incisions are near the vagina, and contamination from urine and feces is almost impossible to completely avoid during healing. I recommend (in addition to using antibiotics) that you wash the entire operative area with soap and water, in the shower, following every bowel movement and urination. Incision line infections still occur occasionally, but they appear to be significantly reduced if you take these precautions.

Buttock lifts

Buttock lifts do exactly what they describe: lift your sagging buttocks into a firmer and more youthful position. You look better in and out of clothes — except for the scar.

Buttock lifts can be designed with a curved horizontal incision above the buttocks, or with a scar in the inferior buttock crease. Over the years, plastic surgeons have largely switched from the lower buttock excision to the above-the-buttock incision. By placing the scars above the buttocks, a more natural look is achieved, and the scars are easier to hide under panties or bathing suits. The lower buttock crease incisions sagged with time, making them very hard to hide in short shorts or bathing suits.

Lower body lift

Lower body lift is an operation that combines a total thigh lift with buttock lift, hip lift, and lower back lift. If you're of normal weight, but have excessive skin in all of the above areas, you may want to consider this procedure.

Lower body lifts are often performed after dramatic weight loss (see Chapter 13). The main reasons to consider a lower body lift are excess skin and sagging thighs, but excess fat may also be an issue. Liposuction (see Chapter 11) and tummy tucks can be combined with lower body lifts.

Lower body lifts (see Figures 12-7 and 12-8) are big surgeries involving extra surgical time, more complex recoveries, and added risk of healing delays or complications.

Lower body lift is such an extensive procedure that you will want to search for a surgeon who has been there before. No one performs this surgery every day. If a surgeon has performed this operation 10 to 20 times over a period of years and can show you good results, he has enough experience.

Figure 12-7: Incisions are made from the pubic area up to the waist and around the back for a circumferential lower body and thigh lift.

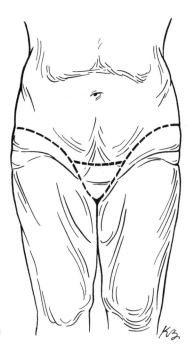

Upper arm lift

Saggy upper arms sometimes develop in normally thin people due to aging and genetics, but usually they're seen in people who have had weight shifts. After the excess skin has developed, exercise doesn't help, and surgery is the only alternative to doing nothing. If you have both excess skin and excess fat, liposuction of the upper arms will help reduce the overall volume but will not totally correct the problem.

Figure 12-8:
This patient was able to reduce her excess fat and lift her skin to greatly improve her overall appearance through a circumferential lower body and thigh lift.

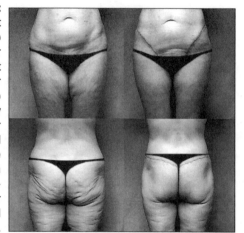

A standard upper arm lift *(brachioplasty)* involves making an incision from the inner elbow to the armpit in order to excise the extra skin. The incisions are planned so that the resulting scar is along the back of your inner upper arm, placed in the least visible location possible. A smaller type of upper arm lift can be performed by excising an ellipse of skin from the area where the inner aspect of the upper arm joins the armpit. This procedure tightens the loose skin but doesn't remove very much of it. Adding some liposuction to this procedure can produce significant improvement and cause very little visible scarring.

Although virtually all the excess skin on your arms can be removed surgically, you don't want the skin tightened excessively. The vessels and nerves for your entire arm run under the area of skin excision. If your arm skin is pulled too tightly, problems with circulation and nerve function can occur. Your surgeon will be walking a thin line and, more often than not, may not be able to take as much tissue as either of you would like.

Combining body contouring with other procedures

Because of advances in anesthesia, intraoperative and postoperative techniques, and postoperative care, plastic surgeons are safely combining multiple procedures. Television programs have helped popularize makeovers that frequently combine several surgical procedures.

Safety is the most important consideration in combining surgeries. So, if your doctor wants to do your surgery in two, three, or more surgeries because of safety issues, listen to him.

Liposuction (see Chapter 11) is very effective for removing excessive fat and is easily combined with body contour surgery when indicated. Liposuction, which can be incorporated into any of the abdominoplasty procedures, is usually used to thin the abdominal flap or to reduce the hips so that the overall contours will be better.

Almost any procedure can be performed with any other, providing certain criteria are met:

✔ You must be healthy.

✔ You must have a normal blood count.

✔ The combination of procedures shouldn't take more than six hours.

The best way to manage your wish list is to discuss with your plastic surgeon the areas that you want to have improved and then allow your plastic surgeon to prioritize the areas into logical sequencing so that you end up with excellent results. In general, I try to complete the surgeries that will provide the biggest emotional benefit to the patient first.

Multiple procedures at the same time can be efficient and good medicine provided that you're healthy and young enough, have no anemia, and the projected blood loss is small.

Deciding Whether Body Contouring Surgery Is for You

Almost everyone who has excess body skin wishes it were gone. For some people, the excess skin makes it impossible to exercise, have sex comfortably, or wear shorts, bathing suits, and normal clothes. Most people who have lost large amounts of weight feel very strongly that dealing with the excess skin is simply another step in the weight-loss program. The motivation to return to "normal" is very strong. Plastic surgeons who do body contour surgery on a regular basis all know at least a couple women who have chosen to do their own extreme makeovers — body lifts, tummy tucks, arm lifts, breast lifts, facelifts, and so on — and emerge as very attractive, sexy women.

Benefiting in more ways than one

Paula, a medical office manager, found herself carrying extra weight around her middle as she recovered from having three vertebrae in her lumbar spine fused. She had difficulty walking, and her spinal surgeon agreed that removing the excess skin and fat would help her recover. Paula decided to have abdominoplasty and belt lipectomy.

In describing the surgical procedure, Paula said, "My surgical experience was great. I was up and walking that evening, and I did 15 laps around the hospital unit. My surgeon left orders for pain medication and I was very comfortable. I walked several blocks everyday starting about the fourth day post-op."

Perhaps more surprising than her relatively pain-free recovery was her actual result. "I am a patient who did this for my health and had never thought about the cosmetic results. I was absolutely stunned when I saw the results! I have a waist and hip bones for the first time in 30 years! I have never owned a pair of jeans before, and now I am in a size 8! I can wear bikini panties and they look very good, according to my husband. I am buying tight tops and pants and turning heads wherever I go! I never thought about what cosmetic surgery could do for a girl but am thrilled to pieces with my surgeon's artwork! Now I want a facelift to match my new body."

What body contouring can and can't do

The goals for body contouring surgery involve improving overall contour, reducing bulges, and improving your appearance both in and out of clothing. This surgery does have its limitations, however. Your surgeon can't eliminate all stretch marks and probably can't ever remove as much skin as you might like. Muscle strength will not be improved by tightening skin. The resting tone of the abdominal wall, however, will be improved by tightening the rectus abdominus muscles. Tightening your muscles also helps to flatten your abdomen.

If you haven't participated in an honest program of calorie management, dieting, and exercise and you have a large amount of intra-abdominal fat, body contouring procedures may not be for you at this time. The best results are obtained after weight loss has been achieved. Your surgeon can then determine where your excessive skin is located and how much extra skin he can safely remove.

An alternative for treatment can be to do nothing at all. Many heavy people have a tendency towards diabetes and increased elevation of cholesterol and, therefore, an increased potential risk for heart attacks and strokes. If this is the case, you may be better off to live with the excess skin. Many people have very loose skin that does not show under clothes. Their faces and necks may look good. Having lost the weight and looking better in clothes may be satisfaction enough.

Assessing the risks

The more involved the body contouring surgery, the greater the risk for complications. Healing delays are more common when the procedure is more complex, the incision lines are longer, and a large amount of tissue is removed. Even the best results sometimes require a secondary surgery or additional liposuction. Check out Chapter 17 to read up on the risks generally associated with cosmetic surgery.

All body contour surgeries may have temporary healing problems, including the following:

- **Discoloration:** Usually temporary and clears up with time.

- **Swelling:** Occurs to some extent after any surgery. In body contour surgery, swelling most commonly follows abdominoplasty.

- **Discomfort in the form of pain and sensitivity:** Almost all pain is usually gone within a month.

- **Numbness for a period of time:** Most common in lower abdomen.

- **Infection:** Generalized infection is very rare. Localized incision line infections occur occasionally and are treated with antibiotics, ointments, and dressings. If you experience this complication, it would most likely occur with thigh lifts and abdominoplasties.

- **Fluid collections:** Fluid collections under the skin are called *seromas*. They are most common following abdominoplasties, but can occur after any body contour procedure. If this happens, your surgeon removes this excess fluid with a syringe and needle or replaces suction drains. Seromas usually disappear within two to four weeks.

- **Skin loss:** In body contour surgery, very small areas of skin loss occur occasionally along the incision lines in the areas of maximum tension. Usually, the area heals over a period of several weeks.

- **Surface lumps and irregularities:** Surface lumpiness usually decreases or disappears over a period of several months. Special treatment or secondary surgery is seldom required.

Permanent trade-offs following contour surgery may involve the following:

- **Asymmetry:** Incisions may not heal exactly the same. Large amounts of asymmetry of either the scars or of the contour may require secondary surgery.

- **Chronic swelling, caused by a seroma:** The swelling usually disappears over a period of a month or more. Occasionally, some of the swelling may be permanent.

- **Possible need for secondary touch-up surgery:** The more surgery you have, the greater the possibility of the need for a touch up, especially after massive weight loss (see Chapter 13.)

An embolism (blood clot to the lungs), fat emboli, and ileus (temporary inactivity of intestines) can be significant complications but rarely occur. Most temporary complications resolve themselves fairly quickly, but final contouring results may not be evident for up to six months. Pulmonary emboli, discussed in Chapter 17, frequently require hospitalization and occasionally cause death. Pulmonary emboli occur more frequently in body contouring procedures than in other cosmetic surgery procedures.

Direct risks and complications involve excessive bleeding during or after surgery that makes blood transfusion necessary. If I suspect prior to surgery that blood loss during surgery may be a problem, I prefer to obtain autologous blood (the patient's own blood) ahead of time to help avoid the risks of blood bank transfusions.

Considering your health

If you're anemic, speak to your personal physician and, if appropriate, get started on therapeutic iron before surgery. If you have low hemoglobin before surgery and you lose blood during surgery, a transfusion may be required. All responsible cosmetic surgeons want to make every effort possible to avoid the need for blood bank transfusions.

If you're overweight and diabetic, lose more weight and get on an exercise program. Your diabetes problems may improve or go away. Diabetic patients have a slightly higher than average chance of infections following any surgery.

If you have a history of heart problems, see your cardiologist and discuss your desires for body surgery. He'll tell you whether you're in good enough cardiac health to proceed and, if you are, will give you clearance for your plastic surgery. If you're not in good enough cardiac condition, he may be able to get you there with new medication or an exercise program or both.

Factoring age into your decision

Age isn't the determining factor as to whether you can have body surgery. Health is. If you are older and have concurrent health issues, your personal physician, your surgeon, and the anesthesiologist will determine what surgery you can tolerate and how much you can have at one time.

Exploring gender-specific issues

There are no differences between men and women regarding usefulness of body contour surgery. Naturally, men won't need breast lifts, but occasionally, skin excision from male breasts can provide great improvement and make it easier to wear T-shirts or go to the beach.

Making Sure Your Surgeon Is a Pro

Finding the right plastic surgeon for body contour surgery requires greater attention to detail than most procedures. This procedure is major and complicated, with significant recovery issues. You certainly want to be sure that a plastic surgeon has experience doing your surgery. The vast majority of plastic surgeons are also general surgeons and have had two residencies devoted to training them to work in this area of your body. You should select a surgeon who has experience and has demonstrated that he can get the results you want. Also, the chemistry between doctor and patient is important because you'll be seeing a lot of each other if the recovery is prolonged. Check out Chapters 4 and 5 to get the complete lowdown on finding a surgeon.

Find out whether the surgeon has privileges perform the operation in a local hospital. Most cosmetic surgery is done in the physician's office-based surgery center or in other outpatient surgical centers. Privileges to perform the same surgeries in local hospitals are critical because hospital committees comprised of the surgeon's peers determine whether he is qualified to perform certain surgical procedures. If he doesn't have those privileges, find another surgeon.

Evaluating before-and-after photos

When looking at photos, you need to be brutally honest. A surgeon isn't going to show his worst results, and if his best results don't make you feel good about having similar results for yourself, try elsewhere. Photos show you reality, so look at them critically.

When evaluating pictures, remember that all of these procedures require long incisions and that the resultant scars end up being more the result of body location than the surgical skill of the surgeon. Evaluate the pictures more for contour results and whether the overall body appearance has been improved, rather than scar width. Here are some things you want to see in the photos:

 ✔ Changes that make the patient look much better

 ✔ Results that you would like to have for yourself

 ✔ Scars that look symmetrical from side to side

You don't want to see low scars on one side and high scars on the other. You want to see good evidence of competent preoperative planning coupled with great surgical skills.

Envisioning change

Imaging can be useful in giving you an idea of your new contours, but it's not capable of showing you exact results.

A surgeon needs a sensitive eye and experienced hands to sculpt the body so that you're happy with the result. The real art of cosmetic surgery is to bring the body back into proportion. Your plastic surgeon should truly have an interest in body contouring surgery. He must have enough experience so that he can realistically predict your final outcome. If the surgeon tells you that you will have absolutely no scars, that he can transform you from a size 16 to a size 8, or other similar unlikely promises, you probably should go elsewhere and deal with a surgeon who understands reality. Imaging doesn't work very well for body contouring surgery with the possible exception of showing new contour possibilities. For more on imaging, see Chapter 10.

Considering facilities and anesthesia

Your operation must take place in an accredited facility in order to assure your safety (see Chapter 3). Most body contour procedures are performed in office-based surgery suites or in outpatient surgery centers. The cost of doing these procedures in hospital operating rooms is higher, so most patients and their surgeons want to be in a safe setting but with lower facility costs.

All multiple body contour procedures are performed under general anesthesia administered by board-certified anesthesiologists or nurse anesthetists.

Getting Set for Surgery and Recovery

Body contouring surgery involves much more significant recovery than most of the procedures described in this book. You need to plan accordingly: Making the decision, getting emotionally prepared to show up at the operating room, and planning for recovery all require careful consideration.

Preparing for surgery

Some patients just aren't physically ready for surgery when they want it. Preparing for surgery may involve a change in your diet and increasing your exercise routines in order to lose those last few pounds. If you smoke, stop. Some surgeons refuse to do large body contouring procedures on patients who smoke. Your surgeon may require a preoperative evaluation by your personal physician concerning the health of your heart and your lungs.

With the help of your primary care physician, you must get diabetes and high blood pressure under control. Certain patients may have to take antibiotics before surgery or may even have to use injectable mini-dose blood thinners to avoid blood clots if they have a prior history of clotting disorders or pulmonary emboli.

At the time of your preoperative visit, you'll be told what to do in preparation for surgery. Chapters 6 and 7 let you know what you can expect.

Recovering from body contouring surgery

Because body contouring is a large operation requiring a somewhat prolonged recovery period, you must be prepared for a moderately difficult recovery period. You also need to accept the fact that, even after such a major surgery, you still probably won't be perfect.

Body contour surgeries have long incisions and leave long scars. You may have an increased risk of healing problems, small areas of superficial skin edge blistering, or even small areas of skin loss.

The dressings used, supporting garments you need to wear, and the need for drains are all important considerations that you should understand before going home. Make sure that your caregiver has a clear understanding of how to deal with dirty or bloody dressings, loose dressings, continued bloody oozing, and other similar problems before leaving the hospital or facility. After body contouring procedures, surgeons usually place drains that are pulled or withdrawn within a week.

In certain cases, such as abdominoplasty or combined procedures, you may need to recover in a hospital, at least for the first day or two. After you're at home, you need adequate nursing care (from a nurse, friend, or relative). Being comfortable and able to rest or sleep is important during your recovery. You must restrict your activities both at work and home.

Before your surgery, make all the necessary arrangements for transportation to and from the surgery center or hospital. Arrange for help at home or wherever you're going to recover.

Getting through the pain

Body contour surgeries tend to be more painful than facelifts, nasal surgeries, or liposuction, particularly if muscles need to be tightened or a thigh lift is being performed. If you don't tolerate pain well, discuss this with your surgeon and his staff at the preoperative visit so that you can have the correct pain medications on hand when you go home.

Taking it easy

After you're home, you need to take it easy, but you still must get out of bed and walk several times per day. Doing so reduces your chances of getting blood clots in your calves and also aids in your general recovery. As you feel better, you can be up more and do more nonstrenuous activities.

After the first few days, you'll be allowed to shower. If you have a thigh lift, you need to shower and cleanse yourself with antibacterial soap following each bowel movement and urination. Your surgeon will have his preferred postoperative instructions, which you should follow carefully. For more details about recovery in general, see Chapter 18.

Generally speaking, you'll be able to move around and possibly drive within 10 to 14 days, and you can resume all normal activities approximately six weeks after body contouring surgery.

Knowing what's normal

You'll see results immediately, but the swelling and bruising won't diminish and disappear for several weeks or months. The ultimate result also depends to some extent on your diet and exercise program.

Some areas may not heal as well or quickly as others. Even though abdomino-plasties are probably the most uncomfortable or painful operations I do, you'll be surprised at how quickly discomfort starts to fade.

Some bruising and swelling are normal, but call your doctor if you have extreme bruising and swelling or if you have

- ✔ An elevated temperature (above 100 degrees)
- ✔ Bleeding
- ✔ Separation of wound edges
- ✔ Pus-filled drainage
- ✔ Extreme pain

Judging the result

Large body contouring procedures take at least six months to heal com-pletely. Scars can be red or pink for a year or more. Results from the same operation may vary depending on the severity of the skin excess problem and on the patient's age and health. At your consultation, have the surgeon be specific (with pictures) about what you can expect when healed.

Dealing with disappointment

After six to nine months of healing, you'll be able to identify any areas that may benefit from touch-up surgery. Discuss them with your surgeon. Most surgeons can give you a good idea of what can be changed and what can't be fully corrected. More skin can be removed and slight asymmetries corrected, but any such procedures require a second healing period.

Surgery can't eliminate all the ravages to your skin that result from pregnancy, weight gain, and weight loss. If you understand ahead of time what the best results in your particular situation can be, you'll be much more pleased with the results.

Keep in mind that the practice of medicine and surgery isn't an exact science. Surgeons and patients can certainly expect good results, but no one can offer a guarantee or warranty, expressed or implied, as to the results that may be obtained. Unlike wood and stone, which can be perfectly carved and retain the shape, your skin may and probably will continue to stretch after the operation.

If you're really unhappy because of asymmetry, laxity, or bad scars, talk about the issues with your surgeon, who will help you if possible. If he doesn't communicate well, talk to the office administrator or staff. Working out problems calmly and rationally is almost always better than becoming angry or searching for an attorney. See Chapter 19 for more about dealing with a disappointing result.

Turning back time after childbirth

After the birth of her first baby, Colleen says that her body was just not the same but that she lacked the discipline to exercise her way back into shape. She and her husband decided after their second child was born that they would have no more children, and Colleen then felt the time was right to get her body back.

Never having had any type of plastic surgery before, Colleen found herself becoming anxious and nervous before the procedure. The communication and education she received before her procedure were extremely important in letting her know what to expect. The staff was extremely important to her. "I'm from a customer service background, so my expectations are pretty high."

Colleen said that her recovery experience was definitely not what she thought it would be. "I was prepared to be in the worst pain I have ever been in. It was all painless, and I was given all the proper medication to make my experience as comfortable as possible."

Two months after her procedure, Colleen says that she's very pleased with the results. Every day gets better and better for her. She says she can't wait to reach the six-month mark. People who know her notice how her body has changed as well as her newfound confidence. Before the surgery, she hated shopping for clothes, but now she loves to try on one thing after another. Though she's happy now, Colleen admits, "I did experience a little breakdown during my recovery. With all the swelling, I wasn't sure what the results were going to be like. Thanks to my husband, I was able to overcome it. He reminded me of everything I had read before my surgery."

Reflecting on her new outlook on life, she says, "I'm a little bit vain. When I got pregnant, I gained 35 pounds. I knew I wouldn't get back to my pre-pregnancy shape. A lot of people say I took the easy way out, but I don't care because I feel good about myself. It was worth every penny."

Chapter 13

Restructuring Your Body after Massive Weight Loss

*I*f you've lost 75 to 200 pounds or more, you may be experiencing an unexpected surprise. You've found that losing a very large amount of weight hasn't solved all your problems. You may be surrounded (literally) by your excess and sagging skin, and exercise isn't helping at all. You look down and see large and sometimes massive folds of skin hanging from everywhere on your body. You don't fit into the clothes you've been longing to wear because you have all this extra skin that has to be stuffed somewhere.

Well, the procedures you need to make your skin fit snugly onto your new body are similar to those discussed in Chapter 12, but with some major differences. This chapter deals with the variations required to achieve good results with the massive-weight-loss patient, but it doesn't repeat the basic information found in Chapter 12.

Knowing If and When You're Ready for Body Contouring Procedures

You're probably eager to get your body into its best shape after all the hard work you put into your weight loss, and you may be somewhat frustrated that the hard work (and cost) isn't over. You now need to deal with the excess skin that surrounds you. Some people determine that weight loss is the end point and live with the excess skin under their clothes. Others want the excess skin gone; if that's you, read on.

If you've lost weight, you've lost more weight in some areas than others, and your metabolism will be altered and in flux until your weight stabilizes. Ideally, you should maintain your goal weight for at least one year before considering surgery. However, if you're like many massive-weight-loss patients, you're anxious to keep moving toward your goal, and many surgeons are willing to operate on you sooner than one year after weight loss.

You need to be patient before you have the excess skin excised so that you can obtain the best result in the safest manner possible. Before embarking on the long process of reconstructing your body, make your goal realistic: Strive for the lowest weight that you can maintain for at least several months.

You need to prove to yourself and your surgeon that you can maintain a goal weight. If you have surgery before your weight is stabilized, everyone's efforts may be doomed to failure, and you and your doctor will be disappointed.

Calculating your body mass index

Your body mass index (BMI) is a calculation that physicians use that relates your total body fat to your height. You may have lost a tremendous amount of weight and still be considered obese based on your BMI. The formula works this way:

$$BMI = \text{Weight in kilograms} \div (\text{Height in meters})^2$$

And for those who don't use the metric system:

$$BMI = \text{Weight in pounds} \div (\text{Height in inches})^2 \times 703$$

If you'd rather avoid the math altogether, look up your height and weight in Table 13-1 and find your BMI without having to dig out your abacus.

Table 13-1 **Figuring Your Body Mass Index**

Height (inches)	19	20	21	22	23	24	25	26	27	28	29	30	31	32	33	34	35
	Body Weight (Pounds)																
58	91	96	100	105	110	115	119	124	129	134	138	143	148	153	158	162	167
59	94	99	104	109	114	119	124	128	133	138	143	148	153	158	163	168	173
60	97	102	107	112	118	123	128	133	138	143	148	153	158	163	168	174	179
61	100	106	111	116	122	127	132	137	143	148	153	158	164	169	175	180	185
62	104	109	115	120	126	131	136	142	147	153	158	164	169	175	180	186	191
63	107	113	118	124	130	135	141	146	152	158	163	169	174	180	186	191	197
64	110	116	122	128	134	140	145	151	157	163	169	174	180	186	192	197	204
65	114	120	126	132	138	144	150	156	162	168	174	180	186	192	198	204	210
66	118	124	130	136	142	148	155	161	167	173	179	185	192	198	204	210	216
67	121	127	134	140	146	153	159	166	172	178	185	191	198	204	211	217	223
68	125	131	138	144	151	158	164	171	177	184	190	197	203	210	216	223	230
69	128	135	142	149	155	162	169	176	182	189	196	203	209	216	223	230	236
70	132	139	146	153	160	167	174	181	188	195	202	209	216	222	229	236	243
71	136	143	150	157	165	172	179	186	193	200	208	215	222	229	236	243	250
72	140	147	154	162	169	177	184	191	199	206	213	221	228	235	242	250	258
73	144	151	159	166	174	182	189	197	204	212	219	227	235	242	250	257	265
74	148	155	163	171	179	186	194	202	210	218	225	233	241	249	256	264	272
75	152	160	168	176	184	192	200	208	216	224	232	240	248	256	264	272	279
76	156	164	172	180	189	197	205	213	221	230	238	246	254	263	271	279	287

Doctors classify BMI according to the following scale:

Less than 18.5	Underweight
18.5–24.9	Normal weight
25–29.9	Overweight
30–39.9	Obese
40 and up	Morbidly obese

You're an ideal candidate for body contouring procedures if your numbers are in the normal weight range. If you're in the overweight category, you may still be a good candidate. Don't forget that at least a few pounds will be carved off during surgery. So even if you're defined as overweight, having surgery may boost you into the normal range when all is said and done.

If you're in the obese range, however, things get a little more complicated. The procedures take longer, and the risks go up. If you truly can't lose more weight, all is not lost. A thoughtful and cautious surgical plan can usually be devised to rid you of some of that excess tissue, but because of your BMI, the surgical team must be extra careful.

Understanding your skin's limits

When you gain weight, your skin stretches by growing new cells. This phenomenon occurs naturally during pregnancy and during normal growth during childhood and adolescence. Gaining weight produces the same result. After you reach a certain size (the limit varies according to age and genetics), the skin no longer contracts when the weight is lost. If this describes your case, you may find that the weight loss isn't making you as happy as you thought it would.

The procedures discussed in this chapter won't reduce the fat within your abdominal cavity. If you have a large amount of intra-abdominal fat before surgery, it will still be there afterward, and you won't get as good a result as someone who doesn't have that fat.

Pinch your abdominal skin and see for yourself how thick the fold is. If your belly is round and protruding and the layer of outside skin and subcutaneous skin is thin, then you have a large amount of fat around your internal organs. You have what's commonly known as a "beer belly." Your surgeon can't remove internal fat; she can remove only the excess exterior skin and fat.

Considering metabolic and health issues

If you lose weight after gastric bypass surgery, a liquid diet, or any other diet, your metabolism will be altered. Metabolism is defined as the sum of all chemical and physical changes that take place within the body that enables it to continue growing and functioning.

To be on the safe side, you should live with and adjust to your new weight and get your body chemistry into normal ranges before having surgery. You may also have become anemic, so you don't want to have additional body reconstruction surgery until your blood count is normal. If you remain slightly anemic, the length of each surgical procedure may need to be reduced, resulting in shorter and more numerous operations. You may think that these guidelines seem somewhat picky, but they're important to your health and, above all, safety. The doctors who guide you through a weight loss process are most likely willing and able to work with you and your plastic surgeon in preparing you for surgery.

Factoring in your attitude

A positive and realistic attitude is extremely important when facing weight-loss surgery. The surgical and healing processes you need to go through are daunting. In losing your weight, however, you probably developed some inner strengths and resources that you'll need to call on as you move toward the next phase of creating or finding the real you.

If you're going to reduce your skin envelope following weight loss, it will take one to four operations. You'll see fabulous changes along the way, but the total process can take a year or more. Optimism makes the whole process easier for everyone, particularly you. Having and accepting realistic goals may be the most critical issue of all. If you have what seem to be yards of extra skin around your thighs, torso, upper arms, neck, and face, you need to accept that the best results in the world won't make you look perfect.

You can expect to experience emotional ups and downs. Your feelings of elation, self-esteem, excitement, and pride will alternate with impatience, disappointment, frustration, and sometimes depression. Keep in mind that this range of feelings is normal. You've probably gone on this roller coaster ride throughout your weight loss program.

You must maintain your vision of the end goal. People who expect disappointment along the way and view it as a temporary pause along the path do better than those who crumple and give way to pessimistic despair, losing sight of future success.

Looking into cost

You can expect to pay for these procedures yourself — your insurance won't be chipping in except in unusual cases. When all is said and done, you're usually looking at several tens of thousands of dollars. These are most often huge procedures that require not only hours of time in the operating room with assistant surgeons involved but also many follow-up appointments. Minor complications are common and require attention and supplies. Your surgeon will see you more often than the typical body contouring patient. All of these procedures and services translate to expense.

Don't compromise on surgical quality because you find someone who charges less. Discounts on fees often come with a discounted result. You may need to explore financing options, spreading the surgeries out over time or doing a smaller amount of surgery at each session.

Patients having this type of surgery frequently need revisions, so discuss this possibility upfront with your surgeon. You don't want to be surprised to find out that you'll have additional costs that you can't afford or don't want to pay. No matter how carefully and beautifully surgery is performed, after you heal, you may still think that your skin still isn't tight enough (it will have stretched more). If you want secondary surgery to retighten the skin, you can't expect to have it done for free, although your surgeon may offer reduced rates for these procedures.

Finding herself again

Sometimes loss in one area of life translates to gain in another. In the case of weight loss after gastric bypass surgery, people often "gain" excess, hanging skin that just won't go away — without a little help. For Sherri, excess skin became an issue when she went from 245 pounds to 140 pounds. Explaining her decision to have gastric bypass surgery, Sherri said that for two years, her weight just kept going up: "I was out of control. Although I'm a tall girl of 5-foot-9, I was miserable. Nothing fit. The only clothing store I could shop in was Lane Bryant. Cute clothes, but *big* cute clothes."

As her weight started to fall off, Sherri says, "I went shopping in a normal store and put on a pair of size 10 jeans just off the rack that fit! I stood there and cried — oh yeah, I bought the jeans!"

Once down to her goal weight, Sherri was thrilled with her new shape, but her husband told her she had "80-year-old thighs" because of the sagging skin on her legs from the rapid weight loss.

Sherri underwent a breast lift and extended lower body lift, which corrected the problem with her thighs. Of her results she told us, "I'm seven weeks post operation. I'm happy with the result, but I'm still a work in progress. Now my weight is 137, and I look like the woman I want to be. Tall and lean, with young girl thighs and a tight butt."

There's one exception to the rule of self-pay. Your insurance plan may include payment for belt lipectomy (an operation that removes abdominal and lower back skin, as well as lifting your buttocks) because this procedure, which I discuss in more detail in Chapter 12, relieves stress from your lower back and improves back pain in some cases. Some insurance companies understand that the massive amount of excess skin that can be present following big weight loss can interfere with normal life activities. Unfortunately, fewer and fewer plans include payment for these procedures, but check with your insurance company. An accompanying letter from your physician and, eventually, even from your attorney may help with your request for approval.

Checking Out Your Options

Several types of operations are available for removing loose skin in different areas of your body. Unwanted skin can be removed anywhere — if you're willing to trade the excess skin for scars. Many of these procedures are performed on average-weight patients as well (see Chapter 12), but for people who've lost a lot of weight, the procedures are usually more extensive, with longer incisions to eliminate the excess skin frequently seen. Secondary or revisionary surgery is much more common.

Looking at your face and neck

Facial and neck skin may become very lax following massive weight loss. Even if you're young, you can find yourself in need of a facelift and/or neck lift. See Chapter 9 for more detail about these procedures. And if you find yourself with a saggy neck or face at age 35, don't worry. Facial surgery works beautifully at any age.

If a moderate amount of excess facial and neck skin is present, the incisions can be placed in the standard locations (see Chapter 9) within the temporal area and behind your ears. If you have an excessive amount of facial and neck skin, placing the incisions in front of the hairline above and in front of the ear and within or below the hairline behind the ears may be a better approach. Your surgeon may extend your incisions all the way around the back of your head and add a vertical incision in the midline at the junction of your neck and scalp to excise all the extra skin that is present. You and your surgeon can easily resolve these issues during a presurgery discussion.

Figure 13-1 shows you the results of a facelift after massive weight loss.

Figure 13-1:
Massive
weight loss
left this
patient with
an excess of
sagging
facial skin,
which was
removed
with a
facelift.

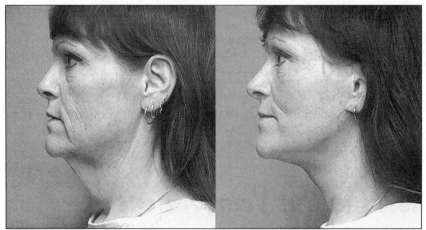

Lifting your arms

Arm lifts *(brachioplasties)* work very well if you've lost a large amount of weight and your arm skin is very saggy. If you're the typical patient for arm lift surgery, when you hold your arms out, you have so much extra skin that your arms resemble wings. In fact, patients frequently refer to their arms as "bat wings." If you have this condition, your extra skin won't fit into the sleeves of your blouses or shirts, and you probably avoid sleeveless attire because of embarrassment.

Surgery can eliminate the excess skin on your arms. You have to accept the fact that you'll have scars that run from the inner elbow up into your under-arm area and even beyond. The incisions can be placed so they're in the least visible location, but the scars will be there forever.

If you have lost a large amount of weight and have excess upper arm skin, you probably also have excess skin in your underarm, side, back, and chest areas. Standard upper arm lifts (see Chapter 12) usually have an incision that extends from the elbow to the armpit area. In your case, however, you may need to continue the excision of excess skin down your side. Having an arm lift and a breast lift at the same time (see Figures 13-2 and 13-3), with the incisions connected, can reduce or eliminate the excess skin in that entire area.

Lifting your breasts

Even if you've had success in losing weight, you may be discouraged when you look at your breasts. You're likely to see droopy breast skin that is flat and empty-looking and nipples that point down toward the floor. Well, all is not lost. Most often, standard mastopexies, or breast lift procedures (discussed in Chapter 16), with breast implants will restore the perkiness and volume of your breasts.

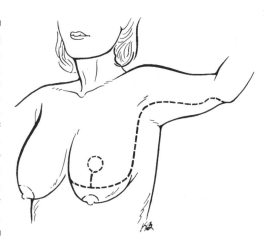

Figure 13-2: An incision stretching from the breast to the elbow is the trade-off when trying to get your arms and breasts up where they used to be.

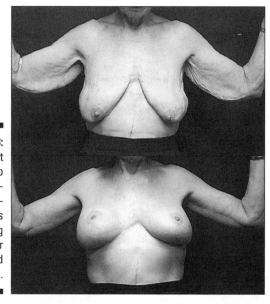

Figure 13-3: This patient returned to pre-weight-gain measurements after having both her breasts and arms lifted.

Keep in mind that, as a result of your weight loss, your breasts probably now sit lower on your chest wall. It is nearly impossible for surgeons to raise the fold beneath your breasts in a manner that lasts. When your surgeon lifts your breasts, she determines the location of your nipples in relationship to the fold beneath it. Thus surgeons frequently advise their patients to add an implant that gives fullness in the upper breast that the lift alone will not achieve. In many instances, the placement of high-profile implants accomplishes this result nicely. Figure 13-4 shows a patient who had a breast lift and augmentation following massive weight loss.

Figure 13-4:
A breast lift and augmentation can help breasts that hang low.

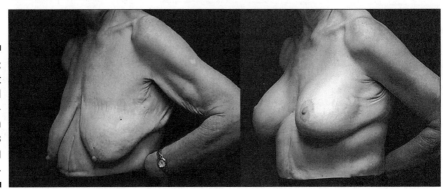

If you and your surgeon agree that you need both a breast lift and breast augmentation, your surgeon may choose to lift your breasts first and perform your augmentation as a second surgery at a later time. Dividing the surgery into two stages increases safety, because of issues of blood supply to the skin.

Following massive weight loss, your back and side skin may be almost as loose and saggy as your breasts. In that case, the incisions for your breast lift can continue around your side (through your underarms) toward your back so that excess skin in those areas can also be removed.

Another word of caution: Be realistic about the breast size that you really want. Don't get greedy and ask for D-cup breasts. It's a known and well-documented fact that breasts that large sag much more than smaller breasts. Your skin has even less elasticity than those women who haven't lost large amounts of weight, so be realistic about your wishes.

Facing your back

Consider for a moment the skin firmly attached to your spine and your breastbone. As you lost weight, the skin between them got looser and began to sag, but the attachments in the front and back held firm. As a result you now have a "swag" around the side of your chest that looks something like the one over the draperies in your living room.

What to do? Well in more extreme cases, the best solution is to remove the tissue, making the incision along the fold beneath the "swag" (see Figure 13-5).

This procedure leaves you with a long scar on either side of your back, extending toward your breasts, but you may have no other choice. At least you won't have breasts coming *and* going.

Figure 13-5: Even the skin on your back sags after massive weight loss, and a lot needs to be removed.

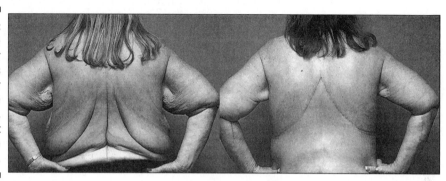

In less drastic weight loss cases, your surgeon can tighten your back with incisions along the side of your chest (see the previous section, "Lifting your breasts"). Depending on your specific needs, your surgeon can design an operation to remove your excess skin.

Looking at your lower body

You may have a huge amount of excess skin hanging from your belly following massive weight loss. In medical terms, this fold of skin is called a *pannus* or *panniculus adiposus*. When it's lifted during an examination, you realize that your pubic area is sagging too. In the rearview mirror (an apt description if ever there was one), you discover that your buttocks have shrunk and are sagging as well. In such cases, surgeons lengthen the standard tummy tuck (see Chapter 12) incision to encircle your trunk like a belt. Hence it is called a belt lipectomy (*lipectomy* meaning excision of fat).

If you're having a belt lipectomy, your excess abdominal and back tissue will be pulled down, and the front and sides of your thighs as well as your buttocks will be pulled up. Your lower back rolls will disappear. Although a belt lipectomy will help tighten your buttocks and outer thighs, it won't help with your inner thighs. See the next section, "Solving your thigh problems."

If you had gastric bypass surgery, any hernias (out-pouching of abdominal contents through a weak area in the abdominal scar) from that surgery may need to be repaired. Hernias are much less likely in patients who have lost weight through diet and exercise and have not had a surgical incision.

If your surgeon didn't perform your gastric bypass with a laparoscope, you may have an incision down the center of your abdominal wall. When the abdominal tissues are pulled lower to do the abdominoplasty, the scar from the bypass may not stretch. It may need to be excised or revised in order to achieve the best result. In extreme cases, a wedge of skin can be removed from the center of your abdominal wall. This wedge can be very useful in helping to tighten your abdomen skin from side to side (horizontally). Horizontal looseness can be as much of a problem as vertical looseness following massive weight loss. Adding a vertical wedge excision will add approximately an hour or more to your surgery but usually doesn't increase postoperative pain or recovery time.

Solving your thigh problems

Standard or medial thigh lifts tighten excess skin on your *inner* thighs, and to a lesser extent, the front and back of your thighs. Your surgeon places an incision that starts above your pubic area and then curves down your groin crease and onto your buttocks.

If you have exceptionally loose inner thigh skin, extending the incision far up and to the outside of the buttocks allows for additional tightening. In extreme cases, making a vertical wedge incision down toward the inner knee may be an option. Doing this decreases the circumference of your thigh and tightens the skin, but at the cost of a permanent scar extending from your groin area toward the inside of your knee. Your surgeon must anchor your thigh tissues to the stronger and deeper tissues in your groin to keep them pulled up tight and to reduce downward movement of the thigh skin due to gravity.

Healing problems in this area are more common because of the likelihood of fecal and urinary contamination with subsequent infection. See Chapter 12 for more details about thigh lifts.

Liposuction can enhance your results at this stage by reducing the volume of your thighs and loosening the tissues so they can be pulled tighter. The tunnels created by the liposuction allow more "give" to the skin.

Total body lift

Total body lift combines circumferential thigh lift, buttock lift, lower back lift, and, frequently, abdominoplasty. Not every plastic surgeon performs this very extensive procedure. This operation is very well suited to patients who have had massive weight loss, and the results can be stunning. The procedure is major enough that it requires an assistant surgeon, and in most cases no other procedures are performed at the same time. You may not be a candidate for this operation for any one of a number of reasons including but not limited to health, anemia, weight, and cost. Most patients require some period of hospitalization following this procedure.

PERSONAL STORY

Breathing life back into a deflated doll

After undergoing gastric bypass surgery, Betty described herself as being left with a ton of excess skin and felt like a deflated blowup doll. Realizing that nothing but plastic surgery could help remove the extra skin and fat, she interviewed five plastic surgeons. She based her choice on the one who provided the most thorough discussion of priorities. They decided to tackle her arms, back, and breasts first.

Of her first surgery, Betty said: "I was so amazed. The day after surgery when she removed the bandages and I saw what she had done, I started crying. I was so amazed what a transformation she had made. Right then I wanted to book the next surgery, but my surgeon said I had to wait for three months until the next one. I decided to have my stomach and rear end lift next." Betty was thrilled when 12 pounds of skin and fat were removed with the next procedure.

Eight months after her first surgery, Betty had a facelift and liposuction of her legs. She says that her new face makes her look 15 years younger. The outcome of all the surgeries has exceeded her expectations, and she can't say enough good things about her surgeon and her new body: "My life is changing daily. I get very emotional when I stop and look at myself. Since losing 222 pounds, I sometimes don't see 'me' in the mirror. In fact, one day as I was walking from the parking structure to the surgery center, I looked in the mirrored glass windows and said to myself, 'That woman has the same sweater on that I do.' I finally realized that woman was me."

WARNING!

Never consider redoing your entire body with a surgeon who has no experience with total body lift. This operation is too complex to trust to a neophyte.

Combining and staging your procedures

If you're like most weight-loss patients, you'll be impatient to get everything done and over with. Time off work, money, and help with the house and kids may all be in short or at least dwindling supply. I suggest that you fix first what bothers you the most. If your tummy and breasts are the biggest problems in your mind, you may be able to improve them in one go.

Doing as much surgery at one time as possible is a good idea within limits. Your surgeon wants to avoid giving you a transfusion, so combining multiple procedures if your blood count is low is a definite no-no. Most hospitals frown heavily on transfusing any blood for elective procedures. If your surgeon suggests that you break up one large operation for two or three smaller ones, listen. She has your safety in mind.

If you've had a gastric bypass, anemia may be a limiting factor. The speed of your surgeon and the presence (or absence) of an assistant surgeon also play a role in deciding how much can be done at one surgical sitting.

After each operation, your body needs to recover. Healing takes time, and waiting at least three months between procedures is usually the best approach. Skin often stretches after surgery and may need to be tightened some more at the next step in your reconstruction. The bottom line is that it's not safe to reconstruct your body in one operation, but you and your surgeon will wish to accomplish the final result in as few operations as possible. Financial constraints may force you to spread things out further.

Making the Right Choices

You've been strong enough to lose the weight. Now you need to be smart enough to make the right choice about where and with whom to have your surgery. Of all the seemingly endless cosmetic procedures there are to choose from, none are as large and demanding of skill and knowledge as the ones I discuss in this chapter. The choices you make in the beginning can make all the difference between an excellent result and disaster.

Choosing the right surgeon

Experience is crucial for these procedures. Look for a surgeon who has treated massive weight-loss patients and who can show you results you can accept. The surgeon should have an office and staff you like because you'll be spending a lot of time there. Unquestionably, you must choose a board-certified plastic surgeon. A head and neck surgeon hasn't been trained in surgery of the body. A general surgeon hasn't the aesthetic training of a plastic surgeon. See Chapter 3 for more about these issues.

For massive weight-loss patients, physician and patient referrals can be invaluable. Ask the surgeon that performed your gastric bypass who she recommends.

Be sure that the surgeon you choose is adept at these more complex procedures. You want a surgeon who handles these cases regularly and has experience with the nuances that set your case apart from the more typical body contouring patient discussed in Chapter 12.

Looking at before-and-after photos

Before-and-after photos of body reconstruction following massive weight loss can be very informative. The most critical points to evaluate are whether the reconstructed area looks like a result you would be happy with and whether the patient's body is symmetrical. You also want to consider whether the incisions look the same from side to side.

The surgeon has relatively little control over how wide the scars end up, but she does have control over symmetry. Ask yourself whether you can be happy with the average results that you're shown. Body reconstruction surgeries are complex, making perfect results uncommon. The amount of skin to be removed is much greater than in normal body contouring procedures, such as breast lifts or abdominoplasties.

Selecting the right office

Your surgeon isn't the only person you have to choose carefully. The entire office staff will be involved in your care. The nurses, for example, are the ones who will change your dressings, pull out drains, remove sutures, renew medications, and field your calls. When you interview a surgeon, ask who will be doing these things and meet those people to see whether you like them and feel that they will be caring and competent.

Office location is an important issue for massive-weight-loss patients. You want an office within a reasonable distance from your home. Because of the nature of these procedures, you'll be in the office frequently, and traveling there over a long distance puts a strain on everyone, especially when you're unable to do the driving yourself, which often will be the case.

Unless you plan to live in another city for an extended period of time, surgery in another city is quite unrealistic. Under no circumstances should you plan on flying to your destination. You may read about a surgeon in another state who sounds like exactly the person for you. No matter how good that surgeon may be, she's the wrong choice unless you own a private jet. Period.

Choosing the right operating facility

Many surgeons want to do these surgeries in the hospital setting. This is certainly the safest place to have such large procedures done, but having hospital-based surgery that isn't covered by insurance is usually cost-prohibitive. Check on the costs before you sign up. Your surgeon may have quoted costs that fit your budget, but make certain that you won't be billed for additional operating room and anesthesia charges if your surgery should happen to take longer than scheduled. Some surgeons (usually in groups) are busy enough that they have their own operating rooms.

If you're considering surgery in an office-based surgery suite rather than at the hospital or independent surgery center, be sure to check the operating suite certification (see Chapter 3).

Following most of your procedures, you'll need to recover in a hospital setting. If you aren't having your surgery in the hospital, be sure you understand how you'll be transferred (usually by ambulance) and how much the transfer and the hospital stay will cost.

Be on the lookout for hidden costs. Many hospitals have designed programs for the care of plastic surgery patients in which the costs are bundled into one price that includes the medications, IV fluids, and so on. Try to avoid a situation where you're charged a fee for the room and must pay regular hospital rates for every additional item — from pain pills to pain pumps. Ask the patient coordinator at your surgeon's office for this information.

Considering anesthesia

You'll need a general anesthetic for most of your procedures, and you'll want to make sure that a board-certified anesthesiologist or a nurse anesthetist is administering it.

For the level of surgery involved here and the health issues related to massive weight loss, I recommend an anesthesiologist. Such a doctor has the years of medical training necessary to best judge your overall medical needs and attend to any complications during the procedure should they arise.

Preparing for Surgery

The surgical procedures after major weight loss are very complex, so you need to have all your ducks in a row before surgery. Who's going to take care of you during all these recoveries? What about the kids? How much time can you get off work and when? Little things and not so little things like this all require a lot of planning. Completing your body reconstruction could take a year or more, so planning the entire event deserves thoughtful preparation.

Getting medical clearance

Age and years of strain on the heart from your period of obesity often make an electrocardiogram (EKG) necessary. If the EKG reveals any abnormalities, you may need further evaluation with a stress test or echocardiogram. A cardiologist may need to evaluate your condition and either clear you for surgery or order other tests.

If you've had a gastric bypass, changes in your metabolism need to be assessed and corrected if possible. Chances are, a physician is monitoring your condition and can assure your surgeon and anesthesiologist that you can safely undergo surgery. Don't feel put out by these delays. They're precautions in place to assure your safety and reduce the risk of prolonged and complicated recoveries. Check out Chapter 7 for more information about getting ready for surgery.

Preparing for potential blood loss

If your procedure is a large one and you don't have anemia, you may be required to donate a unit of your own blood before surgery, ideally several weeks ahead of time. You'll take iron supplements after that to ensure that, by the time of your surgery, your blood counts are back up to normal limits. You want to go into the operating room with a "full tank" and some to spare in the blood bank should you need it.

 If you're anemic, designate a donor whose blood matches yours and have the donor give the blood ahead of time — just a few days before surgery. The risks associated with receiving banked blood are very low, but not zero. Nevertheless, plan ahead and leave anonymous blood available to those who need it unexpectedly and in an emergency.

Lining up nutritional support

Good nutrition plays an important role in your general well-being and in your surgical outcome. Complex surgeries such as those following massive weight loss put a strain on your system at many different levels. Following gastric bypass surgery (and even after weight loss from dieting), calcium, vitamin B12, and iron levels all tend to be low. Most such patients are advised to take multivitamins, B12, calcium, and iron for a year or longer after completion of their surgery. Your need for good nutrition is even greater when you're going through a period of multiple large surgeries.

Understanding the Risks

You can read about the risks of all the procedures you'll be having in both Chapter 17 and Chapter 12, but your situation presents some significant variations, and you need to understand how massive weight loss affects known risks:

✔ **Infection:** Infection is a risk with any surgery, no matter the extent. Most likely your surgeon will prescribe antibiotics around the time of your surgery, but in spite of that, infection can still occur, particularly in the following situations:

- If your BMI is high, you'll have a thicker layer of fat in the operative areas. Fat has a relatively poor blood supply, which makes it more prone to infection.

- If you're diabetic, the chances of bacteria multiplying on the excess sugar in your system are higher. If you use insulin, your requirements will go up temporarily. Diligence in monitoring and adjusting your dose is critical.

✔ **Seromas:** Suction drains that remove fluid after surgery will be placed into the operative site. These allow the raw surfaces underneath to heal together as quickly as possible. These drains are usually removed within one week. Sometimes the wound surfaces don't heal as quickly as desired, and fluid continues to collect in that space, forming a *seroma,* after the drains are removed. The seroma fluid has to be removed (aspirated) with a needle or the drain replaced. This is most common with abdominoplasties and belt lipectomies but can occur with thigh lifts, back lifts, or upper arm lifts, as well. The incidence of seromas in belt lipectomies can be as high as 37.5 percent.

✔ **Wound separation:** All of your incisions will be closed in several layers. Infrequently, one of the layers may come apart. Occasionally small separations can be resutured, but more often, dressing changes and time heal the wound. Areas that are more prone to wound separation tend to be the center of your back, the hips, and the groin. Wound separation is much more common among massive weight-loss patients than in patients of normal weight.

✔ **Deep venous thrombosis (DVT):** DVT means that clots form in the deep veins of your lower legs. Circulation of the deep veins of your calves slows under general anesthesia. The flow may be decreased further by the pressure put on your abdomen as the muscles are tightened during surgery. During long procedures, you need to take precautions to ensure that clots don't form in your calves. DVT is the leading cause of death in body contouring surgery. You may need to give yourself small injections of a blood thinner daily for a week or so, but the needle is small and relatively painless. Find out more about DVT in Chapter 17.

✔ **Lymphedema (swelling caused by excess lymphatic fluids):** Your lymphatic system carries the swelling (body or lymphatic fluids) away from injured tissues and circulates it back into your blood system. Given time, the lymphatic system will usually clear away the excess fluid from the tissues. Rarely, the lymphatic ducts remain blocked and cause chronic swelling, which is most likely to happen when the inner thighs are lifted. The main lymphatic drainage of the leg passes through the groin and is at risk for injury.

Coping with Recovery

For the massive surgeries discussed in this chapter, you must make detailed plans for your recovery period. You'll need a lot of rest and a lot of help from your friends and family. Because these operations are large, minor healing problems are more common, and all the incision lines may not completely heal for a month or more.

Enlisting emotional support

You'll probably be on an emotional roller coaster ride after each operation. After all, you'll be uncomfortable, and your body will be hard at work healing itself, which tends to make you exhausted and cranky. You'll be excited (and probably a little impatient) to check out your results, and no doubt you'll wonder whether you made the right decision. All this physical and mental strain can add up to periods of frustration, disappointment, and possibly depression.

Because this process is such a big deal, you need someone on your team to champion your cause. A loving spouse or partner is a good start if you have one. Close friends and family members are wonderful additions. Going this alone is very difficult and, perhaps, unwise.

Enduring complications

Without question, higher rates of complications occur among massive-weight-loss patients because their surgeries are more extensive and more frequent. Most complications are not serious, however, and are usually annoying and prolong healing rather than causing a bad result. Not infrequently, you can anticipate having more than one complication. Expect them, and try to keep a positive attitude, which makes the situation easier on everyone. Major complications can occur even when all the seemingly necessary precautions have been taken, but fortunately, they're rare. Instead of fretting and casting blame in every direction, focus on doing whatever is necessary to get yourself through it and back on the right track. For more on this topic, see Chapter 19.

Planning for revisions

Make revisions part of your overall surgical plan. For example, no matter how carefully your surgeon draws and makes the incisions, they often end up slightly asymmetrical, a problem that's not hard to correct but does require another surgery. Or another possibility is that you may need revisional surgery because your tissues will stretch a few centimeters within six months after surgery, no matter how tight they were pulled during surgery. (Keep in mind that your tissues don't have the resilience of people of normal weight.) These problems are frustrating both to you and to your surgeon, but don't lose faith in your surgeon. Revisions become a part of the next stage.

Adapting body contouring procedures

Procedures for massive weight-loss patients are similar to those for standard body contouring, but they address some additional concerns and can be a bit more extensive. The major difference between body lift procedures following massive weight loss and the same procedures on non-weight-loss patients is the *extent* of the excess skin present.

For example, in the average non-weight-loss tummy tuck, the excess skin is limited to the abdomen, and an abdominoplasty solves the problem perfectly. Following massive weight loss, the excess skin in the same operation may involve the pubic area, the upper thighs, the hips, the back, and the buttocks. Skin is loose in several areas of the body, not just the tummy. Tightening only the abdominal skin may not make you as happy as you want to be.

Chapter 14

Increasing Your Assets: Breast Augmentation

So you want a little help with the size of your breasts but are too scared to ask. Or embarrassed. Or both. Never fear! You've come to the right place for information to help you make a decision about breast augmentation surgery. This chapter is a comfortable, nonthreatening place to get answers to your questions — or most of them anyway, I hope. Though there has been lots of ink spilled and lots of chat online, the reality is that breast augmentation is successful more than 95 percent of the time. However, as a consumer you still need to make an informed decision after considering the risks.

Sorting Out the Silicone Scare

Concerns about the safety of silicone gel implants became a national news issue in 1990. Based on an exposé by a network television reporter and science that has since been disproven, tort attorneys, some women's organizations, the popular press, and the U.S. Food and Drug Administration (FDA) started campaigning against the reported dangers of breast augmentation.

Tracing the troubles and trials

Before the most recent generation of breast implants, some patients had bad experiences with them. Problems included leakage of silicone through intact implant shells or the rupture or tearing of implant shells, allowing large amounts of silicone gel to be free within the breast cavity. These problems led to *capsule formation* (scar tissue around the implants that causes breast hardness), occasional infection, and the migration of silicone gel into lymph nodes near the breast.

A group of attorneys filed class-action lawsuits attacking the Dow Corning company, then the major manufacturer of silicone gel itself and one of the makers of gel implants, alleging that silicone gel caused several connective tissue disorders such as scleroderma, rheumatoid arthritis, fibromyalgia, polymyositis, and lupus. Those lawsuits included thousands of women plaintiffs and were eventually settled for billions of dollars.

The FDA responded to the pressure of the patients who felt that their complications resulted from silicone gel and to the pressure of the negative publicity. Hearings were held, and silicone gel implants were eventually removed from the marketplace with some significant exceptions: Silicone implants can be used as part of a large nationwide study for a variety of reconstructive procedures.

Coming around to silicone safety

The medical community has learned a lot since the implant litigation began in the early 1990s. This new knowledge makes it clear that the entire premise of the litigation and settlements was incorrect. In truth, women who have had silicone implants and women who have not had silicone implants develop connective tissue disorders at the same rate. These findings refute or discredit the entire basis for the lawsuits and the removal of silicone implants from the marketplace by the FDA.

The manufacture of silicone implants (and saline implants as well) has improved dramatically over the past 10 years. The implant shells have become much stronger and less permeable. They don't leak easily. Since this improvement, capsule formation and breast deformity have diminished dramatically. If the FDA lifted its silicone restrictions today, most plastic surgeons would now use silicone implants (rather than saline implants) for all types of breast augmentation or reconstruction. Currently, the two major manufacturers of breast implants (Mentor Corporation and Inamed) are in the midst of new FDA clinical trials for silicone gel implants, and breast implant surgeons consider it only a matter of time before silicone gel implants are once again available for use in all augmentation mammoplasty procedures.

Comparing Implant Options

Saline and silicone implants both have advantages, and both types of implants can and do produce excellent breast augmentation results. Because of current FDA restrictions, for most women having breast augmentation, saline implants are the only option. Silicone implants can be used for reconstructive purposes during augmentation procedures — if you have had previous breast reconstruction or a chest wall deformity, if there's a large difference in your breast sizes, or if you also need a breast lift at the same time.

Saline implants

Before it's placed in a breast, a saline implant essentially feels like a plastic sandwich bag filled with water. It's constructed of an outer shell of several layers of silicone rubber that includes a valve. Saline implants are usually filled to their final size by a disposable tube that runs from a bag of saline to the implant within the breast cavity. When the tube is withdrawn, the valve seals automatically, and a small additional sealing tip attached to the implant is inserted into the top of the valve.

Implants come in various sizes ranging from 150cc (cubic centimeters) to approximately 700cc. The smaller sizes, from 150cc to 400cc are available in 25 to 30cc size increments. Above 400cc, the increments are 50cc.

Here are some facts about saline implants:

- **Cost:** Saline implants are about half as expensive as silicone gel implants.

- **Feel:** Saline implants can be somewhat less soft and feel less natural than silicone gel implants. The best results with saline implants, however, are comparable to the best results with silicone gel implants.

- **Volume:** Saline implants enable surgeons to microadjust the volume in each implant. When the initial breast size isn't the same on each side, the surgeon can microadjust volume to balance the two sides.

- **Wrinkling:** In many augmented breasts, saline implants can be felt at the bottom or along the lower sides as an edge or as slight wrinkles. This effect is normal.

Silicone gel implants

Silicone gel implants have a shell made of several layers of silicone rubber. In prior generations of silicone implants, the wall or covering of the implants was weaker and more porous. The silicone within the implants was runnier, and small amounts of the silicone would bleed through the implant walls. The silicone now used in gel implants is semi-solid (non-runny and less likely to migrate). Reduced silicone bleed has probably resulted in reduced capsule formation.

Here are some other important facts about silicone gel implants:

- ✔ **Cost:** Silicone gel implants cost about twice as much as saline implants, a problem if the cost of surgery is an issue to you.

- ✔ **Feel:** Silicone gel implants feel softer and more natural than saline implants.

- ✔ **Wrinkling:** If capsule formation does occur, silicone gel implants can develop wrinkling. In general, however, silicone implants don't develop the edge wrinkling that is common with saline implants.

- ✔ **Volume:** No microadjustment in volume of the implants can be made. The implants are completely sealed. From the smallest size available up to 400cc, the implants come in 25 to 30cc size differences. Above 400cc, the different sizes vary by 50cc. This has one small disadvantage in that most breasts normally vary in size, from one side to the other. If size variations can't be corrected in 25 to 50cc increments, some slight asymmetry in breast size will remain.

Other implant options

Although 85 percent of breast augmentations are performed with smooth round saline implants, some other types of implants are also being used:

- ✔ *Textured implants* have a rough outer covering. In the past ten or more years, when there was a high rate of capsule formation, surgeons felt that texturing the implant surface reduced the incidence of capsule formation. Textured implants are available in round shapes, but are also available in anatomic, or teardrop, shapes.

  Most plastic surgeons have abandoned textured implants because they are perceived by many to cause increased rippling and a higher incidence of capsules and consequently are much easier to feel than the newest smooth, round saline implants.

- ✔ *High-profile implants* allow you to have more volume in a narrower base width. Many surgeons use breast measurements to determine the maximum width of breast implant that can be used on a patient without causing distortion. If a small woman with small breasts and a narrow chest wall wishes to be a C or D cup size, the appropriate standard profile implant that fits her frame may not have enough volume to achieve the size she wants.

Is there a breast augmentation– breast cancer link?

No. You read that correctly: *no!* Multiple studies have shown that if you're going to die from breast cancer, women with and without breast implants die at the same rate. Nevertheless, you'll want to be more careful if breast cancer is an issue in your family. In any event, after augmentation, tell your mammography technician that implants are present and she will take one or two extra views. Discuss with your surgeon whether you should consider baseline mammography prior to surgery.

Understanding Anatomy

Breasts are made of glandular tissue (which produces milk after pregnancy), ducts that connect the glandular tissue to the nipple, fat, and connective tissue. Breasts sit above the pectoralis muscles and the muscular fascia (the strong thin covering of the pectoralis muscles). The nipple and the surrounding circle of darker skin (areola) are referred to as the *nipple-areolar complex*. Implants may be inserted above or below the pectoralis muscles (see Figure 14-1).

Figure 14-1:
Together with your surgeon, you'll decide whether over or under the muscle placement is the best option.

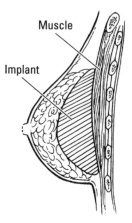
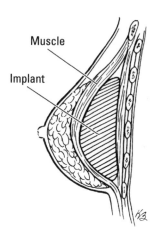

Aging makes the connective tissue looser and stretchier. Gravity can pull the tissue, making breasts sag. We frequently see women around 50 who never had children and who always had small breasts. They often have perfectly shaped, nonsaggy breasts. Since there was little weight in the breasts, gravity was not as effective.

Checking Into Types of Procedures

The procedure that's right for you depends on your specific anatomy and your goals. As you consider undergoing a procedure, be sure that you really understand what the surgeon will be doing in order to address your particular concerns. Armed with this information, you can make the smartest decision.

If you go to consultations with three different surgeons and get three slightly different suggestions, it doesn't mean that one surgeon is right and two are wrong. All three may be right. This is an area of cosmetic surgery where no one knows a single best approach. Many surgeons continue doing a certain procedure because they have found that it works for them.

Incision locations

You and your surgeon will have to make a decision about where to place your breast augmentation incisions (see Figure 14-2) and where to place the implant (under or above the pectoralis muscle). You have four options for incision placement and each involves trade-offs that you must consider carefully. You will have a permanent scar no matter where your incision. Scars usually gradually fade in color over several months, but they never disappear.

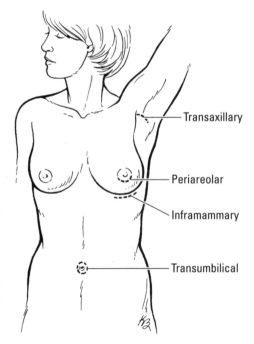

Figure 14-2: Four possible incisions for placement of breast implants.

Transaxillary

Periareolar

Inframammary

Transumbilical

Periareolar

The incision is made around the bottom or the inner half of the edge of the areola (the dark circular area surrounding the nipple). Your surgeon cuts through your breast tissue, and permanent damage to some of your breast ducts may occur. Damaged ducts will not be available for breastfeeding, but because the area damaged is small, you will still be able to breastfeed. These scars are usually thin because the areolar skin heals better than the surrounding breast skin.

Inframammary

Probably the approach used most often, the inframammary incision is made in the crease below the breast. The scars may end up a little wider than those from periareolar incisions, but the dissection for the augmentation doesn't go through the breast tissue at all.

Transaxillary

This incision is made high in the underarm rather than on or near the breasts. Surgeons who are comfortable with this approach can achieve excellent results; however, breast asymmetry after surgery is more common. The scar from this incision is visible when you raise your arms, unlike the previous two methods, which leave scars that are visible only when you're nude.

Transumbilical breast augmentation (TUBA)

This incision is made around the belly button. A tunnel dissection, under the skin and up to the breast area, is made with special instruments. Another instrument is used to make the pockets for the implants. Although the surgical approach seems unusual, the procedure works well in qualified and experienced hands. Breast symmetry is an issue with this approach, and the implants are usually placed above the pectoralis muscle.

Submuscular augmentation

Approximately 85 percent of women who have breast augmentation end up having this procedure. Submuscular placement of round smooth saline implants gives you the best chance of having soft breasts with good shape. It's the most appropriate technique when your breasts are essentially the same size and have normal shape.

During surgery, the implants are placed partially below your pectoralis muscles. The upper part of the implant is under the muscle and approximately the lower third of the implant is covered by breast tissue as well as skin and fat. There are two important advantages to this technique:

- ✔ An extra layer of cover for the implants (the muscular layer)
- ✔ The possibility of reduced chances of capsule formation

You can choose to have your incision either in the crease under your breast or around the lower or inner areolar margin or under your arm. Placing the incision under the breast means that the breast tissue itself is never damaged and no breast ducts are ever cut. This ensures that you be able to make and deliver as much breast milk as possible if you have children. Figure 14-3 shows you the results of a sub-muscular augmentation.

Figure 14-3: This patient chose to have her implants placed under the muscle through incisions around her nipples.

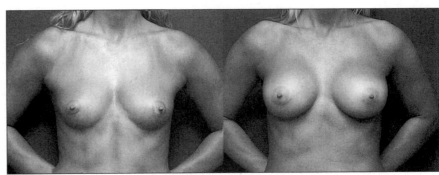

Subglandular augmentation

Some breast surgeons prefer placing the implants on top of the pectoralis muscles and under the breast (glandular) tissue. If your breasts are slightly saggy, sub-glandular placement may be the best way of achieving natural shape because the implants can be placed slightly lower, thereby centering the implants behind the nipple. If the implants are placed higher, the breast tissue can droop over the bottom of the implants.

Placing the implants on top of the muscle increases the chances that you will be able to feel the edge of the implant and that you will be able to feel more wrinkles. Nevertheless, if you have strong reasons to place the implant on top of the muscle (maybe you have slightly saggy breasts but don't want a breast lift), do not fear. You will probably get a good result. Figure 14-4 shows you the results of a subglandular augmentation.

Figure 14-4: To enhance the appearance of her small breasts, this patient had implants placed over the muscle.

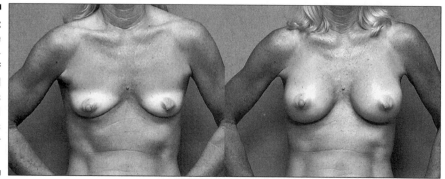

Generally, you can expect to experience less postoperative discomfort if the implants are placed on top of the muscles because this surgical technique involves less dissection. There are sound reasons why most surgeons use the submuscular technique in the majority of patients. If your surgeon suggests the subglandular technique, be sure you understand why. It's easier to dissect the pocket above the muscle, but you don't want your surgeon to use that approach just because it's easier.

Placing the implants above the muscle may lead to an increase in rippling (the ability to feel the implant through the skin) and the telltale appearance of a breast that has been "done" — like a half grapefruit on your chest wall.

Combining augmentation with a short-incision breast lift

For patients with small amounts of sagginess, augmentation may be combined with a short-incision breast lift. If you're slightly or moderately saggy, the removal of an ellipse of skin above the areola or the removal of a "doughnut" of skin around the entire areola can lift the nipple areolar complex. If you choose to have such a lift, the surgeon will place the implants through those incisions.

Any type of breast lift, done for a medical reason in combination with augmentation mammoplasty, allows the patient and surgeon to opt for the use of silicone implants. Many patients wish to take advantage of this loophole in FDA regulations in order to use silicone gel implants rather than saline implants. Obviously, if your breasts aren't saggy, you and your surgeon can't take advantage of this option.

For more about breast lifts, see Chapter 15.

Transaxillary breast augmentation

In this technique, your surgeon tunnels from an inconspicuous incision in your underarm, goes under the pectoralis muscles, and creates a pocket for placement of the implants.

Transaxillary augmentation mammoplasty can be performed with or without an endoscope. (An *endoscope* is an instrument that allows your surgeon to work in the "pocket" where your implant will rest while viewing the area on a television monitor.) Excellent results can be obtained either way. The advantage of the endoscopic technique is that surgeons can see the pocket, making it easier to control bleeding and make the pockets equal.

Historically, obtaining absolute symmetry with this approach has been difficult. Also, if any postoperative problem requires a subsequent procedure, the surgeon needs to make an external incision, usually below the breast tissue. Figure 14-5 shows you the results of a transaxillary breast augmentation.

Figure 14-5:
Incisions through the armpits are a great option for women who want breast augmentation without any incisions on their breasts.

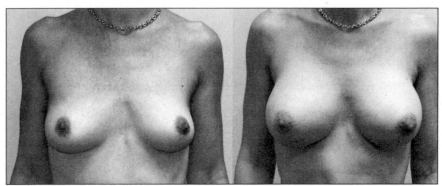

Transumbilical breast augmentation (TUBA)

If you're really concerned with scarring and want to minimize the possibility that a scar will be seen, consider the transumbilical breast augmentation (TUBA) approach. Be sure, however, that you like the look of the surgeon's results in his before-and-after photos before letting him perform this procedure on you. This operation has been available for ten or fifteen years, but many plastic surgeons don't perform it. They view it as an operation that is performed "blindly" (the implant pocket is created without the surgeon being able to see it) and therefore with less control over outcomes. In spite of this, to those surgeons who know how to do this procedure well, the operation is realistic and reliable.

With this technique, breast augmentation can be performed through a small incision at the upper end of your belly button, or *umbilicus*. Usually, the implants are placed above the muscle. If a secondary operation is needed, an incision below the breast will be necessary to provide enough access to the breast cavity. Figure 14-6 shows you the results of a TUBA procedure.

If you have complications after transaxillary or transumbilical augmentation mammoplasty and need another surgery, you may not have a choice about the location of your second incision. It may be necessary to make an incision in the crease below the breast in order to solve your complication issues. This will create more scars, and it's another reason many surgeons recommend periareolar or inframammary incisions.

Figure 14-6:
Implants placed through the navel can offer great results for the right candidate.

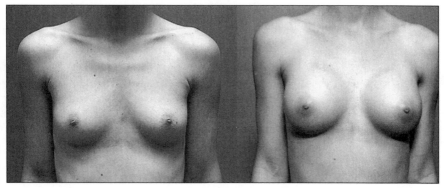

Considering anesthesia

I believe most breast augmentation procedures are best performed under general anesthesia. Years ago, I did most breast operations under sedation and local anesthesia. That approach generally worked well, but some patients were uncomfortable in spite of my best efforts. I now essentially refuse to do breast augmentation (or any major breast surgery) unless the patient is under general anesthesia.

No matter how carefully the breast is infiltrated with local anesthetic agents, eliminating all the pain of placing the implants under the muscle can be difficult. Using general anesthesia is the way to prevent most pain and assure the patient's comfort. See Chapter 3 for more information about anesthesia providers.

Identifying Implant Inspirations

Having breast augmentation will cause some major changes in your life. Evaluating your own feelings about the changes will make it easier to decide whether you want to proceed. In my own experience, patient satisfaction ratings for breast augmentation run in the high 90 percent range. I find that even women who have had problems that require secondary surgery almost never wish to have their implants removed. The level of happiness is sometimes incredible following successful augmentation surgery.

Augmentation is an operation that can be performed on any *healthy* woman. You need to be candid with your doctor if you have any unusual health problems or have used any recreational drugs. No anesthesiologist is going to cancel your surgery because you used marijuana five years ago. If, however, you used cocaine yesterday, he won't want to give you anesthesia today because it may cause a lethal heart problem.

Emotional considerations

Most people suffer some disappointment when reflecting on the difference between what they see in the mirror and society's ideal body. But if you're very sensitive about your breast size, breast shape, or the difference in size between your two breasts, talk to a surgeon and find out what's possible for you. The following sections highlight some of the emotional issues to consider when making a decision about augmentation.

Feeling "abnormal"

If you're like most women, you want to feel "normal." Normal may mean that you want to look like your friend in a blouse or bathing suit or that you want to fit into the larger category of what you believe society decrees to be ideal. You may want to look sexier for your boyfriend, husband, or lover. Your feelings of being different or somehow less than you want to be are powerful psychological forces that drive increasing numbers of women to the surgeon for breast augmentation. If you feel this way, you need to determine how strong the feelings are compared to the risks involved.

Young teens often compare their breast size to others — older sisters, friends, classmates, movie stars, or even their moms. If this is you, you may or may not be pleased with the comparison. But you and your surgeon must be sure you've stopped developing before you consider augmentation. You may be a late bloomer who will come into her own in another few months or so. Most surgeons are reluctant to do breast augmentation on anyone younger than 18, but if a mother brings her 17-year-old daughter for consultation saying that she stopped developing two years ago and asking for help, most of us will.

Intimacy issues

Whether understood consciously or not, breasts in our society are related to sexuality. In France, the ideal breasts are smaller rather than larger. In the United States, however, many people believe bigger is better.

If you're considering augmentation because your sex life is dull or inadequate, look at what else is going on. Is your breast size really the problem? Before deciding that breast size is the cause, try to determine whether your sex life issues are due to natural relationship changes, a new child, financial woes, stress at work, or other relationship problems.

Be sure *you* consider this surgery a potential improvement. Don't be talked into it by anyone — your best friend, mother, boyfriend, or husband. They may mean well, but only you can decide what is right for you. You'll live with the decision for the rest of your life.

Style

Wearing stylish clothes is something that most women enjoy. Whether you're a power dresser, someone who just loves to wear the newest fashion, or a bride-to-be, your shape affects the way you look in clothes. Many women say that the major reason they want augmentation is so that they can wear clothing that fits them better.

If your body size meets the norms, you'll be happily outfitted. If not, shopping and more importantly dressing becomes a disheartening chore. Only you can decide how much of a chore and whether surgery is the answer. The psychologic lift that can occur from looking great in clothes can be dramatic.

Anatomical issues

Most women wanting breast augmentation just want to be larger and look better in and out of clothing. Some women face other issues, including anatomical issues that can be only partially corrected or modified by augmentation surgery. Examples include breasts that are different in size and breasts with unusual placement of nipples. Occasionally, chest wall abnormalities such as *pectus excavatum* (where the breast bone is depressed inward) make achieving a perfect result unlikely. Talk to your surgeon about your options.

Asymmetry

Many women develop with different-sized breasts or wind up with asymmetrical breasts because of a mastectomy. If the difference is not great, placing a larger implant on the smaller side may completely eliminate the difference. If the difference is greater, the smaller breast may not have enough skin, so the shape ends up different (usually flatter) even if the volume is equalized. In these rare occasions, the skin can perhaps be expanded or stretched by placing an expander under the skin for several months. This procedure is frequently used during breast reconstruction following a mastectomy.

Tubular breasts

If your breasts are narrower and perhaps somewhat longer or pointier than you would like, breast augmentation surgery may help to a limited degree. Tubular breasts are extremely difficult to make perfect. Placing an implant behind the breast tissue may cause a "double bubble" effect. The implant causes a wider mound against the chest wall, and the narrower breast doesn't expand to the same width on top of the mound.

Saggy breasts

Your breasts can be saggy because of congenital reasons, childbirth, or aging. Breast augmentation can fill the extra skin, increase fullness in the upper part of the breast (upper pole fullness), and generally make the breasts larger. However, augmentation alone will not lift the nipple height or reduce extra skin. If the amount of sagginess is too great, you need to consider the possibility of a breast lift (see Chapter 15).

Unusual shapes

On some breasts, the nipples point straight forward or are positioned somewhat too far to the side or too low. These findings are almost always congenital, but may result from prior surgery. Although the surgeon can make small adjustments by doing skin excisions or placing the implants higher, lower, farther to the side, or closer to the midline, your breasts will probably continue to have the same problems because such problems can't always be eliminated. You need to discuss these issues with your breast surgeon in detail before surgery.

Doing it again: Reasons for second surgeries

Patients have follow-up breast surgery — secondary breast augmentation procedures — for several reasons. If you have had breast augmentation in the past and now want to be a different size or want to correct hardness (capsule formation), sagginess, or a deformity problem, you may want or need secondary surgery. Your surgeon can address all these issues, and most women who deal with these issues choose to have secondary surgery rather than removing the implants.

Changing size

No, changing your breast size isn't like changing your hair color, but it is possible to do, even after your first surgery. If you want to change the size of your breasts after your implants are in, secondary augmentation with a change of implants to a smaller or larger size is usually straightforward. If your breasts are large and pendulous, replacing larger implants with smaller may not look ideal without reducing the amount of skin present, reducing the size of the pocket, or both. (See Chapter 15 for more about breast lifts.) If you've had a successful augmentation and you later decide that you want your breasts even larger, you're going to be responsible for the costs of making the change. Therefore, be sure that you and your surgeon communicate well about the breast size that you want prior to your surgery.

Correcting capsule formation

Sometimes women need another surgery because of a hardness or lumpiness problem. If capsule formation occurs, a lining or capsule forms around the implant that is thicker and harder than normal tissue in a soft breast. Your surgeon can remove the capsule completely, partially remove it, or surgically score it to release tension, depending on the circumstances. Unfortunately, your chances of a recurrence are higher with secondary surgery than in a primary augmentation, but the incidence is still low. Having a *capsulectomy* (total removal of the scar tissue or capsule) usually works well.

At the time of capsulectomy, your old implant can be reused, or you can replace your implants with larger or smaller new ones. Having secondary surgery also gives you the option of changing from saline to silicone gel implants because of the FDA regulations.

If you're having secondary surgery to correct capsule formation, you may also want to consider changing the location of the implants from above the muscle to below or vice versa. It allows the surgeon to place the implants into an area of fresh tissue with minimal residual scar tissue.

Fulfilling a dream (and filling a bra)

Alice, who was not even an A cup and described herself as having no bust line, was frustrated about not being able to wear pretty bras, but finances were an issue as she considered breast augmentation. She and her husband talked it over for about a year, and then one day her husband said, "Here's some available cash," knowing exactly what she'd want to do with it. And she went to work on fulfilling her dream.

Alice describes her initial recovery as very painful for about ten days, but "it was really speedy after that!"

Alice is extremely happy with her results: "I look and feel natural, and I have little to no scarring around the nipples. I no longer have to wear padded bras, which I wore my entire life. I feel more confident and look good in tops. One regret I have is not doing it sooner. My husband can't get enough of me!"

Coping with sagginess

If sagginess is your biggest concern, a breast lift (mastopexy) is probably required (see Chapter 15). Whatever the issue, you can have your implants exchanged and your concerns about breast size addressed at the same time by placing larger or smaller implants.

Avoiding the magic wand syndrome

All surgery doesn't produce perfect results. If you're considering breast augmentation surgery, you and your surgeon must discuss what outcome can be realistically achieved with your breasts. There are many types of breast shapes, and your anatomy will to some extent determine your surgical outcome. You will want to take the whole of you into account — your shoulder width, hip size, waistline, and height. Consider how you want your whole body to look following augmentation.

If you have small but otherwise normally shaped breasts, you should expect an excellent result. If your breasts have an unusual shape or look different from side to side, you'll almost certainly get a dramatic improvement, but you may not end up with completely symmetrical breasts or achieve an ideal breast shape.

Evaluating Before-and-After Photos

Before you decide on a surgeon, you need to look at his before-and-after photos critically. Symmetry is perhaps the most important aspect of a successful augmentation surgery. As you look through each surgeon's photos, ask yourself the following questions:

- ✔ Are the folds under the breasts at the same height?

- ✔ Do the breasts fill out the same near the midline and at the sides?

- ✔ Do the examples look attractive or, asked a different way, do the breasts look like you would want them for your own?

- ✔ Do the photos show a range of sizes that appeal to you? If they're all larger than you would personally like, discuss with the surgeon how he chooses implant size at the time of surgery.

- ✔ Are both breasts equally full or rounded at the top of the breast? Is the fullness symmetrical from side to side?

Understand that any surgeon is going to show you the best examples of his results. If his best examples don't pass the sniff test, go elsewhere.

Assessing the Risks

The risks of breast augmentation are real, and you need to consider and accept the risks before having surgery. No one likes to dwell on the dark side, but being realistic is a winning strategy when making decisions about surgical procedures.

The two most significant risks that occur most often are bleeding and infection. They both fall into the 1 to 2 percent range. An even more common "risk" is that you may return to your surgeon after a month or more and ask how difficult it is to change to a different (usually larger) size.

You need to know about the following risks of breast augmentation surgery:

✔ **Capsule formation:** Scar tissue can form and contract around the breast implant immediately or much later following surgery, creating a hard capsule that may cause distortion and discomfort. The reasons capsules develop are still somewhat obscure. Infection, postoperative bleeding, and leakage of silicone in older silicone implants may all play some part. Capsule formation sometimes occurs without any apparent stimulating event. If the problem is severe (the breasts are extremely hard, or have some breast deformity or distortion), you may need secondary surgery unless you're willing to live with firm or hard breasts. If the breast is only slight firm and there's no shape distortion, you may want to try massage and pharmaceutical treatments in order to avoid surgery.

In the past, capsules occurred in at least 30 to 40 percent of cases. These days, they show up in only 5 percent of patients. Plastic surgeons attribute this enormous change to the newer and better implants available today.

✔ **Postoperative bleeding:** The operation isn't considered completed until bleeding blood vessels (bleeders) have been controlled. In spite of good surgical technique, a vessel may open up later and bleed again. This leads to an accumulation of blood clots within the breast cavity. If there's only a small amount of blood within the cavity and the breast size looks normal, no treatment is required.

If excess blood causes a difference in the size of the affected breast or causes pain, you'll probably need to go back to the operating room and have the blood removed and the bleeding point *cauterized* (burned with an electrical spark) or *ligated* (tied off). If the excess blood isn't removed surgically, it will gradually be absorbed by the body, but your chance of developing a capsule becomes much higher.

✔ **Loss of sensation:** Nipple, areolar, or skin sensation can be reduced or lost following breast augmentation. The nerves that supply the sensation aren't visible, so it's impossible for a surgeon to avoid them. If you experience some areas of reduced sensation, the problem usually improves or clears up within a year or two. Probably about 5 percent of patients experience some permanent sensory loss. Interestingly, some patients experience increased nipple sensation following breast augmentation.

✔ **Failure of the implant:** Saline implants, which are filled after they've been implanted, leak if a pinpoint hole develops in the shell (outside cover of the implant), if valve failure occurs, if a wrinkle develops and there's constant rubbing of the folded area, or if the implant has some other flaw.

✔ **Formation of "bad" scars:** Even when surgeons use the best plastic surgery techniques, some scars on the skin don't end up looking like either you or your surgeon would like. If, in spite of the best available scar treatment methods, the scar looks lumpy, thick, wide, or uneven after 6 to 12 months, excision and revision (cutting out and resuturing the skin) may be the best course.

✔ **Asymmetry:** After surgery, you may notice a slight difference between your breasts. One breast may look larger or smaller than the breast that you think looks perfect. The fold below one breast may end up slightly higher or lower than the other. One breast may hang to the side more or less than the other. Very few women have totally symmetrical chest walls or breasts before surgery, and surgery sometimes can't entirely correct these differences. Most patients would rather live with a minor difference in size than have another surgery. If the asymmetry is major, you need to discuss revisional surgery with your surgeon.

✔ **Infection:** Thanks to antibiotics, postoperative infections occur infrequently. Virtually all breast surgeons order intravenous antibiotics during breast augmentation surgery and prescribe oral antibiotics for several days thereafter. Nevertheless, if antibiotics don't immediately clear an infection, your surgeon may need to temporarily remove the implant or implants. If that's the case, the surgeon will replace the implant approximately six months later, assuming normal healing has occurred after removal of the infected implant. This scenario is temporarily devastating, but the final outcome is usually excellent.

Insuring implant success

Implant failure occurs less often since the newer and stronger implants have been available. The implant companies will replace your implants if they fail and pay toward coverage of your costs for up to five years. You can purchase additional implant failure insurance that covers all costs of replacement for up to ten years for approximately $120. I urge all patients to purchase that coverage.

Big, bigger, biggest: Finding the right size

You and your surgeon should decide on breast size. Your surgeon must consider anatomical issues, and you need to be aware that what you want may not be possible. If you say you want to be a large C cup and the surgeon says okay without any other effort to quantify what a C cup is, be wary.

If your friend had a breast augmentation and had 300cc implants placed and you like her look and size, should you ask your surgeon for 300cc implants? The answer is almost universally *no*. Your current breasts may be a different size than hers, your chest wall may be wider or narrower, and you may weigh more or less. All these variables influence what size implants you will need to achieve whatever size you choose.

Years ago, as a less experienced surgeon, I discussed sizing issues at length with patients, but ended up with about a 10 percent unhappiness rate over the issue of size. After I asked patients to bring pictures of breasts they would like for themselves, the size issue essentially disappeared. Other surgeons use measurements of breast width in order to determine the largest size of implant that will fit. No matter what method your surgeon uses, ask him how often he needs to reoperate on his patients because of miscommunication about size issues. To get the real

scoop, ask the nurses in the office about this issue when the surgeon is not around.

In our own practice, we have used the following personalized system for several years: You come for a consultation and a sizing appointment, during which you meet with the surgeon to determine your breast size options. We take front- and side-view photos of you in clothing showing your current breast size. Next, you put on a sports bra to which we add "sizer" implants until you get the look you want. We take more photos, and then you can check out your new shape as compared to your before pictures. We even provide a link to a private area of our Web site where your pictures are displayed, so you can show them to your friends and family. Both surgeons and patients understand that this method is for educational purposes because it offers a means for discussion of desired breast size and is not in any way a guarantee of results.

The only minor problem with any use of sizers in this system or any other is that your surgeon must translate what you say you want into what will actually produce that look when the implant is in your body. Most surgeons adjust the size upward from 10 to 15 percent more than the volume of the implant stuffed in the bra, in order to achieve the look you want in real life.

Recovering from Breast Augmentation Surgery

Just as with any surgery, you can optimize the result of your breast augmentation surgery by preparing properly for surgery and following your surgeon's guidelines and postoperative instructions. (See Chapter 7 for general information about preparing for surgery.)

The rub: Does massage aid recovery?

Many patients have been told or have read that massage of the breasts is mandatory if you've had augmentation mammoplasty. The assumption is that massage prevents capsule formation and hardness. In my opinion, this assumption is left over from times past when capsule formation was almost the rule instead of the exception. Massage doesn't harm anything, but it's not the reason for soft breasts. Newer and better implants are the real reason. (I work with four other plastic surgeons. Two insist their patients massage, and two don't. Our incidence of capsule formation among the five of us is the same.) Nevertheless, if your doctor tells you to massage, go ahead and do so.

All recoveries from surgery take time. If you plan to use the few days away from your job or normal lifestyle to catch up on your reading, make sure to buy or borrow the books you want to read in advance! If you want to watch TV for the first time in months and catch up on the soaps, have a *TV Guide* available. Try and make recovery a fun experience that will be a bonus of having surgery.

Dealing with dressings

After surgery, you'll likely be placed in a bra or an elastic wrap with light dressings covering the incision lines. If the surgical bra placed on you in the operating room becomes too dirty, is torn or lost, wear any bra that you already have that fits. If you have several choices, choose a sports bra.

Usually within a few days, the dressings can be removed, and you can shower. You may have been sent home with extra gauze pads with instructions to change them, or you may have been told to leave them alone until you return to the office. Follow your physician's instructions. If you have concerns, call the office for clarification.

Getting through the pain

Surgery involves cutting through tissue, so recovery is bound to hurt! Prepare for this feeling in advance by accepting the fact you'll experience some pain after your surgery. Pain makes you aware and keeps you from overdoing it. Understand that all surgery, including augmentation, leads to some postoperative discomfort. If you've had surgery before, you may have some idea of what your response will be.

For some women, the pain is mild, while others report really suffering. Take heart, though. Your doctor prescribes pain medication to help you through this phase of recovery. Some patients feel that taking pain medication is an admission of weakness, but nothing could be farther from the truth. Your best recovery occurs when you don't suffer unnecessarily. Have a positive attitude and take your medication! Taking pain pills following surgery won't make you an addict unless you continue them after the normal pain is gone. Most patients report that significant pain is usually gone within a few days.

Taking it easy

You won't need to be bedridden more than a day or two, and you can use your arms except when the motion causes pain. Follow your surgeon's instructions. If you have a complication, your surgeon may restrict your activities.

All recoveries from surgery take time and rest, which can vary from patient to patient. Most women can do office work, manage their homes, care for their children, and be out and about within a week or less. All people aren't the same, though, and some feel less pain than others. This difference doesn't measure your worth or your personality. Listen to your body. If you aren't up to driving the carpool or entertaining the boss, don't.

PERSONAL STORY

Getting through a rough patch

Sometimes when life gives you lemons, you need to figure out your own recipe for lemonade. Kelly, a marketing manager, was dealing with an unexpected divorce and sought augmentation to give her an extra boost of confidence that she needed to get through the rough patches. She says it worked and that her confidence boost has been invaluable in coping with her divorce.

Kelly gives the following advice to cosmetic surgery shoppers: "Be sure that you research your doctor thoroughly. Don't be shy to ask to see his work — even other women's breasts. Take pictures of what you want your results to look like (in and out of clothing) and what you *don't* want your results to look like. Explain your reasons behind both to the doctor. This will help him gain a more well-rounded view of what you are after." Even after communicating what she thought she

wanted — to feel more feminine and to be more proportionate — Kelly was hesitant about the size of the implants being recommended, which were larger than she thought she wanted.

Now she's glad she listened because she's perfectly proportionate and says surgery has boosted her self-image and self-confidence. She says, "A proportionate person, whether it's the face, breasts, or another part of your body, is a subconscious thing in the eye of the beholder, which tends to equate with external beauty. I love the reaction I get from men now, and I know that it's not my breasts that are drawing the attention — it's something more. I think it's the newfound confidence that radiates around me when I walk in the room. I feel the positive energy around me now more than ever."

Most women can return to exercise at the gym in about three weeks and start more aerobic exercises such as running, walking, bicycling, or rollerblading, as tolerated, at the same time. In general, allow your body to tell what you can or can't do. If some activity causes pain, stop the activity until it no longer hurts. You'll start feeling like yourself in time.

Knowing what's normal

The key to recovering healthfully and happily is knowing what is normal and what isn't. Understanding these things and knowing that you can call your doctor if you become concerned will give you peace of mind. Your surgeon and his staff are there to listen and support you.

Having some appreciation of what happens to your emotional state following surgery can also be very useful. Understanding that some temporary depression can occur may also be part of the prevention.

The following are normal symptoms that should not alarm you:

- **Swelling:** You'll feel discomfort and pain for a few days following surgery, and your breasts will feel swollen and heavy. Your breasts probably won't feel entirely normal for several months, but all pain is usually gone within the first month.

- **Tightness:** Your breasts may feel tight and too firm. It will take several weeks or longer for your muscles to stretch (assuming your implants have been placed under the muscles) and for the postoperative swelling to decrease. The breasts will achieve maximum softness within one to three months.

- **Nerve numbness or irritation:** Tingling, burning, shooting pains, and numbness are temporary symptoms (in most cases) that will reduce and disappear in time as the sensory nerves heal. Gentle massage is usually helpful in reducing temporary discomfort.

- **Breast shape:** Immediately after surgery, the implants sometimes sit too high on the chest wall, but they usually drop into a normal position over the next days or weeks.

- **Bruising:** A small area of visible bruising is not unusual below or to the side of one breast or both breasts. This symptom means that you have oozed a small or larger amount of blood inside the breast tissue after the operation was completed. If this happens, patients usually have no long-term effects. Larger amounts of blood within the breast cavity may stimulate the formation of a capsule. See your cosmetic surgeon if one breast remains larger and there's external bruising.

Chapter 15

Getting a Pick-Me-Up: Breast Lift

*N*eed a lift? For women with sagging breasts, the lift in question is not just a change in mood but a procedure that changes the shape of their breasts.

If you're considering a breast lift, you probably want your breasts to be higher and to look better in and out of clothing. Breast lift, or *mastopexy,* is an operation that lifts the breasts to a prechosen height, tightens the skin, and reshapes the breasts as needed.

Breast lift procedures come in different sizes to solve different problems. In this chapter, I describe the various operations available so that you can understand your options. For example, you can combine a breast lift with breast augmentation. You can also use the breast lift as an opportunity to reduce large areolar size.

Breast lift procedures do have limitations. The crease or fold under your breasts (inframammary fold) cannot be elevated on your chest wall. This means that if your fold has slipped downward, along with the development of breast sagginess, your newly lifted breast may not end up as high as you might hope for.

Understanding the Anatomy of the Breast

Breasts are made up of glandular tissue, fat, and connective tissue surrounded by skin. The tightness of the connective tissue depends on age, health, and what you inherited from your parents and ancestors. With time and aging, the connective tissue within your breasts begins to sag (see Figure 15-1). Gravity and the weight of your breasts contribute to this cosmetically unhappy situation.

The breasts sit on top of the pectoralis muscles (except for the bottom part of the breasts). The pectoralis muscles attach to the upper inner part of your upper arm and pull your arms toward your chest wall. If breast implants are used as part of your breast lift, they may be placed either above or below the pectoralis muscles.

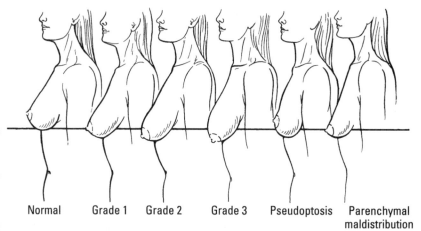

Figure 15-1:
The varying degrees of sagging, or ptosis.

| Normal | Grade 1 | Grade 2 | Grade 3 | Pseudoptosis | Parenchymal maldistribution |

The glands within the breast are connected to the nipples by a duct system. The nipples are surrounded by an area of darker skin called the *areola*. The areolar skin better resists the abrasion caused by nursing than would normal breast skin.

Breasts may become droopy for any of the following reasons:

✔ **Congenital reasons:** Breasts occasionally develop with a saggy shape. Although women with such breasts can breastfeed normally, these breasts don't fit into society's definition of "normal." Many teenage girls are embarrassed by congenitally saggy breasts, especially saggy breasts with downward pointing nipples. Young women with this problem essentially always wish for help but are frequently embarrassed to discuss the issue with their mothers or friends. Plastic surgeons, however, notice that correction of these problems frequently improves the social development of these young women.

✔ **Childbirth:** The natural process of having babies is frequently very hard on breasts. The breasts become engorged during pregnancy, remain enlarged during nursing, and then become smaller as the lactating tissue shrinks (involutes). After women have one or more babies, their breasts often become saggier.

When severe sagginess (called *ptosis*) occurs in a young mother who is struggling with her maternal responsibilities while trying to keep her marriage exciting and happy, the perceived loss of attractive breasts can be a powerful stimulant for change or improvement.

✔ **Weight gain and loss:** If you gain and lose weight, sagginess of the breasts may occur in the same manner that your abdomen or buttocks may sag. Both the skin and the connective tissue support within the breasts stretch during weight gain, and when weight loss occurs, your tissues don't have enough elasticity to tighten your breasts back to normal.

This loss of elasticity appears to be an inherited characteristic and varies from person to person. Many people can gain and lose weight without developing sagginess, but some people can't. For those who can't, mastopexy may be very helpful.

✔ **Aging:** Probably the worst culprit of all is Father Time. The skin surrounding the breast and the connective tissue within the breast (suspensory ligaments) all stretch. This process may begin as early as the 20s and certainly accelerates after menopause. A combination of gravity and the aging process makes this a universal factor of life.

Checking Out Your Breast Lift Options

Many people with saggy breasts hope that having breast augmentation alone can fill the extra skin, increase upper breast fullness, and generally make the breasts larger and higher. Occasionally, a simple augmentation can accomplish this, but to raise nipple height, some type of breast lift usually needs to be done.

Everyone wants perfect breasts with no scarring, but breast lift is a procedure that requires almost every patient to make some sort of compromise. Even the smallest lift leaves some scarring, and larger lifts almost always mean more scarring. Many women are willing to accept the scars as a trade-off for breasts that have better shape and position.

In most breast lift procedures, your excess breast skin is removed (excised) using a special design (similar to a dressmaker's pattern), and your remaining skin is wrapped around your breast tissue, holding your breast in its new location and shape. Figure 15-2 shows you the process.

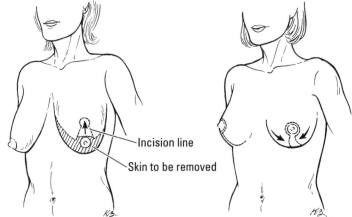

Figure 15-2: Steps for a standard breast lift procedure.

Incision line

Skin to be removed

In some types of breast lifts, the breast tissue itself is reshaped with sutures so that the lift isn't entirely provided by skin support. The most common examples are the vertical breast lifts described later in this chapter.

Some breasts surgeons won't do any breast lift procedures without also placing an implant under the breast even if the implant is very small. Placing an implant increases *breast projection* (the amount that your breasts project away from your chest wall), and many people believe that it improves the final shape. Other surgeons will explain your options and lift you without an implant if breast projection isn't an issue for you. If you and your surgeon have done careful preoperative planning and you both clearly understand what you hope to achieve and what can't be achieved, then you should end up satisfied with the outcome.

Breast lifts for minimal sagginess

If you have breasts that sag only a small amount, or if your only problem is that your nipples are a little droopy, then two operations are available that will help correct those problems and leave only small scars.

Although these operations provide only limited benefits, they can be wonderful when used for small problems or for patients who are unwilling to accept the scars of bigger breast lifts.

Crescent mastopexy

A crescent lift is appropriate if you have breasts with small sagginess problems (minimal ptosis). If you're like most women with saggy (ptotic) breasts, you probably want the problem solved with little or no scarring. Unfortunately, this outcome isn't possible in most cases. If, however, your breasts sag only a very little, your surgeon can do a minor procedure called a *crescent mastopexy* that removes (excises) skin from above the upper or superior margin of the areola, leaving a scar that extends from the 9:00 to the 3:00 positions or perhaps the 8:00 to the 4:00 positions along the upper areolar margin (if you think of the areolar margin as a clock face).

Breast implants can be inserted through these incisions if the patient chooses augmentation mammoplasty as part of the operation. Crescent lifts are done so that the nipple areolar complexes can be raised or elevated slightly, and so that the nipples don't point downward if that has been the tendency. This operation allows the nipple areolar complex to be raised a centimeter or two (less than an inch) at most.

Concentric, or doughnut, mastopexy

A concentric, or doughnut, mastopexy is appropriate if you have breasts with slightly more sagginess than can be corrected with a crescent mastopexy. This procedure is usually done for women with slightly saggy breasts who want a breast enlargement. The procedure is also appropriate for women with or without implants who wish a small lift.

In this procedure, your surgeon uses a skin-marking pen to mark an ellipse or circle of skin for excision around the margin of the areola. She plans what skin should be removed after measuring carefully and basing decisions on her surgical experience. More skin is almost always taken from above the nipple areolar complex than below because the purpose of the operation is to move the nipple areolar complex up. The design and marking of the skin to be removed vary from patient to patient and from breast to breast. The skill of your surgeon is important in making those judgments.

In this procedure, the nipple areolar complex can be moved upward approximately two to four centimeters (one to one and a half inches). In addition, the entire breast envelope becomes tighter. When this procedure is combined with breast augmentation, your breast skin envelope is reduced and, at the same time, filled up with an implant. The combination of larger volume with less breast skin and elevated nipple areolar complexes make it possible for dramatic changes to be achieved.

From a technical perspective, the surgeon needs to widely *undermine* (separate from the underlying breast tissue) the remaining skin (the area around the excised skin) before suturing the skin to the areola so that the area around the nipple isn't flattened. If the surgeon doesn't perform adequate undermining, concentric mastopexy can flatten the front of the breast. Some flattening will occur, even with undermining of the surrounding skin, if the indications for using this operation are pushed too far in an attempt to avoid doing a larger lift with longer scars. In this lift, with or without mastopexy, the only scar is around the areolar margin.

Breast lifts for more extensive sagginess

These procedures have been developed to correct more extensive breast sagginess problems. If your breasts hang very low, for example, removing a small amount of skin around your nipples isn't going to solve the problem.

Two types of breast lifts are available for correction. The standard breast lift works well but has long scars. The vertical breast lift has shorter scars but is frequently considered unacceptable in other ways. Read on for detailed explanations.

Standard mastopexy

Standard mastopexy is the technique that's most commonly performed in the United States. This operation allows correction or improvement of very saggy breasts (where the nipples hang below the fold under the breasts) and, depending on the amount of breast tissue present, can be performed with or without the placement of breast implants. This procedure leaves what is frequently referred to as an *anchor scar,* which circles the areola and runs vertically from the bottom of the areola to the fold under the breast and then horizontally in the breast crease (see Figure 15-3).

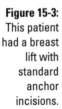

Figure 15-3: This patient had a breast lift with standard anchor incisions.

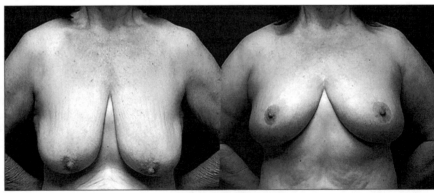

If your surgeon augments your breasts as well, placing the implants under your pectoralis muscle (see the section "Understanding the Anatomy of the Breast," earlier in this chapter) is the safest method (see Figure 15-4). One of the potential complications to breast lift surgery is loss of breast tissue or skin because of inadequate blood circulation. Placing the implant under the muscle reduces that possibility because submuscular dissection of the pockets for the implants has less possibility of injuring the blood vessels that supply the breast tissue and breast skin.

Figure 15-4:
This patient underwent a breast lift with standard incisions and had implants put in at the same time.

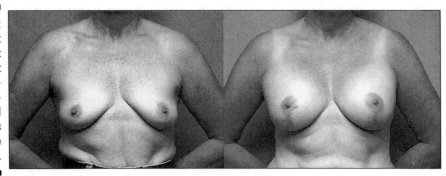

Vertical scar breast lifts

Breast lifts with only a peri-areolar (meaning around the edge of the areola) and vertical scar (resulting in no horizontal scar in the crease below the breast) have been popularized in Europe. Most U.S. surgeons don't perform this operation because, at the end of the procedure, the breast doesn't usually have a normal shape. Patients usually have a small mound of tissue that bunches up at the bottom of the vertical scar, but this tissue smoothes out over several months of postoperative healing. Many U.S. surgeons feel that their patients wouldn't tolerate the deformity because of the time that it takes to become normal. In the hands of surgeons who understand vertical lifts, however, excellent results are possible with that operation.

Another component of the vertical breast lift procedure is that sutures are placed into the breast tissue itself to shape the breast and cause more projection. Proponents of this operation feel that the possible increased projection and reduced tendency for the breasts to sag inferiorly make this the procedure of choice.

Surgeons frequently use smaller versions of vertical breast lifts, with less skin excision below the areola, for patients with less severe breast ptosis but more sagginess than can be solved by a concentric breast lift alone.

Lifting the load

Many women never regain their once perky breast shape after breastfeeding and are left with breasts that tend to head south no matter how much they try to position them otherwise. Raina found that she had lost approximately two cup sizes along with a tremendous amount of volume after breastfeeding her son. Because she's an athletic woman who spends a lot of time in bathing suits, she wanted to recapture the body type that she had in her 20s. Although she's healthy, her recovery time was delayed slightly by a severe muscle spasm. However, she's "very happy" with her results and is ecstatic about not having to wear a bra anymore. She "finally feels sexy again" after having the baby.

Considering anesthesia

Breast lift operations should almost always be performed under general anesthesia, especially if an augmentation (the official surgical name is augmentation mammoplasty; see Chapter 14) is being performed at the same time. No matter how carefully the breast is infiltrated with local anesthetic agents, you can expect to experience some pain when your surgeon places the implants under the muscle. In the past, many breast operations were performed under local anesthesia with sedation, but current practice across the country is to perform these operations under general anesthesia.

See Chapter 3 for more information about anesthesia and why I recommend that either a board-certified physician anesthesiologist or certified nurse anesthetist should provide anesthesia for breast lift surgeries.

Deciding Whether a Breast Lift Is for You

Having a breast lift will cause some major changes in your life. Evaluating your own feelings about the changes will make it easier to decide whether you want to proceed. With the exception of the cost, the biggest decision involves whether having perkier breasts is worth having some permanent scarring on your breasts. Thinking and planning for the anticipated positive changes will reduce preoperative stress and anxiety.

You should have breast lift surgery only if *you* personally really want it. The most important person to please with a breast lift is yourself. Most breast lift patients are women in their 30s and 40s who have had children and lost breast volume and support and whose breasts have become saggy and possibly smaller.

Here are some questions to ask yourself when considering whether to have this surgery:

- ✔ Are you willing to accept permanently visible scars in return for better shape and position?

- ✔ Are you making the decision for breast lift to please yourself? If you're partially making the decision for someone else, is your relationship a stable and loving one?

- ✔ Is having a breast lift something you have thought about for a long time or is it only a sudden whim?

- ✔ If you have decided to have a lift, are you happy with your current breast size or do you wish to be larger or smaller (see Chapter 16 for more about breast reduction)?

If your breasts are saggy, a breast lift may be a very good option for you, but don't take surgery lightly. There are many reasons to have a breast lift — and many reasons not to. Think about your reasons and see where you fit into this scheme. You may want to correct a physical situation or address an emotional issue. Be sure that the surgery you're considering can really meet your desired outcomes.

Feeling abnormal

You may be a woman who had attractive breasts and enjoyed your body image, but after the birth of your children, your breasts drooped and now you want your old look and image back. Or, you may be a woman who has always had saggy breasts and now has the resources to afford a correction. In either example, breast lift surgery can be the solution for you.

Examining the intimacy issue

Flat, saggy breasts are considered unattractive in our society. Some husbands and lovers consider scars to be an equal turn-off. The potential breast lift patient needs to satisfy herself, but she'll probably want to consider the wishes of her significant other on some level. Over the years, I have tended to be less aggressive and am willing to settle for less correction with fewer scars. A partial correction at age 30 can be turned into a full lift at 50 if a woman so desires.

Breast lift surgery is certainly not saving the world, but if you're struggling with emotional issues because of your saggy breasts, you can end up with a lift that makes you feel better about yourself and your life.

Don't let yourself get talked into the procedure just because your husband or lover has read the latest issue of *Playboy*.

Considering your health and age

If you can function in society and have no serious health issues, you're probably healthy enough to have breast surgery. If you happen to have diabetes, heart disease, lung problems, or other health conditions, then you should discuss them with your physician before having surgery.

Make an effort to be as healthy as possible before surgery. For most women having breast lift surgery (who are usually younger, healthy women), health isn't an issue. If you're in good health to start, recovery should go smoothly.

Breast lifts are performed in all age groups, but most women are in their 30s or 40s. Younger patients typically have the surgery to correct congenital problems, the younger middle age group for postpartum problems, and the older group for a combination of aging and postpartum issues.

Evaluating Before-and-After Photos of Breast Lifts

Understand that any breast surgeon is going to show you the best examples of her results. Given that scenario, you need to look at the photos with a critical eye.

Probably the most important things to evaluate are appearance, symmetry, and the appearance of the scars. Ask yourself these questions:

- Are the folds under the breasts at the same height?
- Do the breasts fill out the same near the midline and at the sides?
- Do the breasts look essentially the same and, perhaps even more important, do the examples have shapes that you like?
- How do the scars look? Could you live with them? How do they compare to those being shown by the other surgeons you're considering?

You'll want to look at a number of each surgeon's results to determine how you perceive the quality of scars on her patients. (See the section "Formation of 'bad' scars," later in this chapter, for more information.)

If a surgeon's better examples don't pass the test, go elsewhere.

PERSONAL STORY

Losing the limitations

Tina first considered having cosmetic surgery in high school and always knew she would do it after having children. She says she never felt sexy. All her clothes had to be altered to fit her small bust.

A year after her last child was born, she was at the gym working out, getting thin and getting rid of pregnancy weight, when she realized that she still didn't like what she saw in the mirror. She noticed others who had enhanced their breasts and decided it was time for her to do the same.

Knowing what to expect during the surgical process is sometimes half the battle. Of this process, Tina said, "The communication and education I received during the process were very important to me. Everything that was said to me was also written in a binder that was given

to me. It answered all my questions. A lot of times you forget what was said because of nerves, and I was able to refer to my booklet several times to answer any of my questions. Everything was very organized and professional."

And her results? "They exceeded my expectations," she said. "I feel I'm more intimate with my husband. I have more confidence with him. All in all, I am happier with myself and confident I can do anything I want to."

The fact that she can now wear sexy, low-cut holiday dresses and has a newfound love of shopping for swimwear and lingerie prompts her to tell other people considering the procedure, "Do it! It has been by far the best experience in my life, and I thank my surgeon and his staff for that!"

Understanding the Risks

The risks of breast lift procedures are real, and you need to consider and accept them before having surgery. See Chapter 17 for the general risks of all surgeries.

Because most breast lifts also include breast augmentation, you may want review the risks of the augmentation portion of the procedure in Chapter 14.

Postoperative bleeding

The operation isn't considered completed until all *bleeders* (blood vessels that have been cut during the dissection that are bleeding or oozing) have been controlled and the bleeding stopped. In spite of good surgical technique, a vessel may open up and bleed later, after the surgery is completed. If postoperative bleeding causes a difference in the size of the affected breast or causes pain, you'll probably need to return to the operating room and have the blood removed and the bleeding point cauterized or ligated (tied off).

The immediate symptoms from bleeding are pain and swelling. The longer-term consequences, if untreated, are prolonged swelling, hardness, lumpiness, bruising, and the increased possibility of infection and deformity.

Loss of sensation

Nipple, areolar, or skin sensation can be reduced or lost following any breast surgery. The nerves that supply the sensation are not visible to the naked eye. If you experience some areas of reduced sensation following surgery, you can expect that the sensory nerves will regenerate and that sensation will return over a period lasting up to two years. Occasionally, the damage can be permanent. About 5 percent of patients experience an area of some permanent loss of sensation.

Sensory nerves allow us to feel touch, pressure, pain, and so on. If sensory nerves are damaged or cut during any surgical procedure, they will, to some extent, regenerate and heal over the next several months, and may even keep improving for up to two years.

Sensory change or loss can result from any and all types of breast surgery, no matter what type of incision is used.

Formation of "bad" scars

In spite of the best plastic surgery techniques, some scars don't heal perfectly and don't end up looking the way you and your surgeon want. A fabulous closure on breast skin may well turn into a wide scar, no matter how the incision is taped or whether it's treated with vitamin E oil (or the equivalent) and so on. Scars look and heal differently depending on their location on the body. Breast skin isn't the most favorable for minimal scar formation. For example, facial scars almost always heal better than breast skin scars in the same patient.

You need to understand that the type of scars you end up with on your breasts depends on both your skin and the skill or performance of your plastic surgeon. Dark-skinned people tend to have wider or thicker scars following surgical incisions. If, in spite of the available scar treatment methods, your scar looks thick, lumpy, wide, or raised after 6 to 12 months, removing and revising the scar may be the best treatment.

Before trying scar revision, you and your surgeon may want to consider treatments such as taping, silicone-based creams, silicone sheeting, vitamin E oil (and other similar creams), injections with cortisone, or chronic pressure dressings.

Asymmetry

After surgery, one breast may look larger or smaller than the breast that you think looks perfect. The fold below one breast may end up slightly higher or lower than the other. One breast may hang to the side more or less than the other. Very few women have totally symmetrical chest walls or breasts before surgery, and surgery can't necessarily make your breasts perfectly identical. Most patients don't mind minor differences after surgery. If the asymmetry really bothers you and is very visible, discuss revisional surgery with your surgeon.

Infection

Postoperative infections occur infrequently. Almost all breast surgeons order intravenous antibiotics during any major breast surgery and give you oral antibiotics for several days thereafter. Nevertheless, if an infection occurs that doesn't clear up immediately with antibiotics, temporary removal of the implant or implants (if they have been placed) may be necessary. If that's the case, the surgeon will replace the implants approximately six months later, assuming normal healing has occurred after removal of the infected implant. This scenario is temporarily devastating, but the final outcome is usually excellent.

Removal of implants because of infection is a rare occurrence but is a real risk. Infection can lodge around a breast implant following an infection elsewhere in your body when bacteria are carried in your bloodstream. Almost every busy breast surgeon has seen this complication at least once.

Tissue loss

Breast lift procedures can cause decreased circulation to the skin or nipple areolar complex. In the worst-case scenario, skin, breast tissue, areolar tissue, or the nipple itself can die (necrose) due to reduced circulation. If tissue dies, it turns dark or black and needs to be removed (excised). Should this unlikely complication occur, secondary surgery, such as skin grafting or nipple reconstruction, would probably be necessary.

These serious complications are rare. If such a complication occurs, it will take cooperation between you and your surgeon and the passage of several months before resolution occurs.

In general, the larger the breast lift (meaning the larger the distance the nipple needs to be moved upward), the greater the chance of skin loss or tissue necrosis.

Recovering from Breast Lift Surgery

After a breast lift, most women can do office work, manage their homes and children, and be out and about within a week or less. You may be one of those women who feel good enough to go out to dinner or a movie within a few days. Or you may be at the other end of the spectrum and have a much slower recovery. Your own history should give you some idea of the length of time it will take you to recover. Virtually all pain is gone within a month in most patients.

Recuperating and other post-op issues

At the end of your operation, most surgeons will cover your incisions with light dressings and then place you in a bra. The bra is a perfectly shaped symmetrical dressing. For approximately the first week after surgery, your surgeon will probably want you to keep the incisions covered with gauze or tape or both. The bra you'll receive at surgery is a surgical bra, but it has no magical properties. If your surgical bra gets dirty, torn, lost, or whatever, wear any of your own bras that fit. If you need to choose between a sports bra or an underwire bra, choose the sports bra.

You don't need to be bedridden more than a day or two, and you can use your arms except when the motion causes pain. The amount and degree of pain will vary from woman to woman. If you have a complication (see the section "Understanding the Risks," earlier in this chapter), your activities will probably be restricted.

You'll probably be able to drive within a week. You can probably work from home within a few days if you wish and return to the office within a week or two if desired. If you have small children who require a lot of lifting, you need to plan for additional help during the initial recovery period.

Most women can return to exercise at the gym in about three weeks and start running or doing other aerobic exercise as tolerated at the same time. In general, allow your body to tell you what you can or cannot do. If some activity causes pain, stop the activity until it no longer hurts as much or at all.

Getting past the pain

Most breast lift operations hurt only moderately, and most women can easily control the pain with pain pills. Many patients feel normal after a few days, even though the incisions will not be strong for a month or more.

All surgeries, including breast lifts, will lead to some postoperative discomfort. Understand this ahead of time and be prepared to take pain pills prescribed by your physician to control the discomfort. Taking pain pills following surgery will not make you an addict unless you continue them after the normal post-op pain is gone. Some patients feel that taking pain medication is an admission of weakness, but that's faulty thinking. Take the pain pills if you need them.

Knowing what's normal

Understanding the normal symptoms of breast lift surgery will give you significant peace of mind. If something is abnormal, however, your surgeon will want you to recognize the situation and contact the office. The following are normal symptoms during recovery:

- **Moderate discomfort and pain for a few days following surgery:** If you experience severe or sharp pain in one breast, examine that breast for increased swelling or redness. If either of those symptoms is present, report immediately to your surgeon's office.

- **Swollen and heavy-feeling breasts:** Your breasts are filled with edema fluid, and if you have had implants, the new implants add weight as well. Your breasts will probably not feel entirely normal for several months, but all pain is usually gone within the first month. If you feel that one breast is truly heavier than the other, see your surgeon.

- **Unusually firm breasts:** As swelling goes down and the skin stretches, softness will return — usually within one to three months. You don't want too much softness because that could lead to more sagginess. If one breast remains firmer or harder than the other, discuss this with your surgeon.

- **Healing nerves:** Tingling, burning, shooting pains, and numbness are in most cases temporary symptoms that will reduce and disappear gradually as the sensory nerves heal. Gentle massage is usually helpful in reducing temporary discomfort. Sensory changes may improve for up to two years. Your surgeon will want to know of these symptoms, but no specific treatments will make nerves heal more quickly.

- **Bruising:** Development of a small area of visible bruising below or to the side of one or both breasts means that you have oozed a small or larger amount of blood inside the breast tissue after the operation was completed. This finding usually has no long-term effects and almost never requires secondary surgical treatment.

If you have augmentation mammoplasty as part of your breast lift surgery, your breasts will probably be somewhat swollen, and the breasts may feel tight and too firm. It will take several weeks or longer for your muscles to stretch (assuming your implants have been placed under the muscles) and for the postoperative swelling to decrease. The breasts will achieve maximum softness within one to three months.

You may have been told or read that massage of the breasts is mandatory if you have had augmentation mammoplasty as part of your breast lift. The assumption is that massage prevents capsule formation and hardness. I don't believe this assumption is true. Massage doesn't harm anything, but it isn't the reason for soft breasts. The newer and better implants are the real reason. Nevertheless, if your doctor tells you to massage, go ahead and do so.

No lift is forever. Your skin and breast tissue will continue to stretch and sag over time. Secondary lifts can be performed years later if needed.

Not all of the changes you'll undergo are physical. Your emotions will need to do some healing as well. Understand that you may experience a letdown or some temporary depression following a breast lift or any other surgery. These feelings are a normal part of your recovery process. Incorporation of your new breast shape and position into your body image usually occurs within the first month. For more information about emotions during recovery, see Chapter 18.

Chapter 16

Streamlining Your Form with Breast Reduction

Despite the popularity of jokes and skits about large-breasted women, those with this condition hardly find it humorous. In general, these women suffer from many problems — including physical pain and embarrassment — before surgery, so they're among the most satisfied patients after their surgery.

Breast reduction surgery (also known as *reduction mammoplasty*) makes the breasts the desired size, frequently more symmetrical, and better looking, and it can reduce overstretched or oversized *areola* (the darker circle of skin around the nipple) to a more normal appearance. In addition, back and neck pain associated with large breasts frequently disappears, the chafing under the breasts goes away, and women can purchase smaller clothes and look better in them. Following surgery, women gladly go to the beach or pool for the first time in years.

Breast reduction is one of the few procedures discussed in this book that may be fully or partially covered by your insurance plan. Do your homework on preauthorization.

Understanding Anatomy

Breasts that are very large and heavy *(breast hypertrophy)* usually develop for genetic reasons. Occasionally, breasts become too large following pregnancy.

Breasts frequently become heavy and cause symptoms such as neck, shoulder, or back pain following weight gain. Men sometimes also develop enlarged breasts that make wearing t-shirts or going shirtless psychologically uncomfortable.

Breast tissue is made up of glandular tissue and fat. In some patients, large breasts remain rounded and firm and are minimally saggy. These patients, who are in the minority, have very tight connective tissue that has not stretched with increased breast volume or size. They can be excellent candidates for breast reduction with liposuction, which I describe in the section "Reducing size with liposuction," later in this chapter.

Most patients with breast hypertrophy, however, have breasts that are both too large and too saggy. The extra size and weight is made up of fat and glandular tissue. Sagginess is caused by stretching of the connective tissue within the breasts and may be a result of weight, genetics, or both. Patients whose breasts sag require a standard breast reduction that leaves external scars, usually an anchor-shaped scar (see the section "Standard breast reduction," later in this chapter).

Most women don't have totally symmetrical breasts. In women with breast hypertrophy, this problem is frequently exaggerated. Breast reduction offers a very real opportunity to equalize breast size.

Checking Out Breast Reduction Options

No matter your breast size, shape, or symmetry, there's a procedure that will be helpful to you if your breasts are bigger than you'd like. In most breast reduction procedures, your breasts will be lifted as well as reduced in size. In spite of these cosmetic and physical benefits, however, this surgery involves significant scarring.

If you are considering breast reduction and are in good health, you can assume that you're a candidate for this procedure. Age is usually not a deterrent. Breast reduction is performed from the late teens into the 70s.

Take along photos of what you perceive as an ideal breast size for you when you consult with a surgeon. Keep in mind that photos showing size are usually pictures of perfect breasts and that the results of your surgery may match the size but not the perfection.

Ask any surgeon you're considering how often he performs breast reduction surgery. If the answer is less than six to eight times a year, be somewhat careful. Breast reduction is not the most frequently performed breast surgery (augmentation mammoplasty is). Ask to see photos of breast reductions the surgeon has done both during residency and after.

Standard breast reduction

In a standard breast reduction (by far the most common procedure), your surgeon places an incision around the border of your areola, a second incision extending vertically to the crease under the breast, and a third incision horizontally in the crease below your breast. The three scars form the shape of an anchor.

This procedure removes the extra skin and underlying breast tissue and elevates the nipple areolar complex to a higher position with its own blood supply (and usually its own nerve supply). Figure 16-1 shows you the process, and Figure 16-2 shows the results.

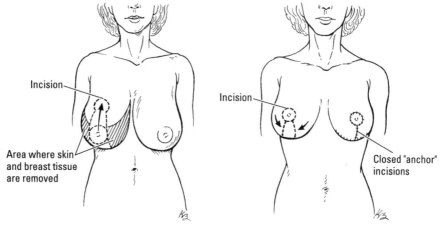

Figure 16-1: A standard breast reduction involves cutting away tissue and moving the nipple and areola.

Incision

Area where skin and breast tissue are removed

Incision

Closed "anchor" incisions

In the standard breast reduction anchor scar, the area where the vertical and horizontal incisions meet may occasionally spread apart during healing and take several additional weeks to heal. In that case, the ultimate scar may be wider than normal and may require later surgical revision.

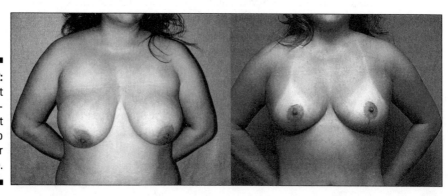

Figure 16-2: This patient had a standard breast reduction to achieve her ideal size.

Vertical scar breast reduction

This procedure uses what is known as a lollipop incision, meaning you won't have the horizontal incision under your breast, but you will have a vertical scar below your areola in addition to a scar around the edge of the areola. The extra or excess breast tissue is removed through these incisions. This technique creates some temporary bunching or gathering of tissue below your breast that lasts for several weeks or months. Occasionally, a small secondary skin excision is required at a later time.

Frequently used in Europe and by some U.S. surgeons, this method can work very well but requires some patience on the part of both patient and surgeon. It works better for reductions in which smaller amounts of breast tissue need to be removed. One advantage of this method is that the breast shape is reconstructed with sutures and the newly shaped breast is not completely dependant on the support of skin.

Breast reduction with nipple transfer

In this operation, the nipple areolar complexes (the nipples and the dark skin around them) are completely removed and later replaced as grafts on the new breast. This operation isn't performed too often, but there are circumstances under which there are no other choices. If your breasts are extremely large and saggy, and if you wish to end up after surgery with B, C, or small D cup sized breasts, it may be impossible to achieve your goal without a nipple transfer (nipple graft). Transferring your nipple areolar complex as a graft may make your nipple area slightly distorted, discolored, or scarred.

There is usually some residual sensation to the nipples after breast reduction surgery. If you have a breast reduction with nipple grafts, however, nipple sensation will not return. In massive breasts, though, most sensation is already gone because of the stretching of the breasts that has occurred. If you fall into that category, having non-feeling nipples will not change your life, and achieving your desired size and shape becomes the most important issue.

Reducing size with liposuction

Because much of the breast tissue is fat, liposuction can be a very useful tool in the right patients. If your nipple height or location is relatively normal, and if your breast shape tends to be more globular or round (with relatively little sagginess), then liposuction can be a wonderful alternative — generally less expensive and with very small scars.

This operation works better if you have "smaller" large breasts. If you start out saggy, your breasts will be smaller but may appear even saggier than before. If your breasts are very large, liposuction may not be capable of making you as small as you hope to be.

Reduction mammoplasty with liposuction is much easier on the patient. There are no long incisions to heal, no drains to be pulled, essentially no sutures to be removed. If you're interested in reduction mammoplasty and have reasonably firm large breasts, discuss this option with the plastic surgeon of your choice. If he feels that your breasts are too fibrous or dense, he may argue that it will be very difficult to suction enough fat to achieve your goals. Liposuction can be very useful in reducing one larger breast to match the size of a slightly smaller one. For more information about liposuction, read Chapter 11.

Reducing male breasts

When men have large breasts, the condition is known as *gynecomastia*. In years past, surgical excision of this excess male breast tissue was performed routinely, but today liposuction (see Chapter 11) has become the method of choice for treating this problem because it works extremely well for most patients and involves minimal scarring. Figure 16-3 shows you the results. Currently, surgical excision of the excess tissue is considered only for men who have very large amounts of breast tissue.

PERSONAL STORY

Feeling masculine again

A self-described optimist, John remembers being in the locker room in junior high school and having one of his fellow teammates comment on his overdeveloped breasts. Because they had been good friends up until that point, the remark really made an impression on him. Although John didn't make an appointment until years later, he was continually reminded of his condition because "We live in a culture that defines us by our appearance and how we project a sense of self confidence in every aspect of our daily lives."

An upcoming summer vacation in Hawaii finally prompted John to go ahead with the male breast reduction procedure. In choosing a surgeon, John says, "The physician's track record with previous patients and his expertise in this area played a large role in my decision."

Reflecting on the surgical procedure itself, John said that he had a very pleasant experience and his results were visible from day one after his surgery, "I was pleasantly surprised with how quickly the swelling went down. I was able to see the new me almost immediately."

John now feels good about his physical appearance and has more confidence taking off his shirt in public. He says he is more apt to choose to go to the beach than the movies these days. "In my opinion, this experience has changed my life for the better, and I would encourage anyone considering cosmetic surgery to trust their instincts, as well as their doctor."

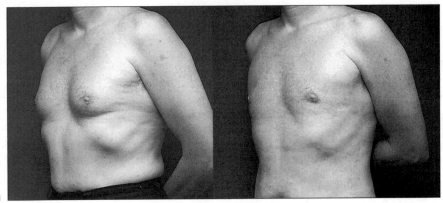

Figure 16-3:
Many men have excess tissue and seek breast reduction, usually by liposuction.

Considering anesthesia

Almost all surgeons prefer to perform surgical breast reduction under general anesthesia. Although it's technically possible to do the surgery under sedation and local anesthesia, eliminating all the pain may be difficult. If your surgeon is using the liposuction technique to reduce your breast size, then you will have more options for anesthesia. Ask your surgeon about the type of anesthesia he recommends for the breast reduction procedure you're considering.

Looking at Common Reasons for Reductions

Having a breast reduction will cause some major changes in your life. Evaluating your own feelings about the changes will make it easier to decide whether you want to proceed or not. Thinking and planning for the anticipated positive changes will reduce preoperative stress and anxiety.

Common reasons for breast reduction surgery include the following:

✔ **Feeling abnormal:** You may feel abnormal because of your breast size. You're not alone if you want to look more average or fall in the range of what society considers to be acceptable. If you're a teenager, large breast size can be a particularly difficult issue to deal with. Being the recipient of wolf whistles or unwanted attention from classmates because your breasts are very large can be embarrassing or psychologically devastating. If you're older, your large breasts may become an annoyance because as they droop, you lose your hourglass figure.

✔ **Social insensitivity:** If you have unusually large breasts, you may be subject to insensitive comments and stares in all kinds of situations. Men may look at your breasts rather than at your face, and you may be the butt of jokes and nasty asides. If you're exposed to this kind of behavior, you may withdraw socially and experience feelings of depression or anxiety. You may find yourself avoiding certain kinds of clothing or staying away from the beach or pool.

✔ **Intimacy issues:** Huge breasts can be embarrassing even in a relationship and may result in problems that affect intimate behavior. Although reduction surgery can't take the place of psychological counseling when a relationship is in trouble, in many cases, it may lead to a happy resolution of intimacy issues.

✔ **Clothing:** If you need triple D-size bras, you may find it hard to find a good fit, and the most beautiful bras are usually not made in the largest sizes. Shopping for a bathing suit can also be a nightmare. The wish to wear more attractive clothes and to look good in them is frequently what motivates women to have breast reduction surgery. Although the desire to look more attractive in clothes is a motivation, I seldom see patients for whom it is the primary stimulus for reduction surgery.

✔ **Sports:** Runners, golfers, tennis players, swimmers, and others find that very large breasts interfere with participation or performance in sports. Wearing more than one sports bra doesn't solve the problem. For women whose breasts get in the way of their golf swing or cause pain when they run, reduction mammoplasty can be a blessing.

✔ **Physical discomfort:** Women with very large breasts are usually unhappy with the size and weight of their breasts and the secondary symptoms of back pain, neck pain, bra strap grooves, and skin irritation and chafing under the breasts. I've seen these symptoms disappear almost overnight following reduction mammoplasty.

Reducing limitations and experiencing life

Cathy first considered having cosmetic surgery about ten years ago because she had very large, heavy, sagging breasts that were out of proportion with her 5-foot-2 petite frame. She was prompted to make the appointment after talking with several girlfriends who had great results and recommended their doctors. Her lifestyle was an important factor in her decision. She's a stay-at-home mom who is very active in sports. Cathy describes herself as a very outgoing person who wants to enjoy life to the fullest.

She says the surgery itself didn't take as much time as she expected and, for her, was a pain-free experience! Cathy was fortunate in that she didn't need the painkillers and wasn't all that uncomfortable during the healing process. She says, "I would rate my surgical result against my expectations as a 10 plus, with 10 being the highest! My back and shoulders don't ache from all that extra weight, and I don't have to wear two bras to play sports. Since I am such an outdoors type of person, my decision for this type of surgery makes my life that much more enjoyable. Clothes fit better, and I can actually go braless. And I'm almost 50 years old! Yahoo!"

Understanding the Risks

Everyone hopes for perfection as the outcome of cosmetic surgery. Breast reduction is no different. The reality, however, is that you will have scars and the shape of your breasts may be slightly different from side to side; you may not end up with perfect shape.

Your surgeon will do his best to achieve an optimum result, but keep in mind that even with the best possible result, it takes time, softening of the operated area, reduction of swelling, and fading of bruises for your breasts to settle into their final shape and size.

The risks of breast reduction are real and need to be considered and accepted before having surgery. Most complications are minor and will not cause a bad result. It may, however, take an extra week or month beyond the normal healing time of approximately one month to reach your final result.

The following potential risks and complications can occur with reduction mammoplasty:

- **Postoperative bleeding:** An operation isn't considered completed until all "bleeders" (blood vessels that have been cut as a part of surgery) have been controlled. In spite of good surgical technique, a vessel may open up later and bleed. Drains are frequently placed into the operative areas before the surgeon closes the incisions. The drain system usually removes the excess blood or fluids.

  If the bleeding is significant enough, then you may need to go back to the operating room to have the blood removed and the bleeding vessel *cauterized* (stopped by using an electrical current) or *ligated* (tied off). If the bleeding is minimal, then you probably will not need secondary surgery. You'll likely develop some visible bruising and swelling that will clear with time.

- **Loss of sensation:** Nipple, areolar, or skin sensation can be reduced or lost following any breast reduction. The nerves that supply the sensation are not visible and therefore are impossible for the surgeon to avoid. Permanent sensory loss occurs in probably 5 percent of patients. If you experience some areas of reduced sensation, the problem usually improves or disappears within a year or two. The larger your breasts, the greater the possibility of sensation loss.

- **Loss of tissue or skin (including nipple and areola):** Rarely, the blood supply to areas of skin or to the nipple-areolar complex itself is reduced to the point that the tissue cannot live. If an area of tissue or skin loses its blood supply, the area turns green, gray, or black, and dark black crusts form. This difficult complication usually requires secondary surgery and certainly involves prolonged healing.

✔ **Formation of "bad" scars:** In spite of the best plastic surgery techniques, some scars don't heal perfectly. Time, the injection of steroids, pressure dressings, and the application of silicone gel strips and Vitamin E oil may all help reduce scarring. If, in spite of the available scar treatment methods, the scar looks bad after six months to two years, excision and revision (cutting out the scar and resuturing it) may be the best course. Scars tend to be darker and wider in darker-skinned patients.

✔ **Asymmetry:** After surgery, you may find that one breast looks larger or smaller than the other. The fold below one breast may end up slightly higher or lower than the other. The scars may not settle in the exact same position. One breast may hang to the side more or less than the other. Very few women have totally symmetrical chest walls or breasts before surgery. Minor differences after surgery are usually accepted by most patients and usually don't require secondary surgery. If the asymmetry is major, discuss the possibility of additional surgery with your surgeon.

✔ **Infection:** Postoperative infections occur infrequently. Virtually all breast surgeons give you intravenous antibiotics during breast reduction surgery and oral antibiotics for several days thereafter. There's no absolute proof that these antibiotics actually reduce infection, but probably more than 90 percent of plastic surgeons think so and act accordingly.

If you develop an infection, an area of breast skin becomes warm and reddish, you may leak pus or cloudy fluid from an incision line, you will start to experience pain, and you will probably run a fever. If these symptoms occur, call your surgeon's office immediately.

Evaluating Before-and-After Photos

Understand that any breast surgeon is going to show you the best examples of his results. When evaluating a potential surgeon, look at his postoperative photos very critically. If the surgeon's better examples do not meet your expectations, look elsewhere. Look for symmetry and overall shape and also ask yourself the following questions:

✔ Are the folds under the breasts at the same height?

✔ What is the position of the nipples? Nipples usually point slightly to the side (not straight forward) and neither point down nor up.

✔ Do the breasts have the same degree of fullness? Stated another way, are the breasts symmetrical?

✔ Do the examples look like breasts you would like to have?

✔ Has there been real improvement between the before-and-after photos?

How much the scars show up following breast reduction is more related to the patient's skin than to the skill of the surgeon. You should, however, look at the symmetry of the scars from one side to the other. The bottom line is that you need to reassure yourself that you're choosing a surgeon whose results you would be happy to live with.

Recovering from Breast Reduction

Reduction mammoplasty is a large operation and it causes some discomfort, but most patients heal quite quickly. At the end of the operation, gauze dressings are placed over the incisions and you are either wrapped up with elastic tapes or placed in a surgical bra. If at any point you're concerned that something is abnormal, however, contact your surgeon. Check out Chapter 18 for more about what you can expect during recovery.

Dealing with dressings

After surgery, you'll likely be placed in a bra or an elastic wrap with light dressings covering the incision lines. Usually within a few days, the dressings can be removed and you can shower. Your surgeon may send you home with gauze dressings to change, or he may ask you to come to the office for dressing changes.

If you have bleeding or fluid drainage that continues for several days, separation of wound edges, blistering of the skin, dark coloration of your nipple areolar complex, or anything else that concerns you, call your surgeon's office. If your surgical bra is too tight, call your doctor. He may instruct you to take it off and wear any bra that fits until you see him again.

Getting through the pain

You'll feel discomfort and pain for a few days following surgery. You'll receive medication to help control the pain, and you should not experience severe discomfort. Taking the pain pills is not an admission of weakness. Your surgeon doesn't want you to experience pain; he wants you to be able to rest and heal. Taking pain pills for a week or so won't make you an addict.

Some patients feel little pain, while others feel a lot. Although breast reduction is major surgery, most patients report that it isn't usually painful. Your pain tolerance to past surgery, if you have had any, may give you an idea of what your response will be.

Taking it easy

You don't need to be bedridden more than a day or two after surgery, and you can use your arms except when the motion causes pain. If you have a complication, your activities will probably be restricted.

If you want, you can probably work from home within a few days and return to the office within a week or two. You'll probably be able to drive within a week. Most women can return to exercise at the gym in about three weeks and start running, as tolerated, at the same time.

Knowing what's normal

Understanding the normal physical symptoms after breast reduction surgery will give you significant peace of mind. Here are some normal symptoms to expect during your recovery:

- ✔ **Bruising:** Some bruising is normal. Large areas of bruising are uncommon and may indicate continued bleeding. Notify your surgeon if large areas of bruising are present.

- ✔ **Numbness:** Almost all surgeries have surrounding areas of numbness that last for several weeks or more.

- ✔ **Swelling:** Your breasts will feel swollen and heavy. They'll probably not feel entirely normal for several months, but all pain is usually gone within the first month.

- ✔ **Firmness:** Your breasts may feel too firm for the first few weeks. As swelling goes down and the skin stretches, softness will return. Too much softness immediately after surgery could lead to more sagginess later. Firmer, tighter, higher — and smaller and lighter — breasts are what this surgery is all about.

Having some appreciation of what happens to your emotional state following surgery can also be very useful. Understand that some temporary depression can occur. For more information about emotions during recovery, see Chapter 18.

Incorporating your new breast size and shape into your body image usually occurs within the first month. It's normal to feel elated and wonderful with your new look. You'll probably feel a powerful urge to head for the lingerie store or the swimsuit department at your favorite department store.

Part IV
Going for It: Preparation and Recovery

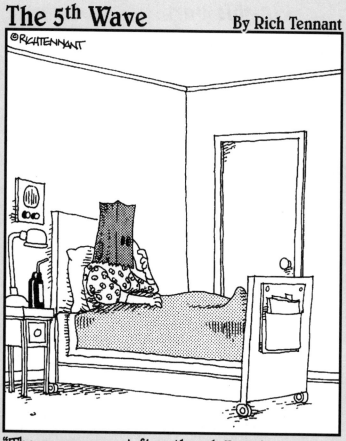

The 5th Wave   By Rich Tennant

"The surgery went fine, though I can't say much for their post–operative sensitivity."

In this part . . .

You wouldn't walk across the street without looking both ways, and you certainly shouldn't decide to have cosmetic surgery without knowing what may lie ahead. In this part, you can find out about the common (and not-so-common) risks of having surgery and then read up on what you can expect from your recovery. Finally, figure out what to do if your results aren't what you'd hoped for — and how to make the most of results that are!

Chapter 17

Assessing the Risks and Preparing for Surgery

*A*fter you decide to have surgery, you need to move into the next phase and begin planning for your recovery. Be an active participant in the decisions that will help determine your outcome. Reviewing the risks of surgery and making sure that your recovery plans are appropriate to your needs are positive steps you should take at this time. For example, don't plan to pick up your medications at the pharmacy on the way home from surgery — you'll be too exhausted and medicated to handle the task.

Assessing the Risks

All surgical procedures have inherent risks that you must understand and accept before going forward. For example, an infection can occur no matter how carefully the surgeon performs the surgery. Some risks are common for all operations, and some additional specific risks are related to specific operations. I discuss the general risks of surgery in this chapter and the specific risks of the individual treatments and procedures in the chapters about each particular operation.

If you are a healthy person who eats well, are not being treated for any illnesses, are not unusually overweight, and can perform normal daily exercises and household tasks, then you can have surgery with the confidence that your risk levels will be average or low.

Age isn't usually a risk factor. If you're in your 70s or 80s, cosmetic procedures are nearly as safe for you as they are for people in their 40s. If you're older, your surgeon and her staff will explore your medical history more aggressively and be more interested in your blood pressure and heart status, but if you're truly healthy, age alone shouldn't stop you from having surgery. The problem with aging is that even though you feel well, your blood pressure may be up a little, your EKG may show some evidence of prior damage, and so on. If you're 70-plus, be prepared for your surgeon to ask you to get clearance from your personal physician or cardiologist.

My experience is that older people heal well after surgery. Nonetheless, if you're over 70, don't be surprised if it takes you longer to heal than your younger friends.

As society has become more accepting of cosmetic surgery procedures, the number of patients with medical problems requesting surgery has increased. Patients who in prior years wouldn't have considered a cosmetic procedure sometimes insist on proceeding even if they're at some increased risk.

Common risks of all operations

Naturally, when you're considering an operation, you never think that a complication will happen to you. After all, you healed beautifully when you had your appendix out at age 12. Nevertheless, risks and complications do occur occasionally, so you should know something about them. The following sections describe the most common problems that all surgeons see in all types of operations. I explain the complications for specific cosmetic surgery procedures in the chapters dealing with those surgeries.

Infection

To help prevent infections, most cosmetic surgeons (around 90 percent) order intravenous (IV) antibiotics during the operation if you're having a major procedure and also prescribe oral antibiotics for a few days following your surgery. Most surgeons believe that these antibiotics reduce infection problems postoperatively, but no actual scientific evidence appears to prove that this is the case. If you develop an infection, appropriate antibiotic treatment by mouth usually solves the problem within a few days. You usually don't need to be admitted to the hospital except in the most severe cases.

Bleeding and hematomas

Before the end of each operation, your surgeon will make sure that all *bleeders* (bleeding blood vessels, veins, or arteries) have been controlled. She does so in most cases by cauterizing the bleeding vessels or, less often, by tying off larger bleeders with a suture ligature.

In spite of these techniques, continued oozing of blood or brisk venous or even arterial bleeding may occur later. In more serious cases, you may need to return to the operating room so the surgeon can control the bleeding and remove excess blood and clots. In more minor cases, the bleeding stops by itself, and you don't need another operation but require another week or more of recovery for the extra swelling and bruising to go away.

Bruising

Bruising occurs when blood seeps into the tissues after an operation or injury. The color of the blood shows through the skin. As the blood is absorbed by the body, the color of the bruise gradually changes from purplish to red to greenish and then to yellow. Severe bruising can take several weeks (or months) to disappear. Some degree of bruising occurs after most operations and isn't considered a true complication. Severe or extreme bruising, when nearly the entire area that was operated on turns dark blue or black, is a complication because it delays a return to normal for weeks if not months.

Abnormal scarring

Even though your plastic surgeon will most likely close your incisions by using the best plastic surgery techniques, abnormally thick or wide scars may occur. These problems may be due to your own skin quality or the location of the incision on your body (some areas are much more likely to make thick or wide scars), or they may be a reaction to sutures or infection.

Patients tend to think that all wide or thick scars are keloid scars, but that's not true. *Keloid scars,* which tend to occur in darker-skinned people, are scars that grow beyond the incision line and are painful. Wide or thicker scars that occasionally occur in people of any color are called hypertrophic scars. The biological process that forms each of these kinds of scars is different, which is why hypertrophic scars can often be improved with steroid injections or revision but keloid scars usually can't.

Numbness or altered sensation

Areas of numbness or altered sensation may occur in or near any incision. Superficial sensory nerves are injured during the operation and frequently require several months to repair themselves. Occasionally, some degree of partial or complete numbness can persist. Persistent numbness may improve for up to two years. No specific treatment is really helpful.

Your body may perceive partial reduction in sensation as altered sensation or increased sensation. An example is the sensation change following many kinds of breast surgery; the nipples become unusually sensitive. The sensory nerves to the nipple have been slightly damaged but instead of feeling numbness, the patient feels increased sensation.

Uncommon but serious risks

Some risks can't be avoided, even with the best possible medical care. You can be reassured that when your surgeon and the medical team can take any steps to reduce the risks, they do. The complications listed in the following sections are less common but more serious than those listed in the previous section. Obviously, other problems not listed here may develop, but they're very unusual. Talk to your surgeon for more information.

Pulmonary embolism

Clots can form in your calves or pelvic area following any operation. If one of the clots breaks loose, it can lodge in your lungs (that's a *pulmonary embolism*) and cause serious symptoms or even death. Long airplane flights have recently been linked to increased incidences of blood clots and emboli. To reduce the risk of blood clots forming in your lower legs, compression stockings or compression pumps should be used during your operation. These methods mimic the effects of walking and utilizing your leg muscles.

If, in the past, you've had blood clots or pulmonary emboli, you need to tell your surgeon, and you may need short-acting blood thinners during your surgery. You'll probably need to consult with a hematologist to plan your medical strategy. These problems aren't common, but they do occur and are potentially serious. If an embolism occurs, you'll probably need to be hospitalized and take blood thinners for months. Women on birth control drugs and chronic smokers have a slightly higher statistical chance to form clots and experience pulmonary emboli.

Heart attack

A heart attack may happen during surgery by chance, or it may happen because you're under stress; either way, it's a very rare occurrence. Should this occur, the surgical team will see the changes on your electrocardiogram (EKG). The surgeon will complete or terminate your surgery as soon as possible, and the staff will begin appropriate medical care in the hospital. If you have any history of heart disease, disclose this fact during your consultation or your preoperative workup. If your medical history indicates heart disease, you'll need clearance from your primary care physician or cardiologist before surgery.

Cardiac arrhythmias

Abnormal rhythms, called *arrhythmias,* can occur during surgery. Minor rhythm problems aren't serious and can be controlled by the anesthesiologist. Serious rhythm problems may require hospitalization and the care of a cardiologist. Rhythm disturbances may develop due to undiagnosed heart problems (such as mitral valve prolapse), medications used during the procedure, or the general stress of surgery and anesthesia. The risk of developing a serious problem during surgery is very rare.

Allergies

Unknown allergies to medications or latex can occur during surgery. Allergic reactions range from simple skin rashes treated with antihistamines to swelling and congestion of the throat or lungs requiring steroids, bronchodilators, and epinephrine. The worst kind of allergic attack is called an *anaphylactic reaction* and can be fatal. However, death from allergic reactions during cosmetic surgery is very rare.

Be sure to report any and all known allergies to your surgeon and the office staff during your consultation or preoperative visit.

Malignant hyperthermia

Very few people having general anesthesia develop a condition called *malignant hyperthermia.* This syndrome can be triggered by some anesthetic agents in patients who are genetically susceptible to the condition. Prior to anesthesia, patients may have no idea that they're at risk unless they have a family history of this condition. It produces an extremely high metabolic rate, and if untreated, your temperature climbs to extremely high levels and can be fatal. A special medication called Dantrolene is available in all certified operating rooms, whether in or out of the hospital. This very rare genetic deficiency is often diagnosed at the time of the first anesthetic, which frequently occurs in childhood.

Anesthesia complications

Most patients worry about anesthesia complications and death. Many patients believe that local anesthesia is much safer than general anesthesia. In truth, all types of anesthesia are amazingly safe, and for most patients, general anesthesia is probably no riskier than local anesthesia with sedation.

In the early 1980s, the risk of anesthesia deaths was 1 per 5,000 anesthetics. Today, the risk is 1 per 250,000 anesthetics. The reasons for this are twofold: First, the medications and anesthesia gases are better than in the past. Second, and most importantly, the monitoring equipment now used during anesthesia is much improved and allows for easier detection of abnormalities in the patient. New technologies that measure oxygen saturation and carbon dioxide levels help prevent wrong placement of the breathing (endotracheal) tube, a major cause of anesthetic deaths in the past. Additional complications that are more minor include nausea, sore throat, hoarseness, and injury to your teeth. Many of these risks can also be minimized by anti-nausea drugs and careful placement of the breathing device by the anesthesia provider.

Reducing Fear and Anxiety

You've evaluated the risks and your personal health with your surgeon. Your surgery is scheduled, and the date is approaching. You're anxious, nervous, and somewhat fearful. How do you cope? Remember the following advice when you start feeling a little nervous:

- ✔ **Go back to basics:** Are you anxious or fearful because you doubt your choice or your decision-making process? Take time to go through it once again. What's bothering you? How badly do you want to change it? Did you choose your surgeon wisely? Is your surgery going to take place in safe surroundings? Do you have a support group in place? If you can answer these questions to your satisfaction, you're ready to move on to the next consideration.

- ✔ **Communicate:** This isn't the time to suffer in silence. Call your surgeon's office and let the staff know about your concerns. All plastic surgeons and their staffs have their own methods of reassuring patients. You may have a genuine concern, or you may be worrying about the smallest issues that your surgeon knows have no bearing on whether you'll achieve the outcome you seek. You and your surgeon's office should be in very frequent communication, and you'll be seen often before and after surgery — even in the middle of the night if there's a problem. A good surgeon should be only a phone call away — 24/7.

- ✔ **Keep busy:** Staying busy may help you feel less fearful and anxious by helping you focus on something besides the surgery itself. One way to stay busy is to plan properly for your recovery. If you're going to recover at home, get your house ready for your convalescence, using the list in the section "Going home," later in this chapter. Make a to-do list for both your surgery and your life in general. Getting as much done as possible *in advance* may help alleviate some of your anxiety and fear about your recovery period.

- ✔ **Do your part:** Follow your preoperative instructions, arrive on time, and leave all the details to the professionals. I tell patients, "Please let us do the worrying for you." Spend your time and energy preparing for and recovering from surgery.

- ✔ **Reach out:** Beyond calling your doctor's office, reach out to friends and family, especially if they've had the same procedure you're having done. Understanding that your concerns are normal helps to bring them into perspective.

✔ **Choose your attitude:** Like most things in life, you have a choice about how you're going to approach surgery — in a positive frame of mind or with fear. You can make your surgical experience more positive just by being positive. If you need information, communication, or reassurance to stay positive, then seek what you need from your surgeon and the people close to you.

You'll have a team of professionals to help you achieve your goals. Although you may not have surgery on a daily basis, surgical procedures are normal, everyday events for your surgeon, the clinic nurses, operating room personnel, anesthesiologists, and surgeons. They're all calm professionals who are prepared to deal with any issues that arise.

If, despite all the above, you're still anxious and fearful and considering canceling your operation, talk to your surgeon or an office nurse and discuss taking a Valium or something similar before surgery. No surgeon wants to get you hooked on medication, but patients sometimes need palliative measures on a temporary basis. You're not alone if you seek this solution. Having surgery frequently prompts last-minute jitters, but simple, safe solutions to calm you down are available.

Going from road rage to reassurance

Everyone has experienced road rage at one time or another, but it's a surprising path to cosmetic surgery. Lucile shared this story: "I first considered cosmetic surgery about 10 years ago when someone expressing road rage called me a 'middle-aged b----.' I had never considered myself middle-aged at 40-something. I felt too good to be in that category. After that, I saw myself differently. I found wrinkles I hadn't noticed before, and each year the drapes grew deeper around my laugh lines and my eyes were not as fresh as they used to be."

While she pondered having surgery, she watched "every cosmetic surgery procedure TV had to offer." She decided on her own extreme makeover — liposuction, breast augmentation and lift, eyelid lift, neck lift, and rhinoplasty. Later,

after she made her decision and the surgery date approached, she began recalling vivid images of scalpels slicing skin, and the images petrified her. "My surgeon and his nurses played a key role in helping to remove my fears by reassuring me and giving me lots of information to read before my surgery," she said. "The material covered everything from what to wear the day of surgery to how my emotions would run amok. I knew ahead of time when I'd see changes in my swelling and bruising. I knew when I was in tears that it was normal. I knew that when my breasts sloshed for a few days after the implant surgery, everything was going as planned. My total experience was greatly influenced by the pre-op education, the clinic staff, and knowing they were always available when I needed them."

Preparing for Your Recovery

Even after you assess the risks and get your emotions under control, you're not ready for surgery. You need to make some important decisions about your recovery phase, which depends on several factors, including the extent of your surgery, general health, family environment, and support systems. Don't underestimate the wisdom of the advice you get from your doctor. She's using her experience to give you advice that has your safe recovery as the primary objective. Don't underestimate your need for help either. Listen carefully to what your surgeon and her staff tell you about your postsurgery needs.

It's better to plan for more help than not enough. You can always tell a friend or relative that you appreciate her offer to help but you're doing well and don't need her help right now. But finding help at the last minute can be difficult, if not impossible.

Evaluating your post-op care options

Decisions about where you're going to recover and who will help you along the way depend on the level of care that you'll need. And the level of care depends on the type of surgery you've had and your personal health factors. For example, if you know that you had strong reactions to anesthesia after a previous surgery or have difficulty taking pain pills, you may want to consider having more help.

If you have general anesthesia, IV sedation, or even heavy oral or intramuscular (IM) sedation, you won't be allowed to go home alone — and, no, you can't call for a cab, either! Someone must stay with you for the first 24 hours after surgery. However, if you have a minor procedure under local anesthesia and your doctor doesn't ask you to make special arrangements for a caretaker or transportation, then after the procedure is over, you may drive yourself home or back to your office. In all likelihood, you won't need post-op assistance in this situation.

Recuperating in a hospital

Following more extensive procedures such as tummy tucks, thigh lifts, facelifts, or breast reductions, your surgeon may want you to spend a night or two in the hospital. Many hospitals have a special program for cosmetic surgery patients with a lower fee schedule than you would normally expect for a hospital stay. My hospital, for example, calls this program the POPS (plastic outpatient surgery) unit.

Whether your operation occurs in your doctor's surgery facility, an ambulatory surgery center, or a hospital operating room, you can be admitted to the POPS equivalent with your catheter and IV tubes in place. This way, you can receive IV or IM pain management. In some regions of the country, the hospital is your only option (other than home) for postoperative care.

Staying at the surgery center

Depending on where you live, your surgeon or surgery center may offer you the option of a "23-hour stay." The advantages are that you don't have to be moved and you have professional caretakers who are familiar with the needs of cosmetic surgery patients.

This service requires special licensure and at least two staff members on hand during your overnight stay. You don't have to be concerned if an independent ASC (ambulatory surgery center) offers this service, but if your surgeon is offering this service, ask about licensure and staffing.

Choosing a post-op care facility

In some communities, your surgeon may recommend post-op facilities that are operated in private homes, hotels, or nursing homes. Either licensed nurses or people with nursing or surgical backgrounds offer services that include picking you up after surgery, taking you to their after-surgery facility, and driving you back to your surgeon for your first postsurgery visit.

These facilities, when run well, provide a wonderful service to the community. You have the choice of staying one night or multiple nights. The cost is usually equivalent to an upscale hotel, but it includes meals and transportation. These facilities can be a blessing if you're planning on having surgery out of town or don't want to expose your family or spouse to the immediate postsurgery phase. Unfortunately, they don't exist in all areas.

When considering this option, the best guide is your surgeon's office. Your surgeon's staff should be well acquainted with the various options and recommend whatever is appropriate for your specific needs.

Arranging for a caretaker

If none of the preceding options are available or necessary for your surgery, you'll be asked to make after-surgery arrangements and designate someone to be responsible for you and your care during the immediate postsurgery phase. (You won't need to do this for minor procedures in which recovery isn't an issue.) Following most cosmetic surgery procedures, you can go home to your own bed and let your friend, spouse, adult child, or professional caretaker remain with you for the first night. After that, except for more extensive or multiple procedures, you often can plan to take care of yourself.

Choose your caretaker as far in advance as possible and give her time to make the necessary arrangements in her own life. If you're undergoing surgery and need anesthesia, your doctor will require someone to pick you up, drive you home, and stay with you for at least the first 24 hours.

Invite your caretaker to come with you to your appointment before surgery. Your doctor may call this visit a pre-op or H&P (history and physical) appointment. Your doctor or an office nurse should discuss immediate postsurgery care and arrangements, and your caretaker will have an opportunity to ask questions and become comfortable with her role.

Hiring licensed nurses or caretaker services

You may want to recover in your own bed, but you don't have a local friend or family member to assist you or someone who wants to take responsibility as your caretaker. Bringing in a capable and experienced caretaker is a wonderful option that reduces stress for everyone. In most cities or regions, registered nurses (RNs), licensed vocational nurses (LVNs), or licensed practical nurses (LPNs) provide this service and also provide transportation. The cost is about the same as for a post-op care facility.

In some areas of the country, you may find caretakers who specialize in cosmetic surgery recovery. Generally, they're unlicensed but frequently very experienced.

Let your doctor's office be your guide about the best choice for you. The key is the experience of the caretaker and the satisfaction of former patients with the caretaker's services. Your surgeon's office will use this information and your specific postsurgery needs to make the appropriate recommendation.

Going home

Whether you're using a professional caretaker or friend or family member, you need to get your home ready for your immediate postsurgery recovery. For example, stock up on the following items:

✔ **Several types of beverages:** To keep hydrated, make sure you have plenty of water; juices; Gatorade or the equivalent; and carbonated drinks such as ginger ale, 7-Up, root beer, or Coca-Cola.

✔ **Bendable straws:** Use these so you don't have to lift your head off your pillow when your caretaker gives you liquids to keep you hydrated.

✔ **Low-sodium crackers or gingersnaps:** These snack choices help with or prevent nausea that may accompany anesthesia or pain meds.

✔ **Soft foods:** JELL-O, applesauce, yogurt, and low-sodium soups are good foods to start with because they're easy to digest while you're taking prescription pain medication and recovering from anesthesia.

✔ **Frozen meals:** You won't feel up to cooking, but you need to keep eating. Frozen foods and convenient snacks maintain nutrition without effort, but watch the sodium content.

✔ **Ice:** Applying ice to the operative area(s) in the first 24 to 28 hours can prevent swelling and provide relief from discomfort. Crushed ice, bags of frozen peas, and gel packs are convenient choices.

✔ **Arnica gel and/or tablets:** Arnica treats bruising and swelling (see Chapter 18). I advise you to confer with a trained health practitioner for proper dosing of Arnica.

✔ **Stool softener:** Pain medications have a tendency to cause constipation, so you'll be glad to have this on hand.

✔ **Extra-strength Tylenol:** Tylenol is effective in treating mild discomfort and doesn't cause the nausea, constipation, or lethargy often associated with narcotics, so as your discomfort diminishes, replace your prescribed narcotics with Tylenol.

✔ **Entertainment:** You may spend quite a bit of time lounging around the house, so videotapes, DVDs, audiotapes, or CDs will be lifesavers.

✔ **Cotton swabs:** These are the best way to deal with possible oozing along your incision lines or to apply antibiotic ointment to your incisions.

Anesthesia medications slow the rate of digestion, so clear liquids in small amounts are your best bet immediately after surgery. When you can tolerate clear liquids, you can usually advance to a soft diet and then to a regular diet.

Your recovery time following cosmetic surgery can be a mini stay-at-home vacation, if you plan well. Assuming that you don't have excessive pain or continuing nausea (both uncommon), you may be able to organize some activities that aren't strenuous but that are rewarding, such as catching up on correspondence, listening to books on tape, or watching those old movies you've been meaning to see. You may also want some company and can encourage visitors when you feel up to it. Don't underestimate how hard it is for a busy, goal-oriented person to just *stop* and let healing take its course. (See Chapter 18 for more about recovery issues.)

Chapter 18

Recovering after Surgery

. . . .

In This Chapter

▶ Doing what your doctor orders

▶ Recognizing normal recovery symptoms

▶ Taking it easy after recovery

▶ Coping with your emotions

. . . .

Your recovery period is one of the most important phases of your surgery. You can help yourself immensely by carefully planning for your recovery and allowing yourself time to heal. If you don't allow yourself the time and conditions that optimize recovery, you run the risk of delaying healing unnecessarily. At worst, failure to follow instructions after surgery can adversely impact the outcome of your surgery.

Every plastic surgeon has a story of a patient who felt so good in the early recovery phase that she decided to clean out a closet, rearrange the books in the den, or head back to work earlier than agreed upon. The second part of the tale is that these patients all set themselves back by not recognizing that boredom and a little burst of energy don't signify that healing is complete.

Your potential and capacity to heal are unique to you. You can influence the healing process positively by choosing to follow your surgeon's instructions and by getting lots of rest. Don't push yourself — allow your body to use its resources for healing. You'll be much better off and have a speedier recovery if you follow this simple advice.

Following Instructions, or Doctor Knows Best

If you're like most people, you think that your surgeon can make you heal. No one can do that for you. The healing process is a natural function of your body. The surgeon will perform your surgery to the best of his ability within current medical standards, but whether you heal well or not is largely up to your body and your own healing capacity (and a little bit of the luck of the draw as to whether you get an infection or create a thick, wide scar). The entire process is a partnership between you and your surgeon.

Your doctor doesn't give you postsurgery guidelines because he wants to torment you or make you more miserable. After-surgery instructions reflect your surgeon's broad experience and knowledge and are designed to help you. Your doctor's instructions reflect a proven course of action that gives you the best chance for an uneventful recovery. When your surgeon tells you to limit your activities, for example, his goal is to facilitate healing and prevent complications.

As a patient, you have the responsibility of following your doctor's instructions. If you decide not to listen, you may well be asking for trouble. Your surgeon and his staff can't be with you 24 hours a day, so they need your sincere participation and cooperation in your own recovery process. If you don't follow the instructions, you aren't fooling anybody but yourself. Your doctor and nurses know what normal looks like.

Healing and recovery are in large part up to you. If you want to put the odds in your favor, then follow the instructions. If you're going to err, then do so on the conservative side. If you're not ready for more activity, for example, then take more time to heal.

Limiting your activities

You need to expect limits on your normal activities and exercise during your recovery. These limits vary according to the phase of recovery you're in, and they're very procedure dependent. For more specific details, turn to the sections on recovery in the procedure chapters in Part III.

You can expect more restrictions if you have multiple procedures or extensive procedures, such as an extended tummy tuck. On the other hand, if you're having your upper eyes done, then you may be out and about very quickly.

Dealing with pain

All surgery involves some postoperative discomfort, so accept this fact ahead of time. Don't regard pain as something negative. Pain is a signal from your body that forces you to restrict activity during the time that your body needs to heal and recover.

For the immediate postsurgical pain, the medications that your doctor prescribes should make your recovery almost painless. Some patients feel that taking pain medication is an admission of weakness, but it's not. Taking pain pills for a short time following surgery will not cause you to become addicted to the drug and will give your body the relief that you need. Later, as you reduce or eliminate the use of pain medication and begin to resume more normal activities, you should be guided by the pain you experience. Don't do any activity if it causes real discomfort in the area that was operated on.

Patiently pursuing a solution

On the eve of her 46th birthday, Bridgette began to think about cosmetic surgery. A self-employed organizational development consultant, she says, "Overall, I thought I was attractive, but a few things about my face bothered me: old acne scars, wrinkles around my upper and lower lips, a droopy brow, and a bump on the bridge of my nose. I thought, 'Hey, I don't have to live with these things anymore. I can get them taken care of.'"

After consulting with three surgeons, she had a gut feeling about one of them, and her research backed up that feeling. She was happy with her surgeon and his staff, but her recovery turned out to be a bigger deal than she had anticipated. "All I can say is you must have patience! It's only at eight weeks post-op that I feel relatively comfortable with my new face and am able to look people in the eyes without wearing tinted glasses or putting on a lot of makeup."

She says she thinks our society has become desensitized to the cosmetic surgery process: "It's still surgery; there are incisions in the skin, stitches to be removed, wounds to heal, hair to grow back, and scars to fade. And there are also strange sensations to get used to, such as tightening of the scalp, nose, and skin. I think it takes a while to 'take ownership' of the process and the new look, even if it is for the positive. I don't anticipate feeling fully healed or considerably more comfortable until I hit the six-month mark."

Although each day Bridgette comes closer to meeting her expectations, she says, "I had an unexpected moderate side effect of the surgery: acne breakouts all over my face, especially my forehead and chin. That has delayed my appreciation of the new look. I also had a bad reaction to the makeup I bought to cover the lasered skin."

What about her new look? "Most people don't even notice that I have made any changes to my appearance, or they can't quite put their fingers on why I look a bit different to them. I actually prefer this reaction (or lack thereof) because it means I look natural."

Your own pain history will give you and your doctor a good clue as to how to best plan for your postsurgical pain. In spite of preplanning, you also need to give your doctor's office good feedback as you take the medications prescribed for you. If your medication doesn't control your pain, your doctor can adjust the prescription for your comfort.

If you're like most patients, you'll want to discontinue the use of prescription pain medications as soon as possible. Nausea and constipation are common side effects, so if you experience either of these problems, let your surgeon know. He may suggest that you stop your pain medication or switch to a different pain medication or to some milder form of pain control, such as Tylenol. Just keep in contact with your doctor so he can use the feedback you provide to find the best solution for you.

Depending on your tolerance for pain or the extent of surgery you're having, you or your surgeon may opt to control your pain with a device known as a pain pump. *Pain pumps* have a reservoir that contains a local anesthetic. The reservoir is connected to small catheters that are placed under the skin in the surgical area that will probably be painful during the healing phase. The pain pumps deliver a measured amount of the local anesthetic over a period of several days. When the extra pain control is no longer needed, the small catheters are withdrawn, and pills are used to control pain, if necessary. Many patients and surgeons find that pain pumps are valuable during postsurgery recovery. They're used commonly with tummy tucks and other invasive body surgeries. Some surgeons use them for breast augmentations as well. Pain pumps have an additional cost of between $250 and $350.

Another kind of self-controlled pain pump, known as PCA (patient controlled analgesia), dispenses narcotics intravenously when the patient wishes. Only a predetermined amount of narcotic can be dispensed at one time, and the amount available to the patient per unit of time is preset. These pumps are only used in the hospital unless a patient has chronic pain or cancer.

Following medication instructions

In addition to prescriptions to help you deal with pain, you'll also receive prescriptions for several other medications. These drugs vary by procedure but commonly include medications to prevent infections or nausea or to enable you to sleep.

These medications have different directions that can be confusing. You'll want to take all of your antibiotics to prevent infection, but if you don't need pills for pain, sleep, or nausea, then you don't need to take them. When in doubt, ask your doctor's office. No medication is prescribed without a reason, so be sure that you understand why you're taking a particular drug and under what conditions you can stop.

Knowing What's Normal

One of the most important ways to have a positive recovery is to know what's normal and what's not. If you choose your surgeon wisely, you'll have a doctor and staff who excel in patient education and communication. They'll let you know in advance and in writing what you can expect as you recover. That way, you'll understand what's normal — so that you'll have a better idea of when to relax and let your body go through the normal healing phases — and what's not normal — so that you know when to be concerned and ask your surgeon for guidance.

I deal with the normal recovery symptoms of specific procedures in the chapters of Part III. In this chapter, I cover more general topics.

Understanding surgery and scarring

Prospective patients regularly call cosmetic surgeons' offices asking for "scarless surgery." No such thing is possible. Surgeons can perform scarless treatments, such as facial fillers, skin peels, and laser surgery, but otherwise, surgery is performed below the surface of your skin, and the scar represents the means of entry. Ideally surgeons leave a scar that's as narrow and short as possible to achieve the surgical goal.

Plastic surgeons understand patient interest in reducing or hiding scars. Depending on the procedure, surgeons can perform certain techniques that are designed to limit scar size or hide scars from public view. For more detailed information about the procedures that interest you, see the specific procedure chapters in Part III and the various techniques associated with scarring.

Reducing bruising and swelling

Almost every surgery may have a small amount of bruising that surgeons consider normal. It's caused by a small amount of blood under the skin that may have oozed after the operation was over. Large areas of dark bruising mean that more than average bleeding occurred under the skin after the surgery was completed. Large amounts of bruising are considered a complication because healing will be delayed for weeks, a month, or more. Swelling usually accompanies large amounts of bruising, but it decreases along with the bruising.

Arnica montana (also know as leopard's bane) is a homeopathic (herbal) drug that has been used for hundreds of years for a number of things, including bruising and swelling. Many doctors think that its use reduces bruising and swelling, so plastic surgeons often prescribe Arnica in pill or gel form for use after surgery. Anecdotally, it frequently appears to help and, even when it's not prescribed by the surgeon, many patients buy this drug at their pharmacies or health food stores and take it.

Newer technologies involve using electromagnetic pulses to treat edema (swelling) and pain. Stimulation of swollen or bruised areas with radio frequencies shows promise.

Your surgeon may recommend a massage therapist to provide lymphatic drainage massage to reduce swelling after surgery. In my experience, many patients find that this procedure not only relaxes them but also contributes significantly to their recovery. Lymph drainage involves a gentle, rhythmic therapy that's intended to cleanse your connective tissues of such things as excess water, toxins, bacteria, proteins, and cellular debris.

Your doctor will recommend a schedule for this therapy. Some surgeons recommend one session before surgery as well as after surgery. Other surgeons encourage only postsurgery appointments. After you know the date of your surgery, make your appointments well in advance because these therapists tend to have busy schedules.

If you seek these services on your own, be sure that the therapist giving your lymphatic massage is a licensed professional certified in lymph drainage therapy. This skill isn't normally included in typical massage training and requires specialized knowledge and techniques.

Healing hardness under the skin

Hardness or lumpiness under the skin, known as *induration,* can occur when the skin in the area has been dissected, or cut. Some level of minimal induration or hardness is present after every surgery. Induration is frequently associated with resolving hematomas (blood clots under the skin that are being absorbed by your body). Ask your surgeon about the following ways to help treat this problem if you're concerned about it:

- Light massage with your fingers
- Ultrasound treatments over the hardened areas, which may be available in your surgeon's office or at a physical therapy office
- Use of a vibrating massager, such as any hand-held device used for neck or back pain relief (use carefully and only with your doctor's advice)

These techniques and the passage of time all contribute to healing and softening. Virtually all induration disappears with time.

Knowing what's normal is important to your recovery, but you also need to be on the lookout for the following conditions that are abnormal and require a call to your doctor. Most of these conditions require an office visit, so ideally you should call your doctor as early as possible so that the office can arrange a visit during normal office hours. But after hours, you still need to call your doctor if you experience

- ✔ **Elevated temperature:** A temperature over 100 degrees could indicate that you have an infection or possibly aren't drinking enough fluids.

- ✔ **Severe swelling:** If you develop severe swelling near any surgical site, call your surgeon as this may indicate bleeding, seroma (collection of fluid), or infection.

- ✔ **Wound drainage:** If you start leaking fluid or blood from an incision site, your surgeon will want to know and will probably need to see you.

- ✔ **Severe rash:** A severe rash is usually an indication of an allergic reaction to one of your medicines, but it can also be an indication of a severe infection.

- ✔ **Severe pain:** A change in the level of pain that you're feeling after surgery, especially a severe increase, may be a sign of a larger complication.

Easing into Activity

Try and make recovery a positive experience that will be a plus in your life. Plan to use the downtime away from your normal work or lifestyle to rest and do things you'll enjoy. You can catch up on those wish-list items that you never seem to find the time for. You're going to have downtime, and you need to choose activities or projects that don't expend too much energy but keep you from getting restless, bored, or depressed. Here are some suggested ways to spend your time:

- ✔ **Get some extra sleep.** Most surgical procedures, even small ones, usually make people feel fatigued. Take the opportunity to really catch up on your sleep, which is one of the best healing strategies. Don't be surprised by the amount of time you can sleep. Don't feel guilty either. You deserve the sleep, and your body needs it.

- ✔ **Watch TV and rent movies.** Recovery offers the opportunity for you to see those daytime TV shows that you never get to watch or rent movies that you kept meaning to see at the theater but didn't.

- ✔ **Read or listen to books on tape.** If you want to catch up on your reading, decide in advance what you want and make sure that you have the books or audiobooks ready. Remember that if you're having any procedure involving your eyes or forehead, books on tape are the best alternative to traditional books.

✔ **Catch up on correspondence.** Whether you write letters the old-fashioned way or use e-mail, make a list before surgery of all the friends you want to connect with. Using your recovery time to write to these people will give you a feeling of accomplishment.

✔ **Organize your photo albums.** Maybe you've been looking for an opportunity to organize all the pictures you took on your last vacation. If so, buy the albums before your surgery so that you'll be prepared.

✔ **Hit the open road.** If you drive a car with power steering, then you can probably drive a few days after surgery — as long as driving doesn't cause pain and you're no longer taking sleeping or pain medications.

✔ **Get some light exercise.** Gentle movement is okay, but more active exercising is not. In other words, easy, slow-paced walking to keep your joints moving is good, but power walking is not. Exercising raises your blood pressure temporarily, which can cause bleeding — a real no-no! You can get up to speed on your exercise program later. If you're going to err here, do so on the side of caution.

✔ **Use recovery time to catch up on work.** At some point in your recovery, you'll probably feel well enough to do some business on your computer or over the phone even though you may be swollen or bruised or even uncomfortable. You shouldn't do anything strenuous or aerobic, but using your mind doesn't usually cause your blood pressure to go up.

If you need to go to the office and work there, doing so isn't usually a problem as long as you limit your time and ease your way back into a full schedule. But a full workday is probably counterproductive to your healing, especially if you've had multiple procedures.

✔ **Go to restaurants, movies, and the mall.** These activities are fine as long as they don't raise your blood pressure — so you may want to see a "chick flick" instead of a war movie. Some patients who are confined to their houses get a little depressed from recovery symptoms, such as swelling or bruising, but also from missing their normal lives. Getting out will help as long as you take it easy. Keep in mind that your energy level will dip more quickly than usual.

✔ **Have sex.** After most procedures, you can have sex after a few days so long as you're not too active, which could raise your blood pressure and increase the risk of bleeding. Be sure that your partner is gentle and that you assume the more passive role. If anything feels uncomfortable, tell your partner and stop or modify the activity.

Dealing with the Emotional Aspects of Recovery

Sometimes you feel a little blue after surgery. It's normal. In addition to the physical aspects of healing, you can expect to face some emotional and psychological issues as well. Cosmetic surgery patients often question their sanity and begin asking themselves, "What have I done? What was I thinking?" Fortunately, for most people this phase is short.

Sometimes you may feel slightly depressed as you go through the recovery phase. Your body is coping with a lot at once, and feeling down at some point as you heal is common. Expectations and excitement are high before surgery, and lows do follow highs. The letdown feelings or depression may last a day or several days but shouldn't persist. You need to know that this reaction is normal and that you'll feel better emotionally as you heal physically. Soon, you'll be feeling better and enjoying your new look, and then you'll be asking yourself why you didn't have surgery sooner.

Surprising emotions

Jill's first cosmetic surgery experience was 15 years ago when she had her eyelids done. A professional woman approaching age 50, she decided she wanted to "combat the effects of life."

"I have a career that I love, and a major part of my profession is speaking in front of hundreds of people and, I believe, presenting myself as a positive role model."

The effects of three pregnancies and nursing her babies took its toll on her body. With the support of her family, Jill decided to have liposuction to "look better and regain her professional image." She is thoroughly pleased with her results and the entire process, including the incredible bond she formed with her surgeon and nurse. She was taken aback, however, by the emotional healing process involved: "A surprising experience I noted was the feeling of guilt. Cosmetic surgery is an elective procedure and requires some physical downtime and a lot of attention — neither of which I was used to needing. I was also very aware of how many of my friends were struggling with illnesses and diseases while I was healthy and 'choosing' to be cut upon. This was something I had to struggle through personally as I evaluated my motivation in the process. This resulted in both emotional and psychological growth for me."

Would she do it all over again? "In a heartbeat!"

If you stay at home and are isolated from friends and co-workers, you may feel cut off from your normal environment, which can contribute to some level of temporary depression. Don't be embarrassed to share your thoughts and emotions, because they're a normal aspect of your recovery. Your surgical support team can usually give you some perspective because many of them have been cosmetic patients themselves and they know just how you're feeling. This is also a good time to call upon your other support systems. Bring in the people who love you. Friends and loved ones are there to talk and provide encouragement. Often everyone else can see the progress you're making better than you can. Focus on things other than your surgery and recovery — start imagining the new you and all the wonderful things you're going to do as soon as you've recovered.

Most patients begin to incorporate their new shapes and sizes into their body images within one to three weeks. If your feelings of anxiety or depression persist beyond this time period, discuss the issue with your surgeon or your nurse so that they can help you. The passage of time is usually all the treatment needed, but in rare cases, some patients may need psychiatric or psychological care.

Chapter 19

Finding Happy Endings

. . . .

In This Chapter

▶ Evaluating your result

▶ Handling disappointment

▶ Capitalizing on your new look

. . . .

*O*n one hand, reality TV shows about cosmetic surgery may lead you to believe that you can find almost instant perfection via cosmetic surgery. On the other hand, media exposés paint horror stories of cosmetic surgery outcomes. The truth, of course, lies somewhere between these extremes.

You're much more likely to have really good results than to reach perfection. The vast majority of patients are very happy with their surgical outcomes, but only a small percentage of patients and surgeons actually describe their results as "perfect." At the other end of the spectrum, a small percentage of patients experience healing delays, secondary surgery, and temporary to permanent complications.

This chapter includes advice about what happens after your surgery, from sizing up your results, to taking action when things don't turn out like you hoped, to working with your surgeon and her staff. Minimizing stress and ending up satisfied with your result is everyone's goal.

Assessing Your Result

If you're like most patients, you're going to be happy with your result and experience an uneventful recovery. Although you'll have some idea about your ultimate outcome immediately after your surgery, healing takes time, and depending upon the procedure, complete healing may take weeks or even months. Allow healing time before ranking your result.

Timing is everything

Three years after having gastric bypass surgery for health and medical reasons, Thea saw her skin sag as her weight declined. When she reached her goal weight, she couldn't do anything about the excess skin. She realized she needed to take care of herself in more ways than one and "look prettier, too."

As the widow of a physician and with two boys out of college, Thea says she realized it was finally her turn: "It was the most life-altering experience I've had. I feel 40 years old, I look 50, and I'm really 63. I've got guys beating down my door, and I feel like I'm in high school or college again. It's given me a second chance to start my life all over again."

Before she decided to have surgery, Thea says, "When I was heavy, I was isolated and not very outgoing. I spent about ten years as a recluse. Now I have a boyfriend, I travel, I go to parties, and I wake up everyday with a smile on my face. I now actually attend and work for the charity events that I used to just send checks to. It's been so life altering, I could get up and write a speech for it."

Her advice to others is to "encourage everyone, not just young people, to get out there and improve themselves. These are the best years of my life now. A lot of women, when they get over 50 or 60 think, 'What's the use?' But I'll tell you there are so many reasons that I can't even list them all!"

Following cosmetic surgery, some patients experience minor complications, and a very few have serious postoperative problems. With good preparation for surgery, you should understand the potential risks of surgery. Complications do occur even with the best of surgeons and optimal safety conditions. You must be prepared to do your part — take responsibility for your decision and follow your surgeon's postoperative guidelines and advice.

Waiting for complete healing

Healing can take a long time. Most surgeries are healed within three to six months, but some take longer. Noses, for example, frequently keep changing for up to a year or more.

If you don't like some aspect of your surgical result, your surgeon may ask you to wait until you've healed completely before considering secondary or revisional surgery. Accept her advice and keep in mind that additional surgery too early in the healing process can sometimes create more problems than it solves.

If you're having some postoperative problems that your surgeon says will clear up with time, smile and keep a positive attitude. Positive attitudes contribute to healing. Everyone loves a winner, and hopefully, you're one of them. As one of my friends says, "If you're going to 'whine,' at least let me get the cheese."

Fending off unwanted opinions

After your surgery, be prepared for lots of feedback from your friends and family. Your girlfriends who come by for coffee, your mother who's helping with the kids, and your frustrated husband who wants to know when you'll be doing the cooking again will all have opinions on the results of your surgery.

It would be nice if everyone were supportive, saying things like "I've never seen anyone look so good this quickly." The reality is that your friends and relatives may point out your problems instead of emphasizing the positives. They may say things like "The right side of your face doesn't look as good as your left side" or "The right breast looks larger than your left," leaving you feeling uneasy. Remember, these are observations made by non-medical people.

Try to let observations roll off your back like water off a duck. If your surgeon says that your recovery course is normal and you're doing well, then you should trust her informed medical opinion. Your doctor knows healing doesn't always occur symmetrically. She can see past the postoperative swelling and bruising, the unevenness, and the lumpiness and know what you'll look like when the healing is complete.

Following post-op instructions

Your surgeon has good reasons for the advice she gives you about what you can and can't do after surgery.

I did a facelift on a good friend several years ago. She felt so good several days after surgery that she decided to reorganize all the books in her library despite her patient education instructions advising her to restrict her activity. The reaching, bending, and lifting that put her library in order also strained her body, causing a blood vessel under the skin to leak and necessitating secondary surgery. She went from no bruising to severe bruising, causing her recovery to be prolonged unnecessarily.

Your surgeon is the expert in cosmetic surgery and associated recovery. Even though you may have a PhD or run a large corporation, you're not an expert about healing and recovering from surgery. Trust your doctor and follow her instructions. Be compliant. You can compromise your own result by doing too much too soon. For more information, turn to Chapter 18.

Trusting your surgeon

In the early days after surgery, you may worry about your result while your surgeon, at the same time, says she's thrilled you're doing so well. Trust in her and her staff's experience and perspective — they've seen many patients at the same phase of recovery, so their assessment is based on broad experience.

Trust is especially important if you experience a complication or delayed healing. If something isn't going the way you hoped and you're concerned, express your feelings to your surgeon or her staff. Presume good intent. Curb expressions of anger, aggressiveness, or hostility and try not to assign blame. You can be sure that your surgeon and her staff want you to have a good result just as much as you do.

Trusting your surgeon doesn't mean that you shouldn't voice your concerns. By expressing your opinion, you can gain insight about what's normal for patients at the same point and get advice about what you can do to help the healing process.

If you end up feeling unhappy with your result or end up looking a way that you can't tolerate, you need to work with your surgeon to find a solution (see the section "Dealing with Disappointment," later in this chapter).

Having realistic expectations

Having realistic expectations applies to all phases of your healing process. If your surgical outcome is in line with the expectations you had before surgery, then all is well. If, however, your results differ from the image you had in mind, then what are you going to do? First, ask yourself where your result falls on a continuum from your starting point to your mature surgical result. Second, listen to what your surgeon and her staff say about how you're doing.

It's easy to forget what you looked like before surgery. If you're discouraged, ask to see your pre-surgery photos and you'll probably be surprised at the positive change that has been achieved.

Most surgeons are very consistent in their surgical techniques and produce predictable results, and most patients are happy with the outcome of their surgeries, but in spite of their surgeon's best efforts, a few are dissatisfied. Sculpting a human body isn't as simple as carving wood or sculpting clay.

Liking your results depends in large part on having realistic expectations. Keep yours in check by doing the following:

- **Know the risks.** Before surgery, both the general risks of all surgery and the specific risks associated with the surgical procedure you're having will be explained to you. If you're among the low percentage who encounter one or more of the known risks, then you need to work through it with your surgeon and not assign blame.

- **Understand that bodies vary.** You may heal faster or slower than the "average" patient. Don't be discouraged if your body needs more time to get rid of that last bit of swelling or bruising. If you've experienced a complication that delays healing, then recovery may take longer but the complication generally doesn't impact your final result.

- **Follow your doctor's instructions.** Your best results come from giving yourself adequate time to heal. Don't take risks with your health, no matter how good you feel.

- **Recognize that your genetic makeup plays a role.** Your surgeon can only enhance your existing features. He will do his best to achieve the result you're hoping for, but he's limited by the innate structure of your body.

- **Understand that you strongly influence your final result.** If you had body contouring surgery when you weighed 120 pounds, then you can't blame the surgeon a year later when you weigh 145 pounds and don't like how you look in jeans.

- **Maintain a positive attitude.** Focus on the positive and presume good intent — no one wants you to have a problem.

Dealing with Disappointment

Even the best surgeon using the best techniques doesn't always achieve perfection. You can accept as truth, however, that your surgeon will do her absolute best to get you the best result possible. Sometimes the result may not be apparent for months. Swelling can take a very long time to disappear — up to six months with liposuction and a year with noses — so be patient. During the healing phase, give your surgeon the benefit of the doubt. Keep the lines of communication open and discuss what your options will be if your procedure doesn't ultimately heal and produce your desired results.

If your surgeon asks you to wait for six months to make a determination about your result, trust her judgment about the time your body needs to fully heal. Certainly you can ask her to explain what will happen if, at month six, you still feel that your result is not ideal. Having a clear understanding with your surgeon will give you psychological relief while you wait and also prevents potential misunderstandings and conflicts. If you're anxious or concerned as you wait for healing, call your surgeon's office and ask for an interim appointment to check on what both of you think about the progress of your healing and outcome.

Complications occur, but they almost always get better, frequently with the passage of time as the only treatment. Understand that patients of the best surgeons have complications, and virtually all surgeons want to help you any way they can.

PERSONAL STORY

Coping with complications

At age 45, Norman started to notice his facial skin sagging and decided he wanted to look better. After about a year of Internet research, he was prompted to pick up the phone when someone he knew had an excellent facelift result.

Norman chose to have a facelift, eyelid lift, neck lift, and liposuction, and although he's now very happy with his results, he thinks that the most important thing for others to know about his experience is that he was ill-prepared for the recovery time: "I think my friend minimized her recovery period. I felt very wiped out and fatigued for about four to six weeks. I am a very physical person, even at age 50, and I (and others) consider myself to be in very good physical shape. I just wasn't prepared for this long of a recovery time — mentally, emotionally, or physically." Norman says that if he had to do it over again he would have gone to a recovery center for the first few days instead of going home. "I live alone, and the person I chose to stay with me for the first 24 hours was not a good choice. He didn't remember the staff's instructions and misplaced some of the medications given to me. I wasn't prepared for the blurred vision. I was unable to read the medication instructions and even the phone number of the surgery center

to be able to call. Nor was I able to see well enough to drive myself to appointments for the next week."

Norman developed a complication (corneal abrasions in both eyes) and had to call his physician, who immediately confirmed that the pain he was experiencing in his eyes was not normal. "I need to add that I was so impressed with my surgeon and the staff and how they handled the complication that occurred for me. He did not try to hide anything about it and had me come in first thing the next morning. My surgeon and his staff were all very open and honest about what probably went wrong and why. They immediately sent me to an ophthalmologist and covered all the costs. There was no permanent damage done, but I must say that the corneal abrasions were the most painful ordeal of my life."

Nonetheless, Norman says he's extremely pleased with his results: "I expected changes in the loose facial skin, but it was an impressive change. My love handles are gone. I just didn't expect the results to be as good as they are." However, Norman also tells people considering surgery to "be prepared for the recovery period. Complications can happen."

Getting second opinions

If you're not satisfied with your surgeon's response to your extreme disappointment, then you shouldn't hesitate to seek advice from another good surgeon, perhaps one who was high on your list of candidates during the research phase. The best way to approach this isn't by casting blame but by discussing this step with your surgeon and telling her who you're planning to see. Ask her if she's willing to discuss your case with that surgeon. That way the medical facts will get transmitted correctly, and the second surgeon you see can be better prepared to give you an informed second opinion.

The second surgeon may tell you that your surgical result is good and that your surgeon is giving you appropriate care and advice. If you sought a second opinion and the second opinion is different from what you're hearing from your own surgeon, ask the two physicians to talk and come to a consensus. If they can't agree, perhaps a third opinion is in order.

In the worst-case scenario, if your surgeon is not or cannot be helpful in dealing with problems, then you may decide to change doctors. If your surgeon is in a group practice, your best course of action is to see another surgeon in the group because a quality practice wants to solve your problem — they want you to be happy.

Most plastic surgeons are highly ethical and speak to you candidly about your concerns about another surgeon's results. Occasionally, an unscrupulous surgeon giving a second opinion will use your visit as an opportunity to undermine your confidence in your surgeon and create new income for herself. Ideally, you want to return to your original surgeon, who is the most likely to perform secondary surgery at lower cost.

Pursuing a secondary operation

Whether you've had a second opinion or not, you and your surgeon may conclude that you need an additional touch-up or revisional surgery. Requesting a revision is clearly appropriate if you've had your eyelids done and one eye still has much more skin than the other, or if you've had your ears done (otoplasty) and one ear clearly sticks out more than the other.

There may also be times when you want a revision and your surgeon thinks that your result falls within normal ranges. For example: You think your scar is slightly wider than you wish or, following any of the breast procedures, one breast is very slightly larger than the other. The situation can become slightly more difficult if you have a problem that your surgeon isn't sure she can improve. If you want a revision and your surgeon is reluctant to do it, then you have to negotiate.

Your surgeon may feel she has achieved a very good result or that further surgery has a chance of making the "problem" worse instead of better. Some patients don't want to settle for very good and want perfect instead, but the surgeon doesn't want to risk turning the very good result into a result that is less good. These kinds of issues come up more with breast surgery but can occur with any kind of cosmetic surgery.

It's important to really discuss the possibility of revisions with the surgeon and the office before surgery, especially if you're having surgeries known to have revisions, such as body contouring after massive weight loss. Not knowing what to expect can bring up a lot of hard feelings during a time of already difficult discussions.

Dealing with the costs of secondary surgery

Unfortunately, if you need additional surgery, you're likely to encounter associated costs, especially if your surgeon operates at a hospital or an ambulatory surgery center. If you have a second procedure within the first year after your first procedure, then most surgeons waive their professional fees, but you're responsible for out-of-pocket costs, the most significant being the cost of the operating room and anesthesia.

If you follow my advice in Chapter 6, then before surgery you should know your surgeon's financial policies relating to revisionary or secondary surgery. Having this information before you make a decision about having cosmetic surgery can make you better prepared for this possibility — both financially and emotionally.

Rarely, a complication occurs that requires a corrective procedure by a surgeon in a different specialty, such as an ocuplastic surgeon. Your insurance often covers most of the cost of such secondary treatment of the complication, and your surgeon may agree to help you with any uncovered costs.

Avoiding litigation

In the worst possible case, you may feel malpractice has occurred. *Malpractice* is defined as illegal, unethical, negligent, or immoral behavior by a physician who has not adhered to the standard of care provided by other physicians in the community. Not liking your result or having a healing complication that was disclosed to you before surgery doesn't constitute malpractice.

If you don't like your result or have a complication, then you should still presume good intent on the part of your surgeon and her staff. Malpractice claims are painful for both surgeons and patients. Each party should do everything they can to avoid getting to that point.

My best suggestion for anyone considering litigation is that, before starting down such a path, you make an appointment with the doctor or the practice manager and discuss your feelings and intentions. You may find that you can reach a solution short of litigation. If some sort of financial remuneration is contemplated, the surgeon's professional liability carrier often becomes involved. Be prepared to sign a full medical release of liability as a part of any financial agreement.

Ending Up Happy

You look in the mirror and you see yourself 10 to 15 years younger. You try on your bathing suit and wonder if *Baywatch* is still auditioning. Perhaps your abdomen now matches your chest, arms, and legs, and you feel like Tarzan. Or, you have a new profile that makes you *want* to look in the mirror.

Is the new you going to function any differently than the presurgery you? In some instances, the answer is a resounding yes. If you have felt a little depressed because of your appearance, have suffered some rejection person-ally, and now feel happier and better about your appearance, then you may well show a new and sunnier face (or body) to the world.

Such transformations take place all the time in plastic surgery patients. A good example is an otherwise pretty 17-year-old girl who comes in for rhinoplasty (a nose job). If she believes, deep down, that her nose is ugly, then neither her mother nor the school counselor can ever talk her out of that belief. Making her nose look acceptable or pretty frequently appears to change her entire personality. If she was withdrawn or a wallflower before, then she becomes outgoing and vivacious. With an improved self-image, she feels better about herself and relates to the world more positively.

If you feel better about yourself, take advantage of your positive feelings. Be more open, allow yourself to live a happier life, and enjoy your relationships on a more fun level. Take as much advantage of your makeover as you can.

I frequently see life changes occur in my patients. I once saw a wonderful young woman who was in for her one-year postaugmentation check-up. She looked stunning and had a perfect result. I asked her what having the surgery had done for her life. She said, "You cannot believe it. No, you really can't understand how wonderful this has been." Clearly, her self-confidence was improved, and her social life had blossomed.

If you restricted your social life because you were flat-chested and felt self-conscious, then breast augmentation may help you come out of your shell. Now that you know your body looks great, you no longer need to hide out. Get a new bathing suit, go to the beach, join a bicycling club, or do whatever it takes to have fun in the sun. If night life appeals to you, then get out that little black dress and head for the disco or Vegas.

When things go well (as they usually do), seize the opportunity and run with it! Although you can't expect that cosmetic surgery will completely change your life, many patients tell me that it's life altering. They're happier with themselves, and the world around them picks up on those good vibes and responds more positively.

Part V
The Part of Tens

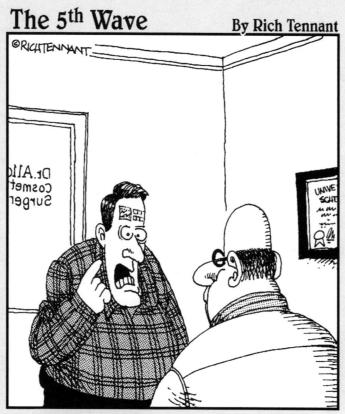

The 5th Wave   By Rich Tennant

"Don't WYSIWYG me, Doc. When I agreed to
the computer image of my facial procedures,
it was never supposed to include the tool bar
and pop-up ad."

In this part . . .

Sort through common myths about cosmetic surgery (sorry — you actually *can't* have scar-free surgery) to get to the facts. Find out about important questions you should consider before deciding to have cosmetic surgery, and figure out what you can do to make your experience as satisfying as possible.

Chapter 20

Ten (Or So) Myths about Cosmetic Surgery

In This Chapter

▶ Recognizing that surgery isn't a cure-all

▶ Understanding that new and famous aren't always better

▶ Getting the real scoop on silicone and anesthesia

*N*ot every myth, especially the ones about cosmetic surgery, can be checked on www.truthorfiction.com. In this chapter, I help you out a bit by discussing and hopefully refuting some of the most common myths out there and uncovering the truth behind the fiction.

Cosmetic Surgery Is the Key to Happiness

Just as money isn't the key the happiness, neither is cosmetic surgery. Many patients who have cosmetic surgery do find that they feel better about themselves afterward — their self-esteem increases and, with it, their enjoyment of life. Cosmetic surgery is about physical changes that I hope you'll enjoy, but you'll have to find your own path to happiness.

Cosmetic Surgery Will Solve All Your Problems

If you can't find a date or have marital or partnership problems, don't look to cosmetic surgery for your total solution. If you eat too much and weigh too much as a result, then looking to your plastic surgeon to liposuction away your excess fat instead of dieting isn't realistic, either. There's no question that cosmetic surgery can solve many physical problems, but you may need a therapist — or an exorcist — to handle the rest of what life throws at you.

You Can Have Scar-Free Cosmetic Surgery

You can't eat a banana without peeling it first. You have to get past the protective coating to get to the fruit. It's the same with cosmetic surgery. If you want your surgeon to deal with problems beneath the surface of your skin, he has to get past your protective layer — also known as your skin. Some procedures, such as lip and chin augmentation, use incisions that can be hidden, and liposuction scars are very small and generally easy to hide. But if your surgeon needs to remove excess skin, then you must understand that you'll have scars. The good news is that one of the key skills plastic surgeons learn and employ on your behalf is minimizing the appearance of scars.

You Can Address Big Issues with Small Operations

The idea that large problems can be solved with either nonsurgical treatments or small surgical techniques is one of the greatest myths that plastic surgeons face. And frequently, other medical specialists who aren't trained to perform the procedure you really need are the ones to suggest seemingly simpler alternatives with little or no supposed recovery time.

The more significant the changes you want, the more surgery you can expect to need. Likewise, if you have small procedures, expect that your results will have a smaller impact and frequently not last as long.

The Newest Procedure Is the Best One

Members of the press love to report the newest and latest cosmetic surgery treatments or procedures. These topics give them something to feature in their magazines, newspapers, and TV shows. But medicine — sound medicine — is based on broad experience, which takes time.

Doctors and researchers make many mistakes as medicine advances. I think you're far better off with the tried-and-true surgical techniques. Choose your surgeon carefully and look at his or her results. You don't want to jump on the bandwagon until the surgeon can show you longer term results, ideally a year or more. And you don't want to go to the only surgeon performing this procedure. Acceptance into mainstream medicine is a good sign, and you're much better off if you wait until that occurs.

The Most Famous Surgeon Is the Best

The surgeon who gets all the buzz in the media may well be the best, but he also may simply be the surgeon with the most effective public relations machine. How can you tell the difference? Get your priorities straight using the shopping guide I provide in Chapter 4. You'll be less likely to fall for hype and more likely to focus on what's important.

Don't let one surgeon's public relations machine obscure the proven skills of surgeons who may be equally competent but are less well known. Ideally, you want both — a well-respected doctor with quality surgical results.

You Get What You Pay For

Although correlations between quality and cost certainly do apply to some things — wines and cruises, for example — you can probably think of many examples where quality is available at lower cost. After all, a two-dollar bottle of wine won a double gold medal in a blind tasting at the International Eastern Wine Competition.

If you see the same jacket in two different stores at two drastically different prices, you're a smart shopper if you buy the lower-priced one. After all, you're getting the exact same jacket. When shopping for cosmetic surgery, however, you can't be sure that two surgeons' skill levels are comparable, so you can't base your decision only on price.

Choose your surgeon by the quality of his surgical results and your estimation of what the quality of your patient experience will be rather than by how much he charges.

Silicone Isn't Safe

Despite the hullabaloo about silicone implants in the early '90s, silicone has been found to be well tolerated within the body. It's used in the manufacture of many medical implants, and the outer shells of all breast implants are made of silicone. Silicone gel implants have been found not to cause the connective tissue disorders that were the root of the lawsuits that made such a splash. Almost all plastic surgeons expect that some type of silicone gel implants will be back on the market within a few years. For more details on the implants, see Chapter 12.

Local Anesthesia Is Always Safer than General Anesthesia

Most patients considering cosmetic surgery worry about anesthesia complications — and death, to some extent. Many patients believe instinctively that local anesthesia is much safer than general anesthesia. In truth, all types of anesthesia are equally safe in the hands of a qualified anesthesiologist. The risk of dying from complications associated with general anesthesia is about 50 times lower now than it was in 1980. The single most important change is the development of sensitive monitoring equipment now used during anesthesia. The slightest deviation from normal in all the important measurements sets off alarms.

There's Plastic in Plastic Surgery

Plastic comes from the Greek word *plastiko,* meaning "to mold"; that's how the surgeons who mold your skin and body became known as *plastic* surgeons. They don't actually use plastic when they operate on you. (Many products that are made of plastic these days are made in molds, hence the use of the term *plastic* to describe them.)

Cosmetic Surgery Lasts Forever

If you could stop the effects of aging and gravity, perhaps cosmetic surgery would last forever — or at least as long as you live. But the effects of these forces can't be controlled, so you just have to be content to enjoy the benefits while you can. The good news is that if you turn back the hands of time by ten years now, you should continue to look ten years younger for the rest of your life. And if you want to further thwart aging and gravitational pull on your body, then you can always opt for additional surgery later.

Chapter 21

Ten Questions to Ask Yourself before Pursuing Cosmetic Surgery

. . . .

In This Chapter

▶ Thinking about what bothers you

▶ Exploring your options

▶ Dealing with the realities

. . . .

Cosmetic surgery offers all kinds of great possibilities, but changing your body is nothing to rush into. Whether you've been mulling over the decision for years or have just started considering your options, taking a good, hard look at yourself and your situation is a good place to start. I can't tell you whether you're ready for cosmetic surgery, but I encourage you to do some soul searching before you pursue it. The following questions will help you determine where you stand.

What Bothers Me?

Start by asking yourself what is it about your face or body that really bothers you. Be extremely detailed in your analysis because if you do decide to pursue cosmetic surgery, then you're going to have to explain your concerns to each surgeon you consult and make your ultimate decision based on their recommendations.

I encourage you to make a list. You may have more than one area of concern: You've never liked your nose, and now you have saggy breasts and a pouching tummy that resists all exercise as well. But, if you're like most people, you must consider the costs of surgery, the downtime, and the reactions of those closest to you. Your self-diagnosis may be larger than your pocketbook. That's why you really have to identify what bothers you most — in other words, establish your priorities.

How Much Do I Want to Change It?

This is really a question about how much your life is impacted by whatever is bothering you. Someone who knows her body isn't perfect but doesn't let it impact her enjoyment of life is a lot less likely to pursue surgery than someone who's avoiding social situations because of a physical problem that embarrasses her. If you won't wear a bathing suit or a sleeveless blouse, then that may be an important factor in your decision to follow through with liposuction. Not being able to buy clothes off the rack is a strong motivator for many women to consider breast augmentation or breast reduction surgery. Weigh your concerns about your body as they affect your life against your concerns about finances, safety, and healing.

What's My Motivation to Change?

Your single most important motivation for surgery should be your own reason — no one else's. If a spouse or partner is pressuring you to do something with your body that you don't agree with, then don't do it. This is about you and your feelings about yourself. Otherwise, you shouldn't be thinking about having cosmetic surgery. Now, it's true that some outside forces — marriage, class reunion, job security — may prompt you to act *at this time,* but you still need to be sure that the course you're contemplating is right for you.

Do I Understand All My Options?

Never forget that your first option is not to have surgery! You can't blithely agree to have surgery without knowing the downside. One of your alternatives is to accept the risks involved and go forward — the other is to *not* have surgery at all.

If you decide to proceed and embark on a series of consultations with a number of surgeons, you may find that different surgeons suggest different solutions to your concerns. Don't hesitate to ask for a discussion of multiple ways of resolving your concerns and to receive fee estimates for each. When you get home, you can go over the range of options, sort through all the advice you've been given, perhaps make some clarifying calls or have second consults, and then make your decision.

Will Family and Friends Accept My Choice?

Families and friends tend to focus on the risks of having cosmetic surgery more than on the positive surgical result. You, as a potential patient in a positive frame of mind, are much more likely to be focusing on the outcome you seek rather than the known surgical risks. Although you need to reach a middle ground where you're considering risks as well as benefits, the chatter you hear from friends and family may be hard to handle.

The opinion of someone close, such as a parent, sibling, partner, or spouse, is going to weigh heavily upon you. You love them, and they love you. Welcome their roadblocks and questions. They can help with your decision.

After Surgery, Can I Hide Out or Do I Have to Tell All?

You may be tempted to keep your surgery under wraps — even after the bandages come off — but hiding out can be more difficult than you realize. Being open about the procedures you've had is a lot easier. You don't have to stay out of sight until every last bruise heals or worry about coming up with a plausible explanation for your suddenly tight tummy.

Keeping this secret is really very tough. The more you have done, the less practical it is to keep it to yourself. If you want to hide out, then you need to do some stealthy planning. Taking a vacation soon after surgery is one way to keep it private. You can come back looking rested with a new hairstyle or tan. Going off to the spa after your "diet" can explain why your body looks so much better.

How Am I Going to Pay for the Surgery?

That's the $64,000 question. If money weren't a consideration, most of us probably would be doing a lot of things that we can't afford to do otherwise. But for most of us, money *is* an issue, and the more procedures you opt to have done, the greater the cost. If you have the money saved and are willing to spend it on looking better, great. If you don't have the cash, you may consider borrowing it and paying interest so that you can move forward with your plans now, but putting yourself under additional financial stress could impede your recovery and harm your credit rating. You may need to plan, wait, and save. Chapter 6 tells you about planning to pay for surgery.

Do I Have Time for Recovery?

In truth, few people have time for recovery, but if you're an astute patient, you'll create the time you need. When your surgeon delineates your post-surgery recovery course, listen up. She's not doing it for her health; she's doing it for yours. Postsurgery instructions are based on years of cumulative real patient experiences. No one knows for sure where you're going to fall on the recovery bell curve before surgery. Be happy if you recover faster and your recovery is at the top or middle of the curve. If you take longer to recover, accept it as a known risk, rest more, and keep in touch with your doctor and her staff.

Can I Cope with Complications?

No matter how skilled the surgeon and how qualified his staff and operating suite are, surgery carries inherent risks. You may be among that very small percentage of patients who experience anything from minor delays in healing to a more serious complication that extends recovery or requires additional surgery. If you're not willing to accept the normal risks of the surgery you're choosing, then don't do it. How your body and your specific genetic makeup will respond to surgery is unpredictable to some degree.

If you find a surgeon and support team whom you can trust to take good care of you, then you can move forward with the understanding that if complications or setbacks occur, they'll be with you every step of the way. And if you haven't found that surgeon, keep shopping until you do.

How Do I Find the Right Surgeon?

If you decide that something is bothering you enough to consider cosmetic surgery, the next step is finding a surgeon. I devote Chapters 4 and 5 to this topic because your choice is so very important. Don't shortchange yourself. Take the time to find out how to shop for a surgeon, and talk to people who've had the procedure you're considering. The Internet is a great resource and an easy way to let your fingers do the walking.

Have at least three consultations and try to go through the same group of questions at each one. That way, you'll be able to compare apples and apples because you'll have three answers to the same question. Perhaps all the solutions will be similar. If so, you need to go with your gut and choose the surgeon and practice that makes you the most comfortable, which I call "finding an emotional home."

Chapter 22

(Almost) Ten Ways to Get Great Results from Cosmetic Surgery

As you approach having cosmetic surgery, your ultimate goal is to be happy and satisfied with both your surgical outcome *and* your emotional experience. Yes, you want to look great and feel better about yourself. But you also want to look back at your patient experience and know that you received top-notch care from a surgeon and staff who were thoughtful and committed to your well-being. This chapter gives you some ways that you can help make your surgical experience happy and satisfying.

Know What You Want

Before you make this important choice, you need to define what it is that you really want. Unless you know, you can't communicate it to your potential surgeon, so he's less likely to address your specific concerns and more likely to make recommendations based on what he sees. The result of such miscommunication may not be the best surgical course for you.

Just because a doctor disagrees with you doesn't mean that you shouldn't consider the change you want. But, if *all* the credible surgeons you see disagree with you, then you probably need to rethink your goal. Make sure that several quality surgeons agree that you can benefit from the procedure you're considering before you decide to go for it. You'll be happier in the end if you expose your goals to the test of rational thinking and come out on the other side understanding the realistic changes that are possible for you.

Allow Yourself Time to Decide

Having cosmetic surgery isn't a decision you want to rush. You should approach your decision to have cosmetic surgery in the same way that you would make any other major purchase, such as a new car or new house. You probably wouldn't rush out and buy the first car you test drove or the first house you were shown. Take the same — or more — care with your cosmetic surgery decision. If you've made the wrong decision, then you can always sell the car or house, but if you've made a bad surgical choice, then you may have to live with the consequences for years to come.

You're in charge of your own buying decision. It's your body and your money — you can do what you want and on your own schedule. Cosmetic surgery involves complex feelings about your own self-image, so take your time. If your auto salesperson or real estate agent didn't listen to your criteria for features or price, you'd redirect them or find someone else who would listen to you. You can do the same with your surgeon.

Make the Right Choice

Suppose you conclude that every surgeon you've interviewed is equally qualified, operates in a safe environment, and demonstrates equivalent surgical quality. That's when your emotional side may take over, as it does in any major decision — maybe you realize that one surgeon's bedside manner is what seals the deal. Still, you want to rank your surgeon's skill and experience over his beside manner. Although I certainly want you to *like* your surgeon (it improves communication and makes all contact more pleasant), being able to trust your surgeon's ability and ethics is far more important. After all, you'll live with the surgical outcome for much longer than you'll deal with the surgeon.

Ideally, you want to choose a practice where you don't have to compromise — where you believe that you can have a great surgical outcome *and* a wonderful emotional experience.

Choose a Top-Notch Support Team

Patient satisfaction can just be so many meaningless words on a mission statement, or it can be a natural result of a group of people — surgeon and staff — dedicated to helping you achieve the positive outcome you seek. Keep your eyes and ears open. The staff may well be the deciding factor.

You'll find a strong correlation between service quality and employee satisfaction. So, if the staff is happy with their workplace, they're more likely to take better care of you. Their good feelings and an upbeat environment translate to a more positive patient experience. Watch how the surgeon and staff interact with each other. Is the surgeon kind to his staff and do they enjoy open communication? Does it feel good to be in the office? If so, then that's the kind of treatment you can expect — even if something goes wrong.

Create a Personal Support System

In addition to the support system in your surgeon's office, you need a personal support group. No matter how independent you think you are, having an emotional support system increases your satisfaction. It's good to have a team of caring people — friends and family — to bounce your thoughts off in the decision-making phase and to bring you tea while you're recovering.

Making substantive changes to your appearance involves a lot of emotions and many decisions. Why go it alone when you probably have many people in your life that would be happy to support you in this adventure and only need to be asked? They'll cheer you on and perk you up. Even if you don't need help deciding to have surgery, you'll be glad when they rally around during your recovery.

Avoid Financial Pressure

If you really want to be satisfied with your cosmetic surgery experience, you'll want to reduce every stress that you possibly can, and financial issues can be a real source of stress. Being prepared financially has several advantages. You don't need to spend your recovery being so worried about money that you go back to work too soon and set yourself back or delay recovery. And if everything doesn't go perfectly, you can be ready for any costs of additional surgery. You don't want to put yourself in the position of incurring horrendous finance charges that you really can't afford.

Follow Your Surgical Team's Instructions

You'll be happiest with your outcome if you can give up control and let the professionals take over. After you make your decision to have surgery, you need to surrender yourself to the surgical process — doing whatever it takes to prepare for surgery and to have an uneventful recovery. Do what's asked of you, and don't fight your surgeon or his staff when they ask you for additional tests or clearances. You don't have the knowledge or experience to decide which of the directives you're thinking of ignoring could be potentially harmful. Remember, your surgeon's rules are forged in the fires of experience and have your best interest at heart.

Set Realistic Expectations

Consider a scale of 1 to 5, with 1 being the worst appearance and 5 being the best. Then think of the appearance of the body part you want to change and assign it a number on that scale. Now, think of the result you want and assign it a number as well. In general, it's very difficult to make a 1 into a 5, even with the very best plastic surgery result. You can realistically expect to change 2 points along the scale or, if you're lucky, 3.

Improving your appearance means that you'll look better. It doesn't mean that you can look like a thin movie star if you're 30 pounds overweight. Nevertheless, the person who you are can look dramatically better, and you can be much happier with the new you. Having realistic expectations can make it much easier for you to move forward positively in your life.

Improve Your Lifestyle

You've spent money to make your body better. Consider using your cosmetic surgery decision as a stimulus for other positive changes in your life. Eat better. Exercise more. Have you been thinking about joining a gym? Go for it. You can do your own extreme makeover by restyling your hair, changing your makeup, updating your wardrobe, or switching from glasses to contacts. Join a book club or take an extension course. If you're feeling happy and grateful, why not add some volunteer activities to your routine?

Do whatever you can to enhance your enjoyment of your life and to improve the quality of your entire existence. There's a world of choices out there — you need only embrace them. Take your new self-image and follow it to new heights of personal enjoyment. You'll be glad you did.

Appendix

Internet Resources

Medical Organization Sites

American Board of Medical Specialties: www.abms.org. The American Board of Medical Specialties (ABMS) provides public information about its oversight of specialization and certification in medicine. You can verify board certification by its member boards on this site.

American Board of Plastic Surgery: www.abplsurg.org. This ABMS-recognized board certifies surgeons in the specialty of plastic surgery. The site allows you to view training and education requirements of the specialty along with FAQs about the board.

American Board of Dermatology: www.abderm.org. Recognized by the ABMS, the American Board of Dermatology Web site provides standards of training, education, and qualifications of physicians rendering care in dermatology.

American Board of Otolaryngology: www.aboto.org. Recognized by the ABMS, the American Board of Otolaryngology Web site provides guidelines for certification and scope of knowledge for the specialty that includes many cosmetic surgery procedures of the head and neck.

American Board of Anesthesiology: www.abanes.org. Recognized by the ABMS, the American Board of Anesthesiology Web site provides guidelines for certification and scope of knowledge for the specialty.

Professional Society Sites

American Society of Plastic Surgeons: www.plasticsurgery.org. ASPS's membership is made up of board-certified plastic surgeons. This site includes answers to the most frequently asked questions about plastic and cosmetic surgery, including the average costs of various procedures.

American Society for Aesthetic Plastic Surgery: www.surgery.org. ASAPS is a public information organization, providing accurate and timely information on all aspects of cosmetic plastic surgery and a physician finder.

American Society for Dermatologic Surgery: www.asds-net.org. The site contains patient information on skin care, dermatologic surgery, lasers, facial fillers, chemical peels, vein therapy, and acne scarring.

American Academy of Dermatology: www.aad.org. The site offers a public resource center with news, publications, and a physician finder. It also has information about common cosmetic procedures performed by dermatologists.

American Academy of Otolaryngology: www.entnet.org. This professional association provides information on the ears, nose, throat, and related structures of the head and neck.

American Society for Laser Medicine and Surgery: www.aslms.org. The Web site provides general education and communication about laser medicine and surgery.

American Society of Ophthalmic Plastic and Reconstructive Surgery: www.asoprs.org. This site offers an in-depth patient information page as well general information for society members. The society oversees advance training, education, research, and the quality of clinical practice in the fields of aesthetic, plastic, and reconstructive surgery specializing in eyelids, orbits, and the lacrimal system.

American Society of Anesthesiologists: www.asahq.org. The Web site offers an extensive patient education section with FAQs, questions to ask before surgery, scope of practice, and educational brochures.

Facility Certification Sites

American Association for Accreditation of Ambulatory Surgery Facilities: www.aaaasf.org. This site allows you to search for accredited facilities and also has a patient info area that educates patients on what is required of certified facilities.

Accreditation Association for Ambulatory Health Care: www.aaahc.org. At this site, you can search for accredited facilities. It also has a public/press area with FAQs.

Joint Commission on Accreditation of Healthcare Organizations: www.jcaho.org. This site allows you to search for accredited facilities and also has a general public area that addresses patient safety and explains what the Joint Commission is.

Public Information Sites

Plastic Surgery Research.info: www.cosmeticplasticsurgerystatistics.com. This site offers statistics regarding plastic surgery and risks and complications on each procedure. Also included are before-and-after photos, ballpark fees, and a doctor search.

A Board Certified Plastic Surgeon Resource: www.aboardcertifiedplasticsurgeonresource.com. This comprehensive site offers information on everything related to plastic surgery. Procedure information, a physician finder, articles, and financing information are just a few of the topics covered.

Plasticsurgery.com: www.plasticsurgery.com. Complete information on the different types of plastic surgery, including breast augmentation and liposuction, is what you find here. Visitors can research procedures, look at before-and-after photos, and locate a physician.

Smart Plastic Surgery.com: www.smartplasticsurgery.com. This site provides information on the top cosmetic procedures, including average prices, preparation checklists, recovery tips, and risks and complications. You also can view before-and-after pictures.

Mentor 4 Me.com: www.mentor4me.com. A leading medical device company that manufactures breast implants, Mentor offers this Web site as a complete resource center for patients considering cosmetic surgery, including breast augmentation. It includes a physician finder to help locate qualified plastic surgeons across the country.

Implant Info.com: www.implantinfo.com. This site provides a place for women to share experiences, opinions, and information on breast implants, breast augmentation, breast enlargement, plastic surgery, and recovery. Ask questions and get opinions about breast implants and breast augmentation in the live chat room and discussion forums.

BreastImplants411: www.breastimplants411.com. Here's where you can find plastic surgeons, answers to all your breast augmentation questions, articles written by board-certified plastic surgeons, and hundreds of breast enhancement before-and-after pictures, as well as cosmetic plastic surgery and breast enlargement success stories. The site also has a discussion forum.

U.S. Food and Drug Administration on Breast Implants: www.fda.gov/cdrh/breastimplants. This site provides study-related information on the safety of silicone and saline implants, as well as links to other useful sites.

Liposuction FYI: www.liposuctionFYI.com. This comprehensive site provides information about who is a candidate, types of liposuction, risks, news, and how to find a doctor.

Lipo4me: www.lipo4me.com. Here you find answers to commonly asked questions regarding liposuction surgery, recovery costs, and many other issues. You can also find a plastic surgeon in your area or view before-and-after liposuction photos of actual patients.

RhinoplastyFYI.com: www.rhinoplastyFYI.com. This comprehensive site provides information about who is a candidate, types of rhinoplasty, risks, news, and how to find a doctor.

Washington Facelift: www.washingtonfacelift.com. This site answers questions about facelifts and facial cosmetic surgery in straightforward language and provides advice on how to choose a surgeon.

Researching Patient Financing

Cosmetic Fee Plan.com: www.cosmeticfeeplan.com. This site helps patients achieve the look they desire by providing convenient methods of paying for procedures. Cosmetic Fee Plan provides monthly payment plans for procedures ranging from $1,500 to $25,000.

PFS Patient Financing: www.mentorcorp.com/breastsurgery/augmentation/cs_ba_finance.htm. PFS Patient Financing has partnered with Mentor to offer patients affordable, low-interest monthly payments to finance breast augmentation procedures over a period of 12 to 60 months. You can find out all about it on the Mentor Web site.

Plastic Surgery Financing.com: www.plasticsurgeryfinancing.com. This site offers fast and affordable financing for all cosmetic and noncosmetic medical and dental procedures. Financing options for all types of credit profiles are provided, and loans with payment terms of up to 60 months are available.

Unicorn Financial.com: www.unicornfinancial.com. This site helps patients by providing financing for cosmetic and elective surgery through their participating provider network. Extended payment plans are available, as well as same-as-cash financing of 12, 18, or 24 months interest free.

Index

• S •

USINESS, CAREERS & PERSONAL FINANCE

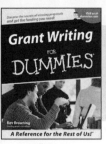

0-7645-5307-0

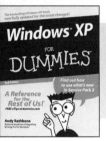

0-7645-5331-3 *†

Also available:
- Accounting For Dummies †
  0-7645-5314-3
- Business Plans Kit For Dummies †
  0-7645-5365-8
- Cover Letters For Dummies
  0-7645-5224-4
- Frugal Living For Dummies
  0-7645-5403-4
- Leadership For Dummies
  0-7645-5176-0
- Managing For Dummies
  0-7645-1771-6

- Marketing For Dummies
  0-7645-5600-2
- Personal Finance For Dummies *
  0-7645-2590-5
- Project Management For Dummies
  0-7645-5283-X
- Resumes For Dummies †
  0-7645-5471-9
- Selling For Dummies
  0-7645-5363-1
- Small Business Kit For Dummies *†
  0-7645-5093-4

OME & BUSINESS COMPUTER BASICS

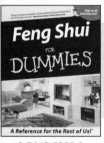

0-7645-4074-2

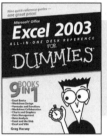

0-7645-3758-X

Also available:
- ACT! 6 For Dummies
  0-7645-2645-6
- iLife '04 All-in-One Desk Reference
  For Dummies
  0-7645-7347-0
- iPAQ For Dummies
  0-7645-6769-1
- Mac OS X Panther Timesaving
  Techniques For Dummies
  0-7645-5812-9
- Macs For Dummies
  0-7645-5656-8

- Microsoft Money 2004 For Dummies
  0-7645-4195-1
- Office 2003 All-in-One Desk Reference
  For Dummies
  0-7645-3883-7
- Outlook 2003 For Dummies
  0-7645-3759-8
- PCs For Dummies
  0-7645-4074-2
- TiVo For Dummies
  0-7645-6923-6
- Upgrading and Fixing PCs For Dummies
  0-7645-1665-5
- Windows XP Timesaving Techniques
  For Dummies
  0-7645-3748-2

OOD, HOME, GARDEN, HOBBIES, MUSIC & PETS

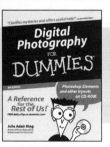

0-7645-5295-3

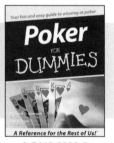

0-7645-5232-5

Also available:
- Bass Guitar For Dummies
  0-7645-2487-9
- Diabetes Cookbook For Dummies
  0-7645-5230-9
- Gardening For Dummies *
  0-7645-5130-2
- Guitar For Dummies
  0-7645-5106-X
- Holiday Decorating For Dummies
  0-7645-2570-0
- Home Improvement All-in-One
  For Dummies
  0-7645-5680-0

- Knitting For Dummies
  0-7645-5395-X
- Piano For Dummies
  0-7645-5105-1
- Puppies For Dummies
  0-7645-5255-4
- Scrapbooking For Dummies
  0-7645-7208-3
- Senior Dogs For Dummies
  0-7645-5818-8
- Singing For Dummies
  0-7645-2475-5
- 30-Minute Meals For Dummies
  0-7645-2589-1

INTERNET & DIGITAL MEDIA

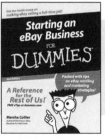

0-7645-1664-7

0-7645-6924-4

Also available:
- 2005 Online Shopping Directory
  For Dummies
  0-7645-7495-7
- CD & DVD Recording For Dummies
  0-7645-5956-7
- eBay For Dummies
  0-7645-5654-1
- Fighting Spam For Dummies
  0-7645-5965-6
- Genealogy Online For Dummies
  0-7645-5964-8
- Google For Dummies
  0-7645-4420-9

- Home Recording For Musicians
  For Dummies
  0-7645-1634-5
- The Internet For Dummies
  0-7645-4173-0
- iPod & iTunes For Dummies
  0-7645-7772-7
- Preventing Identity Theft For Dummies
  0-7645-7336-5
- Pro Tools All-in-One Desk Reference
  For Dummies
  0-7645-5714-9
- Roxio Easy Media Creator For Dummies
  0-7645-7131-1

* Separate Canadian edition also available
† Separate U.K. edition also available

Available wherever books are sold. For more information or to order direct: U.S. customers visit www.dummies.com or call 1-877-762-2974.
U.K. customers visit www.wileyeurope.com or call 0800 243407. Canadian customers visit www.wiley.ca or call 1-800-567-4797.

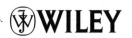

SPORTS, FITNESS, PARENTING, RELIGION & SPIRITUALITY

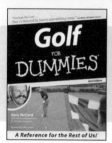

0-7645-5146-9

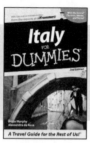

0-7645-5418-2

Also available:
- Adoption For Dummies
  0-7645-5488-3
- Basketball For Dummies
  0-7645-5248-1
- The Bible For Dummies
  0-7645-5296-1
- Buddhism For Dummies
  0-7645-5359-3
- Catholicism For Dummies
  0-7645-5391-7
- Hockey For Dummies
  0-7645-5228-7

- Judaism For Dummies
  0-7645-5299-6
- Martial Arts For Dummies
  0-7645-5358-5
- Pilates For Dummies
  0-7645-5397-6
- Religion For Dummies
  0-7645-5264-3
- Teaching Kids to Read For Dummies
  0-7645-4043-2
- Weight Training For Dummies
  0-7645-5168-X
- Yoga For Dummies
  0-7645-5117-5

TRAVEL

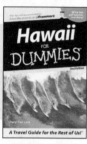

0-7645-5438-7

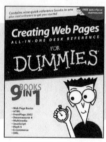

0-7645-5453-0

Also available:
- Alaska For Dummies
  0-7645-1761-9
- Arizona For Dummies
  0-7645-6938-4
- Cancún and the Yucatán For Dummies
  0-7645-2437-2
- Cruise Vacations For Dummies
  0-7645-6941-4
- Europe For Dummies
  0-7645-5456-5
- Ireland For Dummies
  0-7645-5455-7

- Las Vegas For Dummies
  0-7645-5448-4
- London For Dummies
  0-7645-4277-X
- New York City For Dummies
  0-7645-6945-7
- Paris For Dummies
  0-7645-5494-8
- RV Vacations For Dummies
  0-7645-5443-3
- Walt Disney World & Orlando For Dummies
  0-7645-6943-0

GRAPHICS, DESIGN & WEB DEVELOPMENT

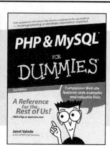

0-7645-4345-8

0-7645-5589-8

Also available:
- Adobe Acrobat 6 PDF For Dummies
  0-7645-3760-1
- Building a Web Site For Dummies
  0-7645-7144-3
- Dreamweaver MX 2004 For Dummies
  0-7645-4342-3
- FrontPage 2003 For Dummies
  0-7645-3882-9
- HTML 4 For Dummies
  0-7645-1995-6
- Illustrator CS For Dummies
  0-7645-4084-X

- Macromedia Flash MX 2004 For Dummies
  0-7645-4358-X
- Photoshop 7 All-in-One Desk Reference For Dummies
  0-7645-1667-1
- Photoshop CS Timesaving Techniques For Dummies
  0-7645-6782-9
- PHP 5 For Dummies
  0-7645-4166-8
- PowerPoint 2003 For Dummies
  0-7645-3908-6
- QuarkXPress 6 For Dummies
  0-7645-2593-X

NETWORKING, SECURITY, PROGRAMMING & DATABASES

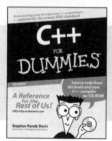

0-7645-6852-3

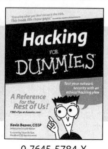

0-7645-5784-X

Also available:
- A+ Certification For Dummies
  0-7645-4187-0
- Access 2003 All-in-One Desk Reference For Dummies
  0-7645-3988-4
- Beginning Programming For Dummies
  0-7645-4997-9
- C For Dummies
  0-7645-7068-4
- Firewalls For Dummies
  0-7645-4048-3
- Home Networking For Dummies
  0-7645-42796

- Network Security For Dummies
  0-7645-1679-5
- Networking For Dummies
  0-7645-1677-9
- TCP/IP For Dummies
  0-7645-1760-0
- VBA For Dummies
  0-7645-3989-2
- Wireless All In-One Desk Reference For Dummies
  0-7645-7496-5
- Wireless Home Networking For Dummies
  0-7645-3910-8